PHLEBOTOMY
H A N D B O O K

Blood Collection Essentials

fifth edition

Diana Garza, EdD, MT (ASCP), CLS (NCA)
Associate Professor
Master's Program in Health Care Administration
College of Health Sciences
Texas Woman's University-Houston Center
Houston, Texas

Adjunct Associate Professor
Division of Laboratory Medicine
University of Texas M.D. Anderson Cancer Center

Kathleen Becan-McBride, EdD, MT (ASCP)
Director, Community Outreach and Education
Coordinator, Texas-Mexico Border Health Services

Professor
School of Allied Health Sciences
Medical School-Department of Pathology & Laboratory Medicine
School of Public Health
School of Nursing
University of Texas-Houston Health Science Center
Texas Medical Center
Houston, Texas

Assistant Director for Academic Partnerships
Greater Houston Area Health Education Center (AHEC)

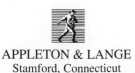

APPLETON & LANGE
Stamford, Connecticut

Notice: The authors and the publisher of this volume have taken care that the information and technical recommendations contained herein are based on research and expert consultation, and are accurate and compatible with the standards generally accepted at the time of publication. Nevertheless, as new information becomes available, changes in clinical and technical practices become necessary. The reader is advised to carefully consult manufacturers' instructions and information material for all supplies and equipment before use, and to consult with a healthcare professional as necessary. This advice is especially important when using new supplies or equipment for clinical purposes. The authors and publisher disclaim all responsibility for any liability, loss, injury, or damage incurred as a consequence, directly or indirectly, of the use and application of any of the contents of this volume.

Prentice Hall International (UK) Limited, *London*
Prentice Hall of Australia Pty. Limited, *Sydney*
Prentice Hall Canada, Inc., *Toronto*
Prentice Hall Hispanoamericana, S.A., *Mexico*
Prentice Hall India Private Limited, *New Delhi*
Prentice Hall of Japan, Inc., *Tokyo*
Simon & Schuster Asia Pte. Ltd., *Singapore*
Editora Prentice Hall do Brasil Ltda., *Rio de Janeiro*
Prentice Hall, *Upper Saddle River, New Jersey*

Garza, Diana.
    Phlebotomy handbook : blood collection essentials / Diana Garza.
Kathleen Becan-McBride. — 5th ed.
        p.   cm
    Includes bibliographical references and index.
    ISBN 0–8385–8141–2 (pbk. : alk. paper)
    1. Phlebotomy—Handbooks, manuals, etc.   I. Becan-McBride,
Kathleen, 1949–   II. Title.
    [DNLM: 1. Phlebotomy—handbooks.   QY 39 G245p 1999]
RB45.15.G37   1999
616.07′561—dc21
DNLM/DLC
for Library of Congress   98–22074
                                                                           CIP

Acquisitions Editor: Lin Marshall
Production Editor: Mary Ellen McCourt
Art Coordinator: Eve Siegel
Interior Design: Mary Ann Dube
Cover Design: Aimee Nordin

ISBN 0-8385-8141-2
90000

9 780838 581414

PRINTED IN THE UNITED STATES OF AMERICA

PHLEBOTOMY
H A N D B O O K

Blood Collection Essentials

fifth edition

To my husband Peter McLaughlin; my children, Lauren, Kaitlin, and Kevin; and my parents for their affection, patience, and constant support.
Diana Garza

To my husband, Mark; my sons, Patrick and Jonathan; my parents; my sister; and my parents-in-law for their support and devotion.
Kathleen Becan-McBride

Contents

V. QUALITY MANAGEMENT AND LEGAL ISSUES / 421

Foreword

The publication of the fifth edition of the *Phlebotomy Handbook: Blood Collection Essentials,* is timely with the increasing emphasis in recent years on the importance of controlling nonanalytic variables that would otherwise impact laboratory results and patient care.[1,2] Nonanalytic variables can be broadly grouped into three categories: specimen collection, physiological factors, and interferences or influence factors. This textbook does an excellent job of covering these categories in a practical and useful fashion.

While a standardized specimen collection technique is a prerequisite to specimen quality, the many steps prior to specimen collection need to be controlled to ensure that the analytic results obtained on the patient's specimen are truly representative of the subject's condition. Thus, the effect of posture during blood sampling, the duration of tourniquet application, the timing of specimen collection, and strenuous exercise the night before a collection can have an impact on the laboratory results. The concentration of many constituents can be dramatically altered with a change in posture, and leaving the tourniquet on for excessive lengths of time during blood collection can result in hemoconcentration. Even common practices that are used excessively can alter the laboratory result, such as repeated excessive fist clenching. Individuals responsible for collecting blood specimens should be knowledgeable about these factors, which are comprehensively delineated in this textbook.

Furthermore, physiological variables, such as age, gender, menstrual cycle, pregnancy, and lifestyle, can influence laboratory results. The effect of a fatty meal can increase triglyceride levels, sustained consumption of alcohol, frequent consumption of caffeine, excessive salt intake, and endogenous interferences due to drugs or circulating antibodies can also alter the laboratory results. Thus, the role of the phlebotomist in capturing an accurate history of the patient is vital to detect preanalytic errors and avoid postanalytic error due to incorrect interpretation or missing information about the patient. Errors in specimen identification and changes in specimen integrity during transport can negate efforts toward achieving standardization of specimen collection.

The authors of the *Phlebotomy Handbook: Blood Collection Essentials, fifth edition,* have skillfully provided the latest information to educate the phlebotomist, not only on the proper use of specimen collection materials and techniques, but on the background needed in disciplines such as basic anatomy and physiology and the circulatory system. Issues that are profoundly important to phlebotomists, such as safety, legal issues, and quality management, are discussed in detail. The use of clear illustrations together with the case studies and appendices provide practical integration of all the knowledge components presented. This textbook is eminently readable and a valuable resource of current and practical information for all health care workers who collect specimens.

Sheshadri Narayanan, PhD
Clinical Professor of Pathology
New York Medical College-Metropolitan Hospital Center
New York, New York

References

1. Guder WG, Narayanan S, Wisser H, Zawta B. *Samples: from the Patient to the Laboratory: the Impact of Preanalytical Variables on the Quality of Laboratory Results.* Darmstadt, Germany: GIT Verlag; 1996.
2. Young DS. *Effects of Preanalytical Variables on Clinical Laboratory Tests.* Washington, DC: AACC Press; 1997.

Preface

This book, *Phlebotomy Handbook: Blood Collection Essentials, fifth edition,* is designed for health care students and practitioners who are responsible for blood and specimen collections (i.e., nurses, phlebotomists, clinical laboratory technicians and technologists, respiratory therapists, and others). The primary goal of the book is to link the phlebotomist (blood collector) to the latest information, techniques, skills, and equipment for the provision of safe and effective collection procedures, for the improvement of diagnostic and therapeutic laboratory testing, for enhancement of customer satisfaction, and ultimately, for the promotion of better health outcomes. It provides a wide range of communcation, clinical, technical, and safety skills that any health care worker will use in the practice of phlebotomy and other specimen collection procedures. In addition, the book provides a background of general knowledge and insights to support the technical skills.

The book highlights trends in the health care industry that have forced greater efficiency, higher quality standards, safer practices and increased cost effectiveness. Also, methods of delivering health care services have continued shifting toward ambulatory care, client-based approaches to empowering patients and families with more information and education, improving customer service and communication skills, streamlining processes, cross-training clinical tasks, such as phlebotomy, and using health care teams in shared decisions about how to meet an individual's needs. The role of the blood collector has expanded to encompass additional patient care duties and clinical responsibilities, a more patient-sensitive role, and improved interpersonal skills to deal effectively with patients, their families, and health care teams. For example, even the traditional title *phlebotomist* has changed in many facilities to *patient associate, patient care technician,* or *clinical assistant.* The practice of phlebotomy is presented in this industry context.

The order in which the material is presented generally follows the way in which a phlebotomist approaches the patient (i.e., beginning with important communication skills, a basic understanding of physiologic aspects, moving to safety considerations in preparation for the phlebotomy procedure, preparation of supplies and equipment, actual venipuncture or skin puncture, and potential complications). Specialty tests and finally a review of quality management and legal issues is presented at the end.

The content is divided into five major parts:

I. The Overview provides a knowledge base of the roles and functions of a phlebotomist in the health care industry and the basics of anatomy and physiology with an emphasis on the circulatory system.

II. Safety Procedures provides information about safety and infection control in the workplace and the documentation and transportation procedures needed for safe handling of biohazardous specimens.

III. Equipment and Procedures provides the most updated information about blood collection equipment, provides a comprehensive description of the actual techniques used in phlebotomy, and reviews clinical and technical complications that may occur during the procedure.

IV. Special Procedures and Point-of-Care Testing provides information about pediatric phlebotomy procedures, arterial and IV collections, and special considerations for the elderly, homebound, and long-term care patients.

V. Quality and Legal Issues covers quality management issues for blood and specimen collection services and legal issues important to phlebotomy practice.

Key features of the *Phlebotomy Handbook: Blood Collection Essentials, fifth edition,* include the following:

- Clinical alert symbols have been added to selected portions of the text to indicate procedures or concepts that have vitally important clinical consequences for the patient. The clinical alert indicates that "extra caution" should be taken by the health care worker to comply with the procedure, thereby avoiding adverse outcomes for the patient.
- Two new chapters: Chapter 13, "Elderly, Home, and Long-Term Care Collections" and Chapter 15, "Specimen Collection for Forensic Toxicology, Workplace Testing, Sports Medicine, and Related Areas."
- Expanded sections have been added to several chapters (e.g., expanded sections on intravenous collection techniques).
- Procedural information is presented in comprehensive descriptions, using an "on the job" perspective.
- Updated information is presented throughout, including blood collection equipment and techniques, legal issues and professional liability, safety and infection control practices, and new health care settings where phlebotomy practices occur.
- Exercises for improving communication skills were designed to "get the feel" of being a patient and being an effective part of a health care team.
- Case studies have been added to the end of each major part.
- Key terms, objectives, and study questions are provided for each chapter.
- A color atlas, including the heart, veins, and artery overviews.
- A color chart indicating blood collection tubes, appropriate color codings, and additives.
- Appendices containing units of measurement and symbols and formulas and calculations used in laboratories.
- Contrasting color tables and figures.
- Larger text format that makes it easy-to-read.

In summary, the authors have created a book that health care professionals and students will use as a compact, central authority of information about blood collection practices. Instructors can also use this as the central body of information to teach specimen collection skills.

Phlebotomy Handbook, fifth Edition, has companion resources that are cross-referenced to the text. One of these is *Appleton & Lange's Quick Review: Phlebotomy/Blood Collection, 5th edition.* This is an aid to students and health care workers preparing for a certification examination. It has four comprehensive, simulated board examinations, consisting of 100 multiple choice questions with referenced explanatory answers. Students can practice taking the simulated examinations in print or computer form. A diagnostic report identifies those topics that need further review and study and provides the score for each content area.

An *Instructor's Guide* that contains a test bank of questions, as well as other instructional materials, is also available.

Acknowledgments

We are indebted to many individuals, companies, and health care organizations for their assistance in preparing the first editions of this textbook. In the spirit of continuous improvement, each version of this book used the previous as a framework to redesign, update, and improve the next.

We are particularly grateful to Becton-Dickinson VACUTAINER Systems, the College of American Pathologists, the American Society of Clinical Pathologists, the University of Texas M.D. Anderson Cancer Center, Texas Woman's University, and the University of Texas-Houston Health Science Center for their support and permission to work on this project. We thank Sheshadri Narayanan, PhD, for contributing the Foreword; Leslie Bardnowski, RN, for input on blood collections from intravenous lines; Estella Woodard, MT (ASCP) and Peter McLaughlin, MD, for their assistance with the venipuncture photography; Willie Singleton, Karen Guidry, and Francis Stovall, MT (ASCP) for their practical expertise in specimen collection; and Jim Lemoine for his photography services. These are exceptional people who worked diligently, often under short time constraints.

We also acknowledge and greatly appreciate our superb editors at Appleton & Lange past and present who have encouraged us and improved our writing through five editions. Special thanks goes to Jane Licht, Cheryl Mehalik, and Lin Marshall.

We are thankful for our families who have tolerated the thousands of hours we spent writing five editions of this textbook. And, we are ultimately grateful to all the health care workers who continue to strive for new knowledge to improve the standards of care for those they serve.

I

OVERVIEW

THE PRACTICE OF PHLEBOTOMY, LIKE ANY other health professional skill, has certain characteristics that balance knowledge and theory with practical expertise. These characteristics include a recognizable definition or identity, a means of assigning tasks and responsibilities, and an established network for communication with other members of the health care team. These skills and responsibilities are now performed in a variety of health care settings, ranging from hospital intensive care units to an individual's home. Furthermore, phlebotomy practice is more widely performed by all types of health professionals, including nurses, respiratory therapists, clinical laboratory professionals, and others. Essential basic functions of the human body must also be well understood before technical skill and expertise can be acquired. Over the years, the practice of phlebotomy has developed these characteristics in sophisticated and elaborate ways. Part I, comprising the first three chapters of this book, defines phlebotomy practice in the current environment and creates a foundation of essential knowledge of the human body. In addition, the color atlas in Part I provides illustrations pertaining to the anatomy and physiology sections.

Chapter 1, Phlebotomy Practice and Health Care Settings, describes a working framework for the phlebotomist (e.g., nurse, respiratory therapist, patient care technician, clinical assistant) in a health care environment that is rapidly changing. Emphasis is on roles and responsibilities, communication, and the vital link that the phlebotomist plays in providing quality health care services.

Chapter 2, Basic Anatomy and Physiology of Organ Systems, provides an overview of the structure and function of each body system. Particular emphasis is on identifying the anatomic regions of the body, the structural levels of the body, the role of homeostasis, and the relation of body functions to testing for diagnostic, therapeutic, and monitoring purposes.

Chapter 3, The Circulatory System, highlights the structures and functions of the circulatory system, as well as describing the specific role of the heart, vessels, and blood. Emphasis is on the arterial and venous system, blood flow and oxygen transport, identification of veins that are used for venipuncture, the cellular and noncellular components of blood, the phases of hemostasis, and blood pressure.

ONE

Phlebotomy Practice and Health Care Settings

CHAPTER OUTLINE

Chapter Objectives
The General Practice of Phlebotomy
- Definition
- Function
- Purpose
Professional Competencies
- Professional Ethics
- Professional Behavior
- Working With Health Care
  Team Members
Communication Skills in the Patient Care
Environment
- Bedside Manner
- Communication Issues in the Home
  and Ambulatory Settings
- Patient Interview
- Teaching Patients
- Communication Strategies
    Verbal Communication
    Nonverbal Communication
    Positive Body Language
    Negative Body Language and
        Distracting Behaviors
    Active Listening

Appearance, Grooming, and Physical
Fitness
- Posture
- Grooming
- Personal Hygiene
- Nutrition, Rest, and Exercise
- Protective Equipment and
  Clothing
Patient's Rights
- Issues in Specimen Collection
- Family, Visitors, and Significant
  Others
Health Care Organizations
- Hospital Inpatient Services
- Ambulatory and Home Health
  Care Services
- The Clinical Laboratory's Role in
  Specimen Collection Services
Self Study
- Key Terms
- Study Questions

CHAPTER OBJECTIVES

Upon completion of Chapter 1, the learner is responsible for the following:

1. Define phlebotomy practice and list the essential competencies for individuals performing phlebotomy/blood collection procedures.
2. Identify health care providers who generally perform phlebotomy procedures.
3. Identify the importance of phlebotomy procedures to the overall care of the patient.
4. List skills for active listening and effective verbal communication.
5. List examples of positive and negative body language.
6. Describe various health care settings, both inpatient and ambulatory, where phlebotomy services are routinely performed.
7. Describe the role of the clinical laboratory in blood collection and testing services.

■ THE GENERAL PRACTICE OF PHLEBOTOMY

The development of modern diagnostic techniques, clinical laboratory automation, computer technology, and changes in the delivery of health care services have increased the variety and number of laboratory testing options available for clinical decisions. As a result, various health care workers (e.g., phlebotomists, laboratorians, nurses, respiratory therapists, medical assistants, and others) are taking greater roles in phlebotomy and other specimen collection processes. Regardless of specific job backgrounds, however, there are common elements about the practice of phlebotomy that should be known by all who perform or are responsible for blood collections.

DEFINITION

The term *phlebotomy* is derived from the Greek words, *phlebo,* which relates to veins, and *tomy,* which relates to cutting. Therefore, the definition can be summarized as the incision of a vein for blood letting (e.g., blood collection). Other synonomous, but less used, words are venesection or venisection.

 The **phlebotomist** is the individual who practices phlebotomy or the "blood collector." The term "phlebotomist" will be used throughout this book even though it is interchangeable with "blood collector." It is also important to keep in mind that phlebotomists often assist in the collection and transportation of specimens other than venous blood (e.g., arterial blood, urine, tissues, sputum).

FUNCTION

Since the role of the phlebotomist has evolved according to specific work assignments and differing environments, individuals who practice phlebotomy may have many clinical, clerical, administrative, or a combination of these responsibilities in addition to blood collection. Regardless of what background the health care professional has, however, the primary function of the phlebotomist is to assist the health care team in the accurate, safe, and reliable collection and transportation of specimens for clinical laboratory analyses.

PURPOSE

Blood and other specimen collections are vitally important to the entire health assessment of patients. Laboratory analyses of a variety of specimens are used for three important purposes:

Diagnostic testing is used to figure out what is wrong with the patient.

Therapeutic assessments are used to develop the appropriate therapy or treatment of the medical condition.

Monitoring of a patient's health status is used to make sure the therapy or treatment is working to alleviate the medical condition.

If specimens are incorrectly acquired, labeled, or transported, laboratory tests are not useful and can even be harmful to patients.

■ PROFESSIONAL COMPETENCIES

Usually, the phlebotomist or blood collector must have a high school diploma or its equivalent to enter a phlebotomy training program. Training sessions may be conducted in a variety of settings, such as hospitals, community colleges, continuing education courses, and technical schools. Typically, the length of training varies from a few weeks to months, depending on the location and size of the facility or the complexity of patients being served, or both. Some organizations require or recommend phlebotomy certification, which is accomplished by passing a national certification examination.

There are professional organizations that recognize phlebotomists independently. All are sponsors of certification examinations for health care workers. (Refer to Box 1–1.)

The **American Society of Clinical Pathologists (ASCP) Board of Registry** has developed competency statements for phlebotomists. These typify the roles and responsibilities for an entry level phlebotomist. (Refer to Box 1–2.)

In the work setting, these types of competencies, along with other measures of ability, productivity, efficiency, and team cooperation are likely to be included in the phlebotomist's performance appraisal.

PROFESSIONAL ETHICS

The principles of right and wrong conduct, as they apply to professional problems, are the ethics for that profession. Professions set standards of conduct for members, and members are expected to adhere to those standards of performance in their work. Standards of behavior are implied in the codes of ethics for each member of the health care team. The three major points common to most ethical standards are:

1. Do no harm to anyone intentionally.
2. Perform according to sound technical ability and good judgment.
3. Respect the patients' rights (which include confidentiality, privacy, the right to know about their treatment, and the right to refuse treatment).

As examples, the ASCP and the **National Phlebotomy Association (NPA)** developed codes of ethics for laboratory professionals and health care workers involved in specimen

BOX 1–1. PROFESSIONAL ORGANIZATIONS FOR PHLEBOTOMISTS

Each of at least five organizations has board certification tests in phlebotomy. A reader intending to apply for one or more of the board examinations should determine which particular phlebotomy examinations are better known or accepted in the local community or state. Other organizations, such as the **American Nurses Association (ANA)** have training materials available for blood collection.

The American Society of Clinical Pathologists (ASCP)

ASCP
Board of Registry
P.O. Box 12277
Chicago, IL 60612-0277
(312) 738-1336

ASCP allows nonphysician members to gain associate membership status. Through the ASCP Board of Registry, a Phlebotomy Technician Examination, PBT (ASCP), is offered quarterly. This is a criterion-referenced examination model. It covers the entry-level skills of a phlebotomist and uses taxonomy levels that assess recall (recognize facts), interpretive skills (use knowledge to interpret numeric data), and problem-solving skills (use applications of specific information to solve problems). Over 13,000 phlebotomists have been certified by ASCP since 1989, when the first phlebotomy examination was administered.

The National Phlebotomy Association (NPA)

NPA
1901 Brightfeat Rd
Landover, MD 20785
(301) 699-3846

NPA was established in 1978 to recognize the phlebotomist as a distinctive and identifiable part of the health care team. NPA offers annual certification examinations.

The American Society for Clinical Laboratory Scientists (ASCLS) and The National Certifying Agency for Medical Laboratory Personnel (NCA)

NCA
P.O. Box 15945-289
Lenexa, KS 66285
(913) 438-5110

ASCLS has recognized clinical laboratory personnel for more than 50 years. Several types of memberships are available, depending on the education and experience of the individual. Currently, phlebotomists join ASCLS as associate members as part of the Phlebotomy Section and take a certification examination through the NCA.

American Medical Technologists (AMT)

AMT
710 Higgins Rd
Park Ridge, IL 60068
(847) 823-5169
(800) 275-1268

American Society of Phlebotomy Technicians (ASPT)

ASPT
P.O. Box 1831
Hickory, NC 28603
(704) 322-1334

BOX 1–2. ASCP COMPETENCY STATEMENTS FOR PHLEBOTOMY TECHNICIANS

In regard to anatomy and physiology, specimen collection, specimen processing and handling, and laboratory operations related to phlebotomy, the phlebotomy technician at career entry:

Applies

- Principles of basic procedures
- Principles of special procedures
- Knowledge to identify sources of error
- Knowledge of fundamental biological characteristics
- Knowledge of standard operating procedures
- Knowledge of medical terminology
- Knowledge of safety measures and infection control

Selects

- Procedural course of action
- Equipment according to established procedures
- Method according to established procedures
- Appropriate quality control procedures
- Reagent according to established procedures
- Site for blood collection

Prepares

- Equipment according to established procedures
- Patient according to established procedures

Evaluates Situation

- Patient situation and specimen appropriateness
- Quality control procedures and specimen appropriateness
- To check for possible sources of error
- To determine possible inconsistencies
- To assess appropriate action
- To determine appropriate method
- To recognize common procedural and technical problems
- To take corrective action according to predetermined criteria

(From The American Society of Clinical Pathologists Board of Registry, 1997, with permission.)

collection. The major themes of the codes involve responsibilities for accuracy and reliability of laboratory test results and patient confidentiality. Also, the concepts of honesty, integrity, and regard for the dignity of other human beings continue to be the personal foundations for the ethical behavior of health care workers.

Many hospitals and health service organizations across the country have also established specific codes of ethics for their employees, statements of organizational values, or both.

Often these codes deal with professional expectations for employees as they relate to the functions or mission of the organization.

PROFESSIONAL BEHAVIOR

Professional behavior cannot be prescribed or calculated in a mathematical equation. Each health care worker has a personal responsibility for providing the best possible care. Important character attributes for health care workers who practice phlebotomy follow.

- *Sincere interest in health care.* Health care workers should be compassionate and possess an intense desire to serve people and become knowledgeable in blood and specimen collection practices. They should also have the emotional stability and maturity to deal successfully with seeing others in pain, handling blood and body fluids, facing injury and trauma, seeing disease sites, and the possibility of observing death. Responses of health care workers to harsh situations must be prompt, professional, and reassuring to the patient, their families, and the health care team.
- *Accountability for doing things right.* Personal integrity, or "doing what's right when no one is looking" (e.g., washing hands between patient collections, observing precautions to gown and scrub in isolation, reporting one's own mistakes, and collecting timed tests at the proper time), reflects a health care worker's personal accountability or individual responsibility for actions.
- *Dedication to high standards of performance.* Health care workers involved in specimen collections, must continually upgrade and maintain the quality of their skills. They must know about new techniques and safety procedures, new supplies and equipment, changing time constraints on tests, computer technology, and changes in scientific knowledge. They should be willing to ask for assistance when dealing with a difficult patient or procedure. They should only collect the specimens ordered and only those that they have been trained to collect.
- *Propensity for cleanliness.* Health care workers must accept that sterile techniques, good personal hygiene, and cleanliness affect patient safety and quality health care. These are more important than saving time or cutting corners to save money.
- *Pride, satisfaction, and self-fulfillment in the job.* Health care workers involved in specimen collection should attain professional satisfaction from continually improving their professional skills and knowledge, from knowing that others are dependent on their work, and from knowing that their skills contribute to the betterment of patients. The most successful, highly regarded phlebotomists are those who are most gratified with their work.

Only the individual dealing with patients on a one-to-one basis knows for sure whether the work that he or she performs each day is based on tenets for optimum professional behavior.

WORKING WITH HEALTH CARE TEAM MEMBERS

In recent years, most health care organizations have reorganized, downsized, or both to provide increasingly efficient services in a more patient-oriented manner. The idea behind this movement was to improve the quality of health care, eliminate unnecessary costs and redundancy, perform duties as a coordinated health care team rather than as individual specialists, and above all, become more sensitive to patient's individual needs. In addition, advanced laboratory technology has enabled laboratory testing to be performed closer to the point of care (e.g., at the patient's bedside, at ancillary or mobile sites, or even in the home). These special testing procedures are more fully covered in Part IV, Special Procedures and Point of Care Testing.

As a result of these trends, shifts in job roles and responsibilities for phlebotomists have been tremendously affected. More than ever in the past, the role of the phlebotomist has become more involved and coordinated with other health care processes. In some cases, health professionals, such as nurses, respiratory therapists, patient care technicians, and others, have been crossed trained to assume phlebotomy duties. In other cases, traditional laboratory-based phlebotomists have been crossed trained to assume other clerical or patient care duties. Whatever the case, the role of health care worker as a team player will continue to evolve and change. Change begins from within and phlebotomists must be flexible enough to work with a variety of health care professionals in a wide range of settings. This type of uncertainty can be unsettling, however, it is important to realize that health care problems have become so complex, a team effort with a mix of skills is needed to solve them. Team efforts have become a necessity.

Teams can improve skills (more talent, expertise, and technical competence), communication (more ideas, mutual respect, crossing departmental lines), participation (increased job satisfaction, combined efforts are greater than individual efforts), effectiveness (solutions are more likely to be implemented, the team has ownership of the shared decisions).[1-3] There are several common sense traits and interpersonal skills that are needed in order for teams to be effective. These are listed in Box 1–3.

■ COMMUNICATION SKILLS IN THE PATIENT CARE ENVIRONMENT

As a vital member of the health care team, the phlebotomist provides the link between the patient and laboratory analytical area. The quality of the blood specimen determines the quality of the diagnostic test result. The ease of collection of these specimens, however, de-

---

BOX 1–3. INTERPERSONAL SKILLS AND TRAITS NEEDED FOR EFFECTIVE TEAMS

1. Understand the mission of the organization
2. Know the basic skills for group process and team dynamics (e.g., active listening, setting norms)
3. Understand relevance and commitment to team goals
4. Be reliable and dependable in work assignments
5. Be able to communicate ideas and feelings
6. Actively participate in decision making
7. Learn how to be flexible in decision making
8. Constructively manage conflicts
9. Contribute to the cohesion of the team
10. Contribute to problem solving strategies
11. Support and encourage other team members

pends on the skills and abilities of the health care worker to perform the collection techniques and interact successfully with the patient.

BEDSIDE MANNER

The climate established by the health care worker upon entering a patient's room. The feeling of confidence that comes from the knowledge that the collection tray is clean and completely stocked is the first step in a good bedside manner. A pleasant facial expression, neat appearance, and professional manner set the stage for a positive encounter with the patient. The first 30 seconds after the phlebotomist enters the patient's room determines how that patient perceives the quality of patient care offered by that hospital. Most patients admit that the procedure they dread most is being "stuck" for blood collection, so phlebotomists should make every effort to minimize the negative effects of the situation.

Upon entering the patient's room, the blood collector should introduce him- or herself and state that he or she is part of the hospital unit or laboratory staff, whichever is the case. The patient should be informed that the specimen is being collected for a test ordered by the physician. A statement indicating that this is routine hospital protocol often reassures the patient. A lengthy discussion of why a certain test was ordered or what tests were ordered is inappropriate. These questions should be referred to the patient's physician.

During all the steps of the venipuncture, the health care worker should remain calm, compassionate, and professional with conversations limited to essential information. Sometimes patients are comforted by letting them know about how the procedure is going (e.g., "this is going well," or "it is almost over"). Care should be taken not to be distracted from the phlebotomy procedure by excessive talk of unrelated issues. Before leaving the room, the patient should be thanked for cooperating.

COMMUNICATION ISSUES IN THE HOME AND AMBULATORY SETTINGS

As previously mentioned, blood collection and testing at the point-of-care is in great demand because of the convenience, reliability, and rapid turnaround time for test results. Various terms are used for laboratory testing in settings outside the inpatient hospital unit. These include on-site testing, alternate-site testing, near-patient testing, patient-focused testing, point-of-care testing, and bedside testing. Because this can take place in different environments ranging from clinics to physicians' offices to mobile vans to an individual's home, the setting may be more casual than in a hospital room. Nevertheless, professional behavior should remain particularly important.

Methods for communication in ambulatory settings or the home usually require more time for the following reasons:

- The phlebotomist must introduce him- or herself and clearly explain the purpose of the interaction.
- The patient should be directed to an appropriate place to sit or recline during the procedure. This may involve walking to a private area, blood collection booth, or special recliner.

- If the phlebotomy procedure is taking place in an unfamiliar setting, such as the patient's home, the phlebotomist must take extra time to find the nearest bathroom (for hand washing, blood spillage) and the nearest bed in case there are complications to the phlebotomy procedure (fainting).
- In a patient's home, the phlebotomist may need to find a phone or bring a mobile phone to clarify laboratory orders or inquire about patient information.
- Information about the procedure should be fully explained (especially if it is a first-time blood collection for the patient, or if it has been a long time since the last blood collection).
- Identifying the patient should be done meticulously and cautiously, using various methods to identify the patient positively (e.g., driver's license or identification card, confirmation of birthday and home address, or social security number, if available).
- The phlebotomist must assure that the puncture site has been appropriately cared for and that the patient is physically fit to leave the area after the phlebotomy procedure. If the patient is homebound, the phlebotomist must assure that the patient is no longer bleeding, the puncture site has been appropriately bandaged, and that the patient is able to stay by him- or herself.

PATIENT INTERVIEW

Health care organizations differ slightly in their guidelines for patient interviews. All agree that proper patient identification is essential. If the patient is hospitalized, this should be accomplished by a match between the test requisition or labels and the armband, and by verbal confirmation from the patient. If a hospitalized patient does *not* have an armband, a positive confirmation must be made by a unit nurse who knows the patient. This process should be well documented by the phlebotomist.

Special identification procedures should also be well documented for ambulatory patients, especially in cases of homebound patients, mobile vans, and other off-site locations. Armbands are not commonly used in ambulatory settings; however, an identification card usually is. It may include some demographic data and other identifying information, such as the patient's identification number, date of birth (DOB), address, or a combination of these. This information should be confirmed by the patient prior to blood collection. The patient should always be asked, "What is your name?" *not* "Are you Ms. Smith?" The first question is a more reliable and direct way of confirming identity. The second question is inappropriate and less reliable because a patient who is heavily medicated will often agree with anything that he or she is asked.

Some health care facilities insist that the health care worker ask for the patient's complete address, whereas others require the mention of the patient's hometown, birthdate, or street name to reinforce and confirm identity. Some prefer that patients spell an unusual last name. This portion of the specimen collection procedure ensures that the remainder of the diagnostic testing protocol provides information on the correct person.

It is important for the health care worker to remember that verbal and nonverbal cues (body language) play an important part in the communication of what the patient perceives and how he or she responds. In addition, listening skills are a valuable part of patient communication. Both of these skills are discussed further later in this chapter.

TEACHING PATIENTS

For most phlebotomy procedures to be successful the patient must participate and cooperate. The phlebotomist must be willing and able to provide sufficient, understandable instruction to the patient for the protocols to be accomplished. For example, in some clinical situations, patients with diabetes need to be instructed on the use of mechanical aids to perform finger sticks on themselves at home to check blood glucose levels.

Nursing staff or unit personnel may have instructed the inpatient that he or she will be fasting or will have "nothing by mouth" until after the early morning blood collections. The health care worker should listen to patients' comments, such as, "I didn't have breakfast yet," and "they won't feed me." Even a question or comment about food may inspire a response to confirm that the patient was truly fasting. When in doubt, simply asking the patient if they have eaten or had anything to drink other than water will confirm that the patient has been fasting.

Even more critical are the timed tests, such as the glucose tolerance test. In this test, patient understanding is essential. For the procedure to yield valid and reliable results, the patient must stay fasting, be in his or her room at the specified time, and drink enough water to provide the timed urine specimens. If the patient is a child, the parents or guardian must receive and understand the instructions. If the patient begins to feel ill or faint, the phlebotomist should know how to cope with the situation, depending on the setting they are in. Usually the appropriate nursing staff should be notified to aid in the patient's care; however, in ambulatory situations, nursing staff may not always be available and the phlebotomist should be trained on how to monitor the patient and cope with the circumstances. A bed and bathroom should be convenient to the collection area to provide for the patient's comfort and safety. Complications in blood collection, such as fainting (syncope), are discussed further in Chapter 10, and other first aid topics are reviewed in Chapter 5.

Other times at which the health care worker is involved with teaching patients about specimen collection involve 24-hour urine specimens, urine specimens for microbiologic culture, sputum, and stool specimens. These are more thoroughly discussed in Chapter 15.

COMMUNICATION STRATEGIES

Communication of information is essential not only for teaching and interacting with patients, but also for everyday effectiveness in all areas of the workplace. Effective verbal interactions can be depicted as a communication loop. The message must leave the sender and reach the receiver (Box 1–4). The receiver usually provides feedback to the sender. Without feedback, the sender has no way of knowing whether the message was accurately received or if the message was somehow blocked by extraneous factors. The factors can "filter out" meaning from a message. Filters can be damaging to effective communication. In the following sections, communication is broken down into its three more detailed components:

1. Verbal communication.
2. Nonverbal communication.
3. Active listening.

BOX 1–4. PATIENT–PHLEBOTOMIST COMMUNICATION LOOP

Sender/Phlebotomist

"Hello, please excuse the interruption, my name is Brenda and I work on this unit as a blood collector. I am here to collect a blood sample."

Filters

(Television is on, patient is about to eat breakfast, two family members are in the room talking about the football game last night, and a volunteer walks in to deliver mail.)

Receiver/Patient

"This is not going to hurt, is it? By the way, why are you doing this?"

Sender/Phlebotomist Feedback

(The phlebotomist should read verbal and nonverbal cues from the patient and family members to discern the patient's comfort level with the request to draw blood. Based on these impressions, his or her questions should be answered and additional issues should be clarified prior to proceeding with patient identification and specimen collection.)

"Would you mind if I turn down the volume on the television while we discuss this? It is important that a blood sample be taken prior to your breakfast so that the laboratory can run the tests your doctor has ordered. The procedure hurts a little, but it should be over quickly. Do you have any other questions about this procedure? Your family members may stay in your room if you are more comfortable with them here."

Feedback Loop Is Completed by Confirmation From the Receiver/Patient

"I don't have any other questions, and you can go ahead with the stick. I would like my family members to stay for moral support."

Verbal Communication

A basic understanding of the language is needed for any health care worker to communicate with all patients, young and old. There are filters or barriers to simple verbal communication, however, that can interfere greatly with the patient–phlebotomist relationship.

Language.   Many members of the health care team use jargon or medical terminology to explain procedures to the patient. This can be confusing to lay people. In addition, the meaning of words varies with the context and age of the speaker. To promote understanding, a vocabulary that is easily understood should be used with patients whenever possible. This is particularly true with children.

Patients must *not* be told, "This won't hurt." Most blood collection procedures are slightly painful; therefore, it is important that the patient be forewarned and prepared. This is even more important when dealing with children. To help ease anxiety, the child can be asked to hold something (e.g., a bandage) while the procedure is taking place. This allows the child to feel helpful and provides a distraction from the procedure.

Hearing Impairments.   The more complex the directions, the greater the need to communicate. Thus, the health care worker should be more sensitive to patients who have impaired hearing. A question such as, "Is there a step you would like me to repeat before we begin?" yields better clues that the patient has heard and understood than saying, "Do you understand?" If it is obvious that the patient did not hear, all efforts should be made to write down instructions for the patient. It is strongly recommended that writing tools be kept at the bedside of these patients and also be accessible in ambulatory settings.

Other distracting noises can also interfere with hearing. A busy hallway, visitors, a television or radio in the room, or headphones can prevent the patient from hearing accurately. In these cases, the phlebotomist should take steps in a polite and professional manner, to reduce the sound level so the patient can hear necessary instructions. Examples might include phrases, such as the following:

- *To visitors:* "Excuse me please, it is important for me to explain this procedure to Mr. Jones. Would you mind if we have a quiet moment together for a few minutes? Thank you for your cooperation."
- *For the television:* "Mr. Jones, I am sorry to disrupt your television show, but would you mind if we lower the volume for a few minutes so we can go over the procedure for collecting your blood sample? Thank you, this should only take a few minutes."
- *For headphones:* "Mr. Jones, it is important that we discuss this procedure before beginning. Would you mind taking off your headphones for a few minutes? I will be brief. Thank you for your cooperation."

English as a Second Language.   The diversity of languages spoken in this country is extensive. In many parts of the United States, one sees signs in multiple languages. Patients who do not speak English can understand some basics from nonverbal cues, such as sign language, but the phlebotomist must know how to locate an interpreter, if possible. Often there may be volunteers to perform language interpretations. If a large segment of the patient population speaks another language, the health care facility should provide interpreters who know the basic use of that language. In the absence of an interpreter, written instructions in other languages may facilitate the process. Printed cards in different languages can be used to transmit information.

In the southern and western United States, it is important to develop some skill in Spanish. It is recommended that the health care worker practice the phrases with someone who can speak the language before attempting to communicate with a patient because mispronounced words may lead to more confusion.

Keep in mind that English language skills and understanding may vary greatly in the United States. The cultural diversity in this country lends itself to language differences. The health care worker should always speak respectfully, in a highly professional manner, and with phrases that are clearly articulated. The dignity of the patient, whether he or she is English speaking or not, is of utmost importance. If a health care worker feels frustrated by an inability to communicate with a patient, he or she should seek assistance from a supervisor, translator, family member, or physician. Each patient should be treated compassionately, fairly, and with the utmost of dignity, regardless of language abilities. (Basic requests in Spanish are listed in Box 1–5.)

Age.   The vocabulary of a teenager is different from that of someone 70 to 80 years old. Phlebotomists should be sensitive to word usage for each age.

BOX 1–5. BASIC REQUESTS IN ENGLISH AND SPANISH

The following translations are designed to present the health care worker with a *very basic* means of communicating with patients who speak Spanish. Before speaking with patients, the health care worker should practice using these phrases with someone who knows the correct pronunciation. Otherwise, the patient may become even more confused. Another alternative is to have the key phrases printed on cards that the health care worker may point to or use as a reference when he or she is communicating with the patient.

English	Spanish
one	uno
two	dos
three	tres
four	cuatro
five	cinco
six	seis
seven	siete
eight	ocho
nine	nueve
ten	diez
twenty	veinte
thirty	treinta
forty	cuarenta
fifty	cincuenta
sixty	sesenta
seventy	setenta
eighty	ochenta
ninety	noventa
one hundred	ciento/cien
Hello.	Hola.
Good day.	Buenos dias/Buendia.
Good morning.	Buenos dias.
Good afternoon.	Buenas tardes.
Good evening.	Buenas noches.
Mother	Madre/mama
Father	Padre/papa
Sister	Hermana
Brother	Hermano
Son	Hijo
Daughter	Hija
Husband	Esposo/marido
Wife	Esposa/marida
Infant/baby	Niño/niña
Grandfather	Abuelo
Grandmother	Abuela
Friend	Amigo/Amiga
Mister	Señor
Mrs.	Señora

(continued)

BOX 1–5. (continued)

English	Spanish
Miss	Señorita
Doctor	Doctor
Nurse	Enfermera
My name is . . .	Me llamo . . . /Mi nombres . . .
I work in the laboratory.	Trabajo en el laboratorio.
I speak . . .	Hablo . . .
We are going to analyze	Vamos analizar
. . . your blood.	. . . su sangre.
. . . your urine.	. . . su orina.
. . . your sputum.	. . . su esputo.
Do you understand?	¿Entiende Usted (ud.)?
I do not understand.	No entiendo.
Please (pls.)	Por favor (p.f.)
Thank you.	Gracias.
You are welcome.	De nada.
Speak slower, pls.	Hable mas despacio, p.f.
Repeat, pls.	Haga me el favor de repetir.
Relax.	Relajese.
What is your name?	¿Como se llama?
What is your address?	¿Que es su domicilio?
What is your birth date?	¿En que fecha nacio?
How old are you?	¿Cuantos años tiene ud.?
Have you been here before?	¿Ha estado ud. aquí antes?
Who is your doctor?	¿Quien es su doctor?
Your doctor wrote the order.	El doctor/la doctora escribio la orden.
Here is the bathroom.	Aquí esta el baño.
Here is the call light.	Aquí esta la luz de emergencia.
You may not eat/drink anything except water.	No debe de comer/beber nada solamente agua.
You may not smoke.	No puede fumar.
Have you had breakfast?	¿Ya tomo el desayuno?
We need a blood/urine/stool sample.	Necesitamos una muestra de su sangre/orina/del excremento.
Please	Haga me el favor de
. . . make a fist.	. . . cerrar el puño.
. . . bend your arm.	. . . doblar el brazo.
. . . roll up your sleeve.	. . . levantarse la manga.
. . . open your hand.	. . . abrir la mano.
. . . sit down here.	. . . sientese aquí.
. . . change your position.	. . . cambiarse de posición.

(continued)

BOX 1–5. (continued)

English	Spanish
. . . turn over.	. . . voltearse.
. . . change to the left.	. . . cambiarse a la izquierda.
. . . change to the right.	. . . cambiarse a la derecha.
I need to	Necesito
. . . take a blood sample.	. . . sacar una muestrade sangre.
. . . stick/prick your finger.	. . . picarle su dedo.
It will hurt a little.	Le va a doler un poquito.
The needle will stay in your arm while I am collecting the blood sample.	La aguja se quedara en su brazo durante el tiempo necessario para obtener la muestra.
I am finished.	Ya termine.
Press this gauze on your arm/finger until I can make sure that the bleeding has stopped.	Comprese esta banda en su brazo su dedo hasta que pare la sangre.
Are you lightheaded?	¿Esta usted mareado/mareada?
Do you feel as if you are going to faint?	¿Se siente como si se va a desmayar?
You must lie down.	Necesita acostarse.
Collect the midstream portion of the urine in the container or bottle.	Coléccione la porción del medio de la orina en el vaso.

Tone of Voice. The tone of one's voice and the inflection used can change a positive sentence into a negative sounding statement. The pitch, or tone, of voice should match the words that are spoken. Sarcasm is usually communicated just by tone of voice. Health care workers can avoid sending mixed messages to patients by practicing a calm, soothing, and confident tone of voice. Box 1–6 is a practice exercise for health care professionals to use in observing their own facial expressions and voice tones.

Emergency Situations. Emergency or "STAT" blood collections are common in emergency rooms and in some complicated surgical or medical cases. These phlebotomy procedures require extra speed and accuracy without jeopardizing the "personal touch." Patients in emergency rooms may not have identification information with them and may be unconscious. All facilities, however, should have documented procedures for the identification process with which phlebotomists should be familiar. Individual patients should be considered in terms of his or her dignity and individual needs, not by nicknames, such as, "Mr. L down the hall," or "the broken leg in 3C." Each is entitled to professional, respectful care in all circumstances.

Nonverbal Communication

Some educators believe that communication is comprised of 10 to 20 percent words and 80 to 90 percent nonverbal cues. These nonverbal cues, or body language, can be positive and helpful to understanding, or it can be negative and hinder effective communication. These cues are summarized in Box 1–7.

BOX 1–6. EXERCISE TO IMPROVE TONE OF VOICE AND FACIAL EXPRESSIONS

The following exercise is useful for improving verbal and nonverbal communication skills. Practice it in front of a mirror or with a co-worker.

Step 1. Using a *nice tone of voice* (i.e., calm, compassionate, clear, professional tone), with a smile on your face, practice saying the following phrases:

- "Please . . . "
- "Good morning."
- "How was your breakfast?"
- "Have you had lunch?"
- "May I check your identification bracelet?"
- "Thank you."

Step 2. Now, using a *degrading tone of voice* (i.e., sarcastic, whiny, angry tone), with a frustrated, disdainful look on your face, repeat the phrases listed in step 1.

Step 3. List the specific features you liked about the first method with those features you disliked about the second method. Try to contrast details of facial features (wrinkled eyebrows or smiling face), how the voice lowers or raises at the end of the statements, and how you feel when speaking in the two manners.

Step 4. Keep a mental impression (or actually take a picture) of the way you look and sound during the first step. *Remember:* A simple smile can often force a positive change in voice tone.

BOX 1–7. NONVERBAL COMMUNICATION, OR BODY LANGUAGE

Positive Body Language

Maintaining erect posture

Having relaxed hands, arms, shoulders

Communicating face to face

Maintaining eye contact

Communicating at eye level when possible

Displaying good grooming habits

Maintaining zone of comfort

Smiling

Negative Body Language and Distracting Behaviors

Slouching, shrugging shoulders

Rolling eyes, wandering eyes

Looking at ceiling or window, staring blankly

Rubbing eyes, blinking excessively

Squirming

Tapping foot, fingers, pencil

Sighing deeply, moaning, groaning

Crossing arms, clenching fists

Wrinkling forehead

Thumbing through books or papers

Chewing gum

Repeatedly looking at clock or watch

Lining up objects on a desk

Stretching, yawning

Sitting backward on a chair (i.e., straddling it)

Peering over eyeglasses

Pointing a finger at someone

Positive Body Language

Smiling.   A simple, compassionate smile can set the stage for open lines of communication. It can make each patient feel that he or she is the most important person at that moment. In addition, most people look better with smiles on their faces than they do with frowns.

Eye Contact and Eye Level.   The most expressive parts of the human face are the eyes. Therefore, eye contact is important in effective communication. Eye contact promotes a sense of trust and honesty between the patient and phlebotomist. It can make the entire procedure less traumatic for the patient if he or she sees a compassionate expression in the phlebotomist's eyes.

Eye level is also a consideration. Bedridden patients must always look up to those in the room, including the health care team members. This can create a feeling of intimidation, of being "looked down on," or of weakness. Most of the time, phlebotomists do not have the extra time to spend finding a chair to sit in so that they are at eye level; however, if a health care worker must explain a lengthy procedure or if it is noted that the patient is particularly nervous about the procedure, the explanation should be done while seated at eye level with the patient. Box 1–8 is an exercise for understanding what it feels like to be bedridden.

Face-to-Face Communication.   Phlebotomists should face patients directly. Otherwise, the patient may feel neglected, that they are being avoided, or that information is being withheld. If a patient turns away from a phlebotomist, however, it should be taken as a cue that the patient is either very frightened, reluctant, angry, or in pain. The phlebotomist should do everything to make the patient feel more comfortable during the phlebotomy procedure.

Zone of Comfort.   Most individuals begin to feel uncomfortable when strangers get too close to them physically. A **zone of comfort** is the area of space around a patient that is private territory, so to speak. When a stranger gets too close, it can cause the patient to feel nervous, fearful, or anxious. Health care workers must be understanding and approach nervous patients slowly and gently to avoid causing feelings of being threatened. This is particularly true with children, many of whom have a wide zone of comfort; that is, they do not like anyone to approach them except close relatives or friends. A skilled health care worker must be aware of his or her threat to a patient and use a calm, professional, and confident manner.

BOX 1–8.   PRACTICE EXERCISE FOR DEVELOPING SENSITIVITY TO BEDRIDDEN PATIENTS

Health care workers should strive to be as compassionate as possible. Bedridden patients often feel intimidated because health care workers must repeatedly "look down" on them to provide care. Sometimes, these patients are depressed because of their condition or prognosis. This exercise will help you imagine yourself in the patient's condition and can make you a more compassionate member of the health care team. Practice the exercise with a co-worker.

1. Lie on a bed while your co-worker stands directly over you, looking down.

2. Have the co-worker go through the motions of a venipuncture procedure, including the greeting and identification process. Try to imagine the anticipation of the needle stick. Have the co-worker maintain eye contact with you while conversing.

3. Repeat step 2, without eye contact.

4. Mentally note the positive and negative aspects of this procedure.

In some cultures, the zone of comfort may be wide, and in others, people naturally speak more closely to each other. How much at ease a person feels with physical closeness can also vary with gender. Some women feel very uncomfortable having a male health care worker standing over them preparing to draw a blood specimen, and vice versa. It is particularly considerate if a phlebotomist recognizes this and responds accordingly. Again, respect for the patient's needs and dignity must be considered. Phlebotomists can practice having the sensation that someone is "too close for comfort" by using role reversal. Box 1–9 provides a brief exercise.

Negative Body Language and Distracting Behaviors

Wandering Eyes.   When people roll their eyes upward, they convey the sense of being bored, inattentive, or unwilling to perform a duty. Because this behavior is distracting, it should be avoided when a phlebotomist is communicating with, listening to, or observing patients, co-workers, or supervisors.

The same can be said about gazing out the window or looking up at the ceiling. If a phlebotomist enters a patient's room and begins addressing the patient while looking out the window, the patient will feel neglected and the phlebotomist will appear unconcerned. If the window is too tempting to avoid a glance, the phlebotomist can include the patient in his or her observations. A friendly comment about the weather might be appropriate; then the phlebotomy procedure can be continued when full attention can be given to the patient. The objective is to make the patient feel at ease through good communication techniques so that the procedure can be successful.

Nervous Behaviors.   Behaviors, such as squirming or tapping a pencil or a foot, can be very distracting. They can make a patient feel nervous, hurried, or anxious about the venipuncture. A calm and confident image maximizes the patient's comfort and trust. It is also helpful to recognize these behaviors in patients, especially children, so that efforts can

BOX 1–9. ROLE REVERSAL EXERCISE

Having respect for an individual's personal space, or zone of comfort, is part of being a compassionate health care worker. The comfort zone of each person varies with sex, culture, and situation. However, most people feel uneasy when strangers are touching them or are "too close for comfort." An example of this uncomfortable sensation is in a crowded elevator. People take great measures to move so that they are not touching strangers, and as people exit the elevator, the remaining people move and shift to provide more space around themselves. This same sense of uneasiness is felt by patients who are approached by unfamiliar health care workers.

To simulate a real patient–health care worker interaction, practice the following exercise with a co-worker who is not a close friend. Eye contact should be made during this exercise.

1. Lie on a bed as if you are a patient.
2. Have the co-worker slowly approach you. He or she should begin 10 feet away and pause between steps.
3. Note at what distance you begin to feel awkward or uncomfortable. (Usually, this distance is about 2 to 4 feet from the bed.) This distance is the boundary of your zone of comfort.
4. Repeat the exercise with the same co-worker. You will probably require a smaller zone of comfort because a person becomes a little more at ease after initial contact with an unfamiliar person.

be made to reduce fear. Allowing a few extra moments of conversation or preparation may help.

Breathing Pattern.   A deep sigh can convey a feeling of being bored or a reluctance to do the job. Phlebotomists should avoid sighing, especially when communicating with an angry, uncooperative patient. Likewise, if a patient sighs deeply or moans at the mere sight of the phlebotomist, this should be a cue that a little extra attention, conversation, or a smile might ease the patient's reluctance for the procedure.

Other Distracting Behaviors.   Many other actions can convey negative or defensive emotions. Among these are crossed arms, a wrinkled forehead, frequent glances at a clock or watch, rapid thumbing through papers, chewing gum, yawning, or stretching. Health care workers should realize that these behaviors can detract from their professional image when they are communicating with patients, families, visitors, co-workers, and supervisors. It is also important to realize what these cues mean if a patient exhibits them. The most effective communicators can detect these signs immediately and deal with them in an honest, compassionate, and professional manner. Regular in-services or continuing education programs can be directed at reminding phlebotomists to be aware of positive and negative body language, both in their own behavior and that of patients.

Active Listening

Another component of effective communication is the art of listening. **Active listening** helps close the communication loop by ensuring that the message sent can indeed be repeated and understood. Listening skills do not depend on intellect or educational background; they can be learned and practiced. Box 1–10 provides tips for becoming an active listener.

■ APPEARANCE, GROOMING, AND PHYSICAL FITNESS POSTURE

Phlebotomists usually perform their work while standing. There are occasions, however, particularly with ambulatory patients, when it is more effective to sit adjacent to the patient for the blood collection procedure. Erect posture conveys a sense of confidence and pride in job performance. Slouching conveys a sense of laziness and apathy.

Good posture is helpful for both the phlebotomist and the patient. It minimizes the health care worker's back and neck strain and eases the patient's mind about the confidence of the phlebotomist. Relaxed hands, arms, and shoulders enable the health care worker to work more freely and to show the patient how to relax their arms and shoulders as well.

GROOMING

Physical appearance communicates a strong impression about an individual. Neatly combed hair, clean fingernails, a clean, pressed uniform, protective garb, and an overall tidy appearance communicate a commitment to cleanliness and infection control, and they instill confidence in a person. This is particularly important in today's health care environment, where patients and employees are deeply concerned about the spread of infectious diseases, such as hepatitis, tuberculosis, and human immunodeficiency virus (HIV).

> ## BOX 1–10. STEPS FOR ACTIVE LISTENING
>
> The following steps are presented as a starting point for the development of listening skills by health care workers. Because individuals can mentally process words faster than they can speak them, a good listener must concentrate and focus on the speaker to keep his or her mind from wandering. Development of these skills can help an individual in professional life as well as in personal life.
>
> 1. Concentrate on the speaker by "getting ready" to listen. Take a moment to clear your mind of distracting thoughts. Begin the interaction with an open, objective mind. Sometimes taking a deep breath can help clear your mind and prepare it to receive more information.
> 2. Use silent pauses in the conversation wisely by mentally summarizing what has been said.
> 3. Let the speaker know that someone is listening. Use simple phrases, such as "I see," "Oh," "Very interesting," and "How about that," to reassure the speaker and communicate understanding and acceptance.
> 4. Keep personal judgments to yourself until the speaker finishes relaying his or her idea.
> 5. Verify the conversation with feedback. Make sure that everything was clarified. Ask for more explanation if necessary.
> 6. Mentally review the key words to summarize the overall idea being communicated.
> 7. Pay attention to body language and ask for clarification. Simple prompts, such as "You look sad," and "You seem upset or nervous," can add more meaning to the conversation and encourage the speaker to verbalize feelings.
> 8. Listen for true meaning in the message, not just the literal words.
> 9. Maintain eye contact to communicate interest or concern.
> 10. Encourage the listener to expand his or her thoughts by using simple phrases, such as "Let's discuss it further," "Tell me more about it," and "Really?"
> 11. Paraphrase the idea or conversation to ensure complete understanding.
> 12. Practice active listening at work and at home.

PERSONAL HYGIENE

A professional appearance is completed by careful attention to personal hygiene. A daily bath or shower followed by the use of deodorant is recommended. Perfume or aftershave lotions should be used sparingly because patients may be allergic or may find some scents overpowering and distasteful when they are sick.

NUTRITION, REST, AND EXERCISE

The role of a health care worker requires physical stamina. Good health improves the health care worker's appearance, attitude, job performance, and ability to cope with stress. Appropriate eating habits, rest during lunch and break periods, and off-duty exercising are essential to an individual's well-being. Practicing a healthy lifestyle while on and off duty will facilitate a return to work with a refreshed and more productive attitude.

In most health care environments, the pace is hectic, and overtime work is common. Therefore, it is helpful to know how to deal with stress. Box 1–11 gives some tips for dealing with stress.

> ## BOX 1–11. TIPS FOR DEALING WITH STRESS
>
> Take time to manage time effectively.
> Plan time to rest, even at work during breaks.
> Associate with gentle people.
> Learn and practice relaxation skills.
> Eat nutritious foods and exercise to improve health.
> Engage in satisfying, meaningful work and hobbies.
> Find time for privacy.
> Read interesting books and articles to get new ideas.

PROTECTIVE EQUIPMENT AND CLOTHING

Employers of health care workers are legally required to provide **personal protective equipment (PPE)** or barrier protection for workers handling biohazardous, infectious substances. This type of garb includes gowns, gloves, masks, laboratory coats or aprons, and face shields. Due to latex sensitivities and allergies, employers must provide an array of sizes and styles of gloves and gowns in order to protect their employees. Careful compliance with safety standards minimizes the risk of occupational exposures to blood-borne pathogens. Safety considerations are covered in more detail in Chapter 5.

■ PATIENT'S RIGHTS

All members of the health care team must recognize that their first responsibility is to the patient's health, safety, and personal dignity. Many organizations, such as the **American Hospital Association (AHA),** have recognized rights for patients in health care organizations. The AHA originally adopted a **Patient's Bill of Rights** in 1973, and it has revised and/or reaffirmed it as needed. The key elements involve a patient's rights to the following:

- Respectful and considerate care.
- Accurate information.
- Informed consent.
- Refusal of treatment.
- Privacy.
- Confidentiality.
- Advance directives.
- Information about the identity and role of personnel involved in his or her care.
- Information about research procedures involved in his or her care.
- Billing information.

ISSUES IN SPECIMEN COLLECTION

There are occasions during specimen collections when a patient's rights are particularly important. The patient may be rude, ill tempered, demanding, uncooperative, or a combination of these. It is important, however, for members of the health care team to always deliver the best quality of care that they can give, while being careful to show consideration, fairness, compassion, and respect for each patient.

Requests for certain laboratory tests and the results of clinical laboratory tests are part of the patient's medical record and are *strictly confidential*. This rule of confidentiality applies in all areas inside and outside of the work site. A health care worker should never discuss patient information with individuals who are not directly responsible for some aspect of patient care. Nor should patient information be discussed in public places, such as an elevator, hallway, or cafeteria. Family members or friends may overhear and would not have the benefit of a full explanation. Joking in the work area about a patient's condition, physical feature, or character trait is completely inappropriate and unprofessional. These situations could be interpreted as a violation of confidentiality and are subject to legal action.

Clinical laboratory requisitions and reports also contain demographic data that should not be exposed to the public, even if the analytic results are not yet recorded. The health care facility is responsible for the security of data in electronic information storage and retrieval systems and for making the information available only to those who specifically need it. Health care workers are, however, also responsible for doing their part in maintaining confidentiality.

In general, the patient's primary care giver, usually a physician, is responsible for discussing information about why laboratory tests were ordered, the results, the testing methodologies, or the medical decisions that will be made based on the results. Health care workers involved in specimen collection should refrain from giving information of this nature to patients, their families, or their friends. This can be correctly handled by saying to the patient or family member, "Your physician ordered blood to be drawn for testing; it would be best to discuss the tests with him or her."

Sometimes, a talkative patient may want to share information of a personal and sensitive nature with the health care worker. It is appropriate to stop the patient politely from disclosure and continue the collection procedure.

As part of the principle of informed consent, the health care worker should briefly explain to the patient the procedures used to collect the blood sample. The patient also has the right to know that the blood drawing team member is part of the organizations' staff and who he or she is. It is important for the phlebotomist to stress that the physician has ordered the tests. The patient also has the right to know if someone involved in his or her care is a student. It is helpful if the student's supervisor can reassure the patient of the student's competency to perform the procedure. Every effort should be made to have student–patient interactions be positive.

If a patient refuses to have a blood specimen drawn, the health care worker is responsible for reminding the patient that the physician ordered the clinical laboratory tests as part of the patient's medical care. If the patient still refuses, the health care worker should inform his or her supervisor and, if possible, the physician. Emotional confrontations or conflicts with the patient should be avoided. All actions and discussions should be documented.

FAMILY, VISITORS, AND SIGNIFICANT OTHERS

Family members and friends of patients are often present when phlebotomists need to acquire specimens. It is important to realize that they can make the patient more secure and comfortable. Sometimes, however, families and visitors are much more difficult to deal with than the patients. They may make requests that are beyond the scope of acceptable or authorized responsibilities for the health care worker. For example, unless specifically authorized to do so, a health care worker should not give food to hospitalized patients. It is better to inform the appropriate health care team member of the family member's request.

If several visitors are in the room with the patient, they may be asked to step into the hall while the blood specimen is being drawn. If the health care worker believes that assistance is required, a family member may be asked to assist. This can make the family members feel helpful, as well as provide reassurance to patients, particularly children.

Physicians, priests, and chaplains have the right to visit privately with patients. Unless the blood specimen is timed, the health care worker should respect that privacy and return to the patient after completing the other draws in the unit or area. If the procedure is timed or stat, the health care worker can apologize for the interruption, explain the nature of the request, and ask permission to collect the specimen.

Families and visitors of patients should not be permitted in the clinical laboratory or provided with patient information, except by prior arrangement and permission. Their safety and the confidentiality of patient records must be considered. Frequently, patients do not want their family members to know test results.

■ HEALTH CARE ORGANIZATIONS

Until the 1990s, health care in the United States was provided primarily in physicians' offices, clinics, and hospitals. Services were provided by highly specialized health care workers (e.g., specialty doctors, nurses with specialized training for specific illnesses, clinical laboratory scientists, respiratory therapists, nutrition and dietary experts, phlebotomists). As technologic advances and pressures to lower health care costs have driven facilities to become more patient-centered and efficient, health care teams constantly try to balance quality and cost-effectiveness. Tasks of team members are becoming more integrated and blended; for example, many nurses are now responsible for collecting blood samples, whereas many phlebotomists have become *clinical assistants* or *patient care technicians* as they help with patient care duties along with specimen collection duties.

Health care organizations have also evolved into different levels of care. **Primary care** is given to maintain and monitor normal health and to prevent diseases by means of laboratory screening tests and immunizations. Blood cholesterol screening and blood glucose screening for diabetes are examples. Other examples of primary care include treatment of minor injuries, diagnosis and treatment of colds or sore throats, well-baby checkups for infants, immunizations, prenatal care during a normal pregnancy, and treatment of chronic illnesses and diseases, such as diabetes mellitus.

Primary care physicians are usually trained in family practice or internal medicine. Other primary health care workers include nurse practitioners, nurse midwives, nurse specialists, and physician assistants (PAs). When patients need a higher level of care, the primary care professionals are responsible for referring patients to the appropriate specialist.

Secondary care refers to specialized care involving a physician who is an expert on a particular group of diseases, a group of organ systems, or an organ. For example, an ophthalmologist is a specialist who diagnoses and treats eye disorders.

Tertiary care is highly specialized and oriented toward unusual and complex diagnoses and therapies. Sophisticated instrumentation and technology or invasive procedures, such as open-heart surgery, are used in an acute care hospital environment. **Acute care** hospitals are characterized by hospital stays of less than 30 days. **Long-term care** refers to care needed longer than 30 days. Hospitalized patients are often referred to as **inpatients.**

HOSPITAL INPATIENT SERVICES

There are approximately 6000 hospitals in the United States. They vary according to the following:

- Mission (patient care, education, research).
- Bed size.
- Ownership (public or nonprofit, governmental, for profit or proprietary).
- Length of stay (short term [e.g., less than 30 days]; long term [e.g., greater than 30 days]).
- Type of care provided (general acute care hospitals; and specialty care hospitals, such as birthing centers, cancer centers, psychiatric hospitals, pediatric hospitals, and rehabilitation hospitals).
- Location (urban or rural).
- Relationship to other health facilities (integrated hospital systems, religious multihospital systems, independent hospitals).

Traditional hospitals have been organizationally structured around departments according to medical or surgical specialties. The typical hospital departments of the 1980s and early 1990s are shown in Table 1–1 and sometimes are still used. Subspecialized departments are usually organized around organs or organ systems as shown in Table 1–2. Sometimes, departments or ancillary services are organized around therapy services or procedures offered to the patient. Phlebotomists should become knowledgeable about these areas of the hospital because patients spend time in them prior to, during, and after their phlebotomy procedures. There are factors that may affect the outcome of the laboratory test that relate to these departments. Typical hospital services are listed in Box 1–12.

Hospitals are in a state of flux due to the shifting health care trends previously mentioned. As a result of reengineering and restructuring, new organizational structures have surfaced in recent years. Many traditional hospital departments have been merged or have been eliminated as needed. Some models now provide for departments around disease sites, such as breast cancer or prostate cancer. Other innovative approaches involve patient centered, family centered, or both types of care with more emphasis on empowering the patient and families to be responsible for the care. Hospitals, in some cases, have taken on nontraditional services, such as hotel management, music therapy, etc. Another trend for hospitals has been to expand their services to provide more of a continuous system from birth through death. Community outreach efforts have also been expanded to reach new managed care markets. New markets sometimes include patients enrolled in **Medicare** (federal program covering health services for the elderly) and **Medicaid** (joint federal and state program covering health services for the poor and other special populations).

In summary, for the next few years, the hospital industry will continue to experiment with new models of health care delivery that will affect all health care workers.

AMBULATORY AND HOME HEALTH CARE SERVICES

Ambulatory care is personal health care provided to an individual who is not bedridden. Trends in the health care industry have led to a wide range of ambulatory services delivered in a variety of settings. The shift from inpatient hospital services to ambulatory or "outpatient" services has been facilitated by technologic advances, computer applications that

Table 1–1.   Departments Found in Most Large Health Care Facilities

DEPARTMENT	BRIEF DESCRIPTION
Internal medicine	General diagnosis and treatment of patients for problems of one or more internal organs
Pediatrics	General diagnosis and therapy for children
Surgery	Diagnosis and treatment in which the physician physically alters a part of the patient's body
Anesthesiology	Preparing the patient for specialized treatment and/or surgery
Pathology and laboratory medicine	Diagnosis, both before and after treatment, using anatomic and/or clinical laboratory test results
Obstetrics/gynecology	Diagnosis and treatment relating to the sexual reproductive system of females, using both surgical and nonsurgical procedures
Psychiatry/neurology	Diagnosis and treatment for people of all ages with mental, emotional, and nervous system problems, using primarily nonsurgical procedures
Radiology/medical imaging	Diagnosis and treatment, primarily through the use of x-ray, ultrasonography, and other internal imaging procedures
Allergy	Diagnosis and treatment of persons who have allergies or "reactions" to irritating agents
Geriatrics	Diagnosis and treatment of the elderly population
Oncology	Diagnosis and treatment of malignant (life-threatening) tumors
Proctology	Diagnosis and treatment of diseases of the anus and rectum
Rheumatology	Diagnosis and treatment of joint and tissue diseases, including arthritis
Family medicine/general practice	Care of medical problems of all family members so that a different physician is not necessary for each family member by age level or sex
Neonatal–perinatal	Study, support, and treatment of newborn and prematurely born babies and their mothers
Physical medicine	Diagnosis and treatment of disorders and disabilities of the neuromuscular system
Plastic surgery	Correction of the deformity of tissues, including skin

allow for portability, and more efficient models of delivering quality care outside the hospital. In addition, with the "aging of America" the fastest growing segment of the population is the elderly. Many health care services have been established to make it more accessible and comfortable for elderly individuals with chronic conditions to seek treatment outside the hospital setting. Long-term care services may involve inpatient and/or ambulatory services.

Home health care services are rapidly expanding. Home health care involves the provision of services in a patient's home under the direction of a physician. Phlebotomists, nurses, home health assistants and aides, and others are employed by companies and hospitals offering these services. These health care workers usually perform multiple tasks at homes throughout the community. They then transport the blood to the clinical laboratory for testing. Box 1–13 describes a range of ambulatory care settings.

Table 1–2.   Medical Departments Listed by Organs and Organ Sysems

DEPARTMENT	ORGANS AND ORGAN SYSTEMS
Orthopedics	Bones and joints
Ophthalmology	Eyes
Otolaryngology	Ears, nose, and throat
Urology	Sexual and reproductive system for males and renal system for females and males
Cardiology	Heart
Dermatology	Skin
Neurology	Nervous system
Hematology	Blood system
Immunology	Immune system
Gastroenterology	Esophagus, stomach, and intestines
Nephrology	Kidneys
Endocrinology	Organs and tissues that produce hormones (e.g., estrogens, testosterone, cortisol)
Cardiovascular	Heart and blood circulation
Pulmonary	Lungs

Many of these settings provide on-site laboratory services. In some cases, however, blood and other patient specimens are sent by courier to a larger independent laboratory or back to a hospital-based laboratory for testing. In other cases, blood tests may be done at the site of the collection, e.g., **point of care** testing.

THE CLINICAL LABORATORY'S ROLE IN SPECIMEN COLLECTION SERVICES

A typical hospital-based clinical laboratory can have two components: **clinical pathology** and **anatomic pathology.** In the clinical pathology area, blood and other types of body fluids and tissues are analyzed (e.g., urine, cerebrospinal fluid [CSF], sputum, gastric secretions, synovial fluid). In the anatomic pathology area, autopsies are performed, and cytologic procedures and surgical biopsy tissues are analyzed. Laboratories can also be independently owned and operated outside the hospital setting. Regardless of the type of laboratory, it is important to understand that the phlebotomist plays a vital role in the process of analysis. Reliability and accuracy of test results depend on the *preanalytic* process of specimen collection.

Personnel who work on the *analytic* phase of laboratory testing may have different educational backgrounds:

- *Pathologists:* physicians who have extensive training in pathology, which is the study and diagnosis of disease through the use of laboratory test results.
- *Administrative staff:* individuals who usually have a graduate degree in health care administration or business. Often these individuals have extensive clinical experience as well.
- *Technical supervisors:* clinical laboratory scientists (also known as medical technologists) with additional experience and education in a laboratory specialty area, such as hematology, microbiology, or clinical chemistry.

BOX 1–12. TRADITIONAL HOSPITAL ANCILLARY SERVICES OR DEPARTMENTS

- *Laboratory medicine/pathology:* uses sophisticated instrumentation to analyze blood, body fluids, and tissues for pathological conditions. Laboratory results are used in diagnosis, treatment, and monitoring of patients' health status.
- *Occupational therapy:* assists the patient in becoming functionally independent within the limitations of the patient's disability or condition. Occupational therapists (OTs) collaborate with the health care team to design therapeutic programs of rehabilitative activities for the patient. The therapy is designed to improve functional abilities or activities of daily living (ADLs).
- *Physical therapy:* assists the patient in restoring physical abilities that have been impaired by illness or injury. Rehabilitation programs often use heat/cold, water therapy, ultrasound or electricity, and physical exercises designed to restore useful activity.
- *Pharmacy:* dispenses medications ordered by physicians. Pharmacists also collaborate with the health care team on drug therapies. Phlebotomists may collect blood specimens at timed intervals to monitor the level of the drug in the patient's bloodstream.
- *Nutrition and dietetics:* perform nutritional assessments, patient education, and design special diets for patients who have eating-related disorders (i.e., diabetes, obesity).
- *Diagnostic imaging/radiology:* uses ionizing radiation for treating disease, fluoroscopic and radiographic x-ray instrumentation and imaging methods for diagnosis, and radioisotopes for both diagnosing and treating disease. Fluoroscopic, tomographic, and radiographic analyses of the human body are performed. In this department, patients and employees are protected from exposure to unnecessary radiation. Sometimes patients are injected with dye that might interfere with some laboratory tests. The phlebotomist should document the circumstances as appropriate. In addition, the phlebotomist should be aware of applicable safety requirements.
- *Nuclear medicine:* uses radioactive isotopes or tracers in the diagnosis and treatment of patients and in the study of the disease process. The radioactive substance is injected into the patient and emits rays that can be detected by sophisticated instrumentation. Phlebotomists should be knowledgeable of special safety requirements for entering this area. Also, the radioisotopes may interfere with laboratory testing so this should be documented.
- *Encephalography:* uses the electroencephalograph (EEG) to record brain wave patterns.
- *Electrocardiography:* uses the electrocardiograph (ECG or EKG) to record the electric currents produced by contractions of the heart. This assists in the diagnosis of heart disease.
- *Radiotherapy:* uses high-energy x-rays, such as from cobalt treatment, in the treatment of disease, particularly cancer. Safety precautions are again important to avoid unnecessary irradiation.
- *Other support services:* housekeeping, physical plant, maintenance, security, information system management, purchasing, personnel, and laundry.

- *Clinical Laboratory Scientists (CLS) or Medical Technologists (MT):* individuals with a bachelor's degree in a biological science. Educational requirements include 1 or more years of study in a CLS program. Licensing is required in some states. Roles and responsibilities include performing chemical, microscopic, microbiologic, or immunologic tests pertaining to patient care; recording and reporting test results; participating in research and development of new test methods; performing preventive maintenance, troubleshooting, and quality control of instruments and reagents; maintaining safety in the clinical laboratory; and teaching residents and fellows in pathology and laboratory sciences.

BOX 1–13.   AMBULATORY CARE SETTINGS

Hospital-based clinics
Hospital-based emergency centers
Physician group practices
Individual or solo medical practices
Specialty practices
Rehabilitation centers
Mobile vans for blood donations
Mobile vans for primary care delivery
Mobile mammography units
Free standing surgical centers
Health department clinics
Community health centers (CHCs)
Rural health clinics
Community-based mental health centers
School-based clinics
Prison health clinics
Dialysis centers
Multiphasic screening centers
Home health agencies
Home hospice agencies
Durable medical equipment suppliers
Health maintenance organizations (HMOs)

- *Medical Laboratory Technicians (MLT) or Clinical Laboratory Technicians (CLT):* these individuals have a 2-year certificate or associate degree. The MLT may perform designated tests and procedures, prepare specimens for testing and transport, prepare reagents, perform quality control measures, and assist the CLS in numerous preanalytic and postanalytic processes.
- *Other laboratory personnel:* laboratory information systems (LIS) operators and programmers, clerical staff, quality management staff, infection control officers, and biomedical equipment specialists.

Large clinical laboratories usually cluster testing processes according to the following subsections:

- Clinical chemistry.
- Hematology and coagulation.
- Microbiology and parasitology.
- Immunohematology (blood banking) or transfusion medicine.
- Immunology and serology.
- Cytology.
- Histology.
- Cytogenetics.
- Urinalysis.

Examples of the types of commonly performed tests in each of these sections are listed in Table 1–3. The importance of specific test procedures will be discussed further in Chapters 2 and 3.

Smaller laboratories can be located in remote locations or clinics, physician offices, and in mobile vans. Health care workers who perform the testing must maintain the same high standards of quality as is found in larger, high-volume laboratories.

The federal government also regulates all clinical laboratories through the **Clinical Laboratory Improvement Amendments of 1988 (CLIA 1988).** Regulations apply to *any* site that tests human specimens, including small **physician's office laboratories (POLs)** or screening tests done at a hospital bedside. The regulations include establishing qualifications for health care personnel who perform the tests, periodic inspections, proficiency assessments, and the investigation of complaints. Laboratory tests are grouped into three categories according to the level of complexity of the testing procedure and the risk involved for the patient if errors are made in performing or interpreting the test. The tests may also be reclassified from one category to another as technology advances. The categories are listed next.

Waivered tests are those tests that are the easiest to perform, the least susceptible to error, and the least risky to patients. Examples include urinalysis, urine pregnancy tests, blood glucose screening tests, rheumatoid factor tests or mononucleosis tests using blood agglutination, occult blood detection from stool samples, spun microhematocrits, and erythrocyte sedimentation rates. These are tests that are commonly done in ambulatory settings, on hospital units near the bedside, and in other remote locations.

Moderate complexity tests are those tests that are simple to perform but may involve more risk to the patient if results are inaccurate. Examples include white and red blood cell counts, hemoglobin, hematocrit, blood chemistries, and urine cultures.

High complexity tests are those tests that are complex to perform and may allow for reasonable risk of harm to the patient if results are inaccurate. These include tests that require sophisticated instrumentation and oversight by a pathologist or PhD-level scientist. Examples include molecular probe analyses, bone marrow evaluations, immunoassays, flow cytometry, cytogenetics analysis, and electrophoresis.

Other regulatory agencies also have oversight of clinical laboratories, depending on the type of testing they do and the reimbursement they receive for the procedures. Among these are the Health Care Financing Administration (HCFA) for Medicare, Medicaid, the Food and Drug Administration, the American Association of Blood Banks, the American Society for Clinical Pathologists, and the Joint Commission for the Accreditation of Healthcare Organizations.

Table 1–3. Summary of Major Tests Performed in the Clinical Laboratory Sections

CLINICAL CHEMISTRY PROCEDURES

Total proteins
Glucose and glucose tolerance
Glycated hemoglobin
Triglycerides
Total cholesterol
HDL cholesterol
Iron
Total iron-binding capacity (IBC or TIBC)
Electrolytes (sodium [Na^+], potassium [K^+], chloride [Cl^-], bicarbonte [HCO_3^-])
Magnesium
Blood gases (pH, partial pressure of carbon dioxide [Pco_2], partial pressure of oxygen [Po_2])
Creatinine
Uric acid
Blood urea nitrogen (BUN)
Enzymes (e.g., lactate dehydrogenase [LD], alanine aminotransferase [ALT], creatine phosphokinase [CPK])
Drug analysis (e.g., gentamicin, tobramycin, primidone, phenytoin, digoxin, quinidine, salicylates, blood alcohol, barbiturates)
Biblirubin
Hormones (e.g., thyroxine [T_4], insulin, testosterone, luteinizing hormone, parathyroid hormones, prolactin, cortisol)

CLINICAL CHEMISTRY PROCEDURES

Acid-fast bacilli (AFB) smear	Fungus direct smear	Ova and parasites
Anaerobic cultures	GC cultures	Pinworm preparation
Culture and sensitivity (C&S)	Gram staining	Stool cultures
AFB culture	Occult blood	Strep screening
Fungus cultures	Nose/throat cultures	Urine cultures
Blood cultures		

HEMATOLOGY AND COAGULATION PROCEDURES

CSF cell count	Hemoglobin	RBC count
Differential	Hemoprofile	Reticulocyte count
Eosinophil count	LE cell preparation	Sedimentation rate
Fecal leukocyte count	Nasal eosinophil count	Sickle-cell preparation
Hematocrit	Platelet count	WBC count
CBC	Partial thromboplastin time (PTT)	Thrombin time
Fibrin split product	Prothrombin time (PT)	
Fibrinogen		

(continued)

Table 1–3. *(continued)*

CLINICAL MICROSCOPY AND URINALYSIS PROCEDURES

Routine UA		Miscellaneous UA
pH	Bilurubin	Hemosiderin
Specific gravity	Nitrites	Pregnancy test
Protein	Urobilinogen	Synovial fluid analysis
Sugar	Ascorbic acid	Seminal fluid analysis
Ketones	Occult blood	
	Leukocytes	

IMMUNOHEMATOLOGY PROCEDURES (TRANSFUSION MEDICINE)

ABO and Rh$_o$ (D) typing	Antibody screen indirect	Rh phenotyping and
ABO grouping	Coombs' test	genotyping
Antibody identification	Antibody titer	Rh$_o$ (D) typing
Hepatitis B core antigen and antibody	Direct Coombs' test	
Hepatitis B surface antigen (HB$_s$Ag) and antibody		
HIV-1 testing		

CLINICAL IMMUNOLOGY/SEROLOGY PROCEDURES

Amebiasis screening	Cold agglutinins	Rheumatoid factor
Antinuclear antibody (ANA)	CSF/VDRL	RPR
ASO screening	Syphilis antibody (FTA-ABS)	RPR quantitative
ASO titer	Infectious mononucleosis	*Salmonella* agglutinins
Brucella antibody	MHA-TP	Q fever
C-reactive protein	*Proteus* OX antibodies	
Borrelia burgdorferi (Lyme disease) antibody	Rubella HIA	
Francisella tularensis antibody		
Legionnaires' disease antibody		

Abbreviations: ASO, anti-streptolysin O; CBC, complete blood count; CSF, cerebrospinal fluid; FTA-ABS, fluorescent treponemal antibody absorption; GC, gonococcus; HDL, high-density lipoprotein; HIA, hemagglutination-inhibition antibody; HIV-1, human immunodeficiency virus—type 1; LE, lupus erythematosus; MHA-TP, microhemagglutination—*Treponema pallidum;* RBC, red blood cell; RPR, rapid plasma reagin; UA, urinalysis; VDRL, Veneral Disease Research Laboratory; WBC, white blood cell.

SELF STUDY

KEY TERMS

Active Listening
Acute Care
Ambulatory Care
American Hospital Association
    (AHA)
American Nurses Association
    (ANA)
American Society of Clinical
    Pathologists (ASCP)
American Society for Clinical
    Laboratory Scientists (ASCLS)
Anatomic Pathology
Clinical Laboratory Improvement
    Amendments of 1998
    (CLIA 1988)
Clinical Pathology
Home Health Care Services

Inpatients
Long-term Care
Medicaid
Medicare
National Phlebotomy
    Association (NPA)
Patient's Bill of Rights
Personal Protective Equipment
    (PPE)
Phlebotomist
Physician's Office Laboratories
    (POLs)
Point of Care
Primary Care
Secondary Care
Tertiary Care
Zone of Comfort

STUDY QUESTIONS

The following questions may have *one* or *more* answers.

1. Which of the following are important trends in health care?

    a. cost containment
    b. the "aging of America"
    c. shift from in- to outpatient settings
    d. restructuring the health care team

2. Examples of nonverbal, distracting behaviors include which of the following:

    a. chewing gum
    b. gazing outside the window
    c. direct eye contact
    d. glancing at the clock

3. Which of the following statements is inappropriate during a phlebotomy procedure?

    a. "This won't hurt a bit!"
    b. "Your name is Mrs. Jones, isn't it?"
    c. "You are required to cooperate with this procedure."
    d. "Could you please spell your last name for me?"

4. Which of the following are key elements in effective communication?

   a. active listening

   b. nonverbal cues

   c. verbal skills

   d. "point of care" procedures

5. The AHA adopted the Patient's Bill of Rights. These include which of the following:

   a. informed consent

   b. refusal of treatment

   c. privacy

   d. confidentiality

6. Which of the following is/are considered primary health care providers?

   a. nurse

   b. nurse midwife

   c. cardiologist

   d. internal medicine doctor

7. Which of the following procedures would be considered primary care?

   a. immunizations

   b. prenatal checkups

   c. blood glucose screening

   d. CAT scan

8. Hospitals differ according to which of the following:

   a. bed size

   b. length of stay

   c. mission

   d. ownership

9. PPE might include which of the following items:

   a. clipboard for requisitions

   b. gloves

   c. gowns or aprons

   d. face shields

References

1. Johnson DW, Johnson RT: *Joining Together, Group Theory and Group Skills,* 5th ed. Allyn and Bacon; Boston: 1994.

2. Mears P: *Healthcare Teams, Building Continuous Quality Improvement.* St. Lucie Press; Delray Beach, FL: 1994.

3. Parsons ML, Murdaugh CL: *Patient-Centered Care: A Model for Restructuring.* Gaithersburg, MD; Aspen Publishers: 1994.

2

TWO

◼

Basic Anatomy and Physiology of Organ Systems

CHAPTER OUTLINE

CHAPTER OBJECTIVES

Upon completion of Chapter 2, the learner is responsible for the following:

1. Describe the anatomic surface regions and cavities of the body.
2. Identify the eight structural levels of the human body.
3. Describe the role of homeostasis in normal body functioning.
4. Describe the purpose, function, and structural components of the 11 body systems.
5. Recognize examples of disorders associated with each organ system.
6. List common diagnostic tests associated with each organ system.

■ ANATOMIC REGIONS

The human body has distinctive characteristics; that is, a backbone, bisymmetry, body cavities, and 11 major organ systems: integumentary, skeletal, muscular, nervous, respiratory, digestive, urinary, reproductive, endocrine, lymphatic, and cardiovascular. This chapter highlights the basic **anatomy** (structural components of the body) and **physiology** (functional components) of each system except the circulatory or cardiovascular system, which is covered in Chapter 3.

Body regions can be categorized in various ways. One way is to begin at the top and work down. In this manner, the body can be described as having the following regions:[1]

- Head and neck.
- Upper torso.
- Lower torso (female and male).
- Back.
- Arms.
- Legs.
- Hands and feet.

The body can also be described by surface regions, body planes, and body cavities. The front, **anterior,** or **ventral** surface of the body is separated into thoracic, abdominal, and pelvic cavities. The back, **posterior,** or **dorsal** surface is divided into cranial and spinal cavities. Each of these cavities houses one or more organs. Areas and directions of the body can be described by their distance from or proximity to one of the **body planes** (Fig. 2–1 and Table 2–1). The **sagittal plane** runs lengthwise from front to back, dividing the body into right and left halves. The **frontal plane** runs lengthwise from side to side, dividing the body into anterior and posterior sections. The **transverse plane** runs crosswise, or horizontally, dividing the body into upper and lower sections. **Medial** means toward the midline, and **lateral** means toward the sides of the body. *Normal anatomic position* refers to an erect standing position with arms at rest and palms forward.

■ STRUCTURAL ORGANIZATION

The design of the human body is elaborate and sophisticated. A human body can be divided into eight structural levels (Fig. 2–2): atoms, molecules (chemical constituents), small structures within cells or organelles, cells (the basic living units of all plants and animals), tissues (groups of similar cells), organs (two or more tissues), organ systems (groups of organs), and the organism (the human body) itself. Trillions of cells make up each individual. Similar groups of cells are combined into tissues, such as muscles or nerves, and tissues are combined into systems, such as the circulatory or reproductive system. These organ systems work simultaneously to serve the needs of the body. No one system works independently of the others.

Before the major organ systems and their functions are discussed, a basic understanding of the human cell is necessary. Figures 2–3 and 2–4 illustrate a basic cell and its structures and some examples of specific cell morphologies. The size and shape of a cell depend on its function. Some cells fight disease-causing viruses and bacteria; some transport gases, such as oxygen (O_2) and carbon dioxide (CO_2); some produce movement, store nutrients, or manufacture proteins, chemicals, or liquids; and others, such as the egg and the sperm, can

Figure 2-1. Body planes.

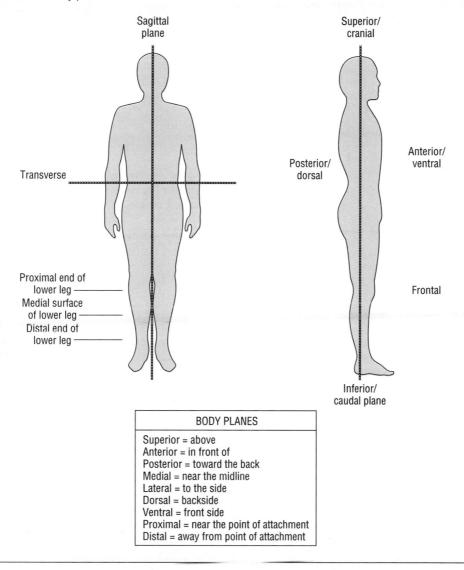

BODY PLANES
Superior = above
Anterior = in front of
Posterior = toward the back
Medial = near the midline
Lateral = to the side
Dorsal = backside
Ventral = front side
Proximal = near the point of attachment
Distal = away from point of attachment

create a new life. At the same time, other cells contribute to thoughts and emotions. Despite such diverse functions, several cells have basic structural elements in common. The cell membrane encloses the contents of the cell. This membrane serves as a protective barrier that selectively allows certain substances to move in or out. Nutrients and O_2 are taken in through the membrane only when needed, and wastes are eliminated as they build up. Most cells also have a **nucleus,** which is enclosed inside a nuclear membrane. The nucleus (*nuclei* for two or more) is commonly thought of as the control mechanism of the cell that gov-

Table 2-1. Directional Terms for Body Position

TERM	DESCRIPTION AND EXAMPLE
Right/left	Toward the right/left side of the body. (Example: The patient has scar tissue on the right arm.)
Inferior/superior	A structure or organ below/above another. (Example: The forehead is superior to the nose. The nose is inferior to the eyes.)
Anterior (ventral)	Front of the body. (Example: Toes are anterior, or ventral, to the heel.)
Posterior (dorsal)	Back of the body. (Example: The spinal cord is posterior, or dorsal, to the heart.)
Proximal	Closer to the point of attachment to the body trunk. (Example: The knee is proximal to the ankle.)
Distal	Farther from the point of attachment to the body trunk. (Example: The toes are distal to the ankle.)
Lateral	Away from the midline of the body. (Example: The hip is lateral to the navel.)
Medial	Toward the midline of the body. (Example: The heart is medial to the arms.)
Superficial	Closer to the outer surface of the body. (Example: Skin is superficial to muscles or bone.)
Deep	Internal or farther from the outer surface of the body. (Example: The heart and lungs are deep organs.)

erns the functions of the individual cell (i.e., growth, repair, reproduction, and metabolism). Inside the nucleus is a **nucleolus** and threadlike chromatin, which also aide in cell metabolism and reproduction. The nucleus contains a blueprint of itself in the genetic material so that it can reproduce itself when necessary. If the nucleus of a cell is damaged or destroyed, in most cases the cell will die; however, even though red blood cells (RBCs) lose their nuclei when they mature, the cells continue to live and carry O_2 for several months. Another component of the cell, the **cytoplasm,** contains mostly water with dissolved nutrients and fills up the rest of the cell membrane. Within the cytoplasm are smaller structures called *organelles.* The names and functions of these organelles are as follows:

- **Mitochondria.** Produce energy for the cell.
- **Ribosomes.** Assemble amino acids into proteins.
- **Endoplasmic reticulum.** Acts as transport channel between the cell membrane and the nuclear membrane.
- **Lysosomes.** Release digestive enzymes into vacuoles, or small pouches, for digestion of food particles.
- **Golgi apparatus.** Stores proteins.
- **Centriole.** Plays a role in cell division.

Cells communicate with each other in sophisticated reactions using electrical impulses (such as from one nerve cell to another) or in chemical reactions that result in the release of hormones or other enzymes and proteins to stimulate a particular function. The study of cellular structures and processes has captivated clinical laboratory scientists for years. With technologies, such as flow cytometry, amplification of genetic material, and specific probing, the ways of seeking information about cellular functions continue to expand.

Figure 2-2. Levels of structural organization.

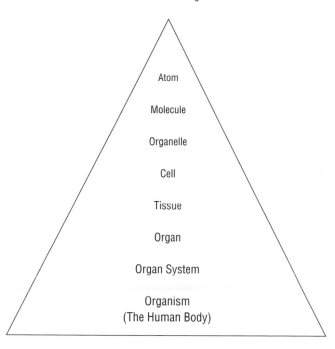

Levels of Structural Organization

Atom

Molecule

Organelle

Cell

Tissue

Organ

Organ System

Organism
(The Human Body)

Deoxyribonucleic acid (DNA) is a long molecule commonly described as a *double helix* or *twisted ladder.* The molecule contains thousands of **genes,** which carry the code for an individual's genetic makeup, such as eye color, sex, and height. An individual's DNA contains the *DNA-coded blueprint* that was inherited from that person's parents. Genes also instruct the body to make the proteins needed to sustain life. Although each nucleus has a complete set of genes (except the egg and the sperm, each of which contains half a set), only certain genes are used in each cell to perform the cell's specific functions. DNA also duplicates exact copies of itself. An individual's DNA directs the development, growth, and functioning of all body systems and makes each individual's body unique, except in the case of identical twins.

Survival is the primary function of the human body, and many complex processes work independently and together to achieve this function. In human physiology, the body strives for a **steady state,** or **homeostasis.** Literally, *homeostasis* means "remaining the same." It is a condition in which a healthy body, although constantly changing and functioning, remains in a normal, healthy condition. Homeostasis, or a steady-state condition, allows the normal body to stay in balance by compensating with changes. For example, if the body is taking in too much water, it responds to this imbalance by excreting water from the kidneys (urine), skin (perspiration), intestines (feces), and lungs (water in expiration) (Fig. 2–5). A

Figure 2-3.   Basic cellular structure and components.

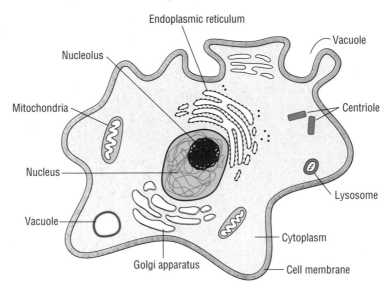

Figure 2-4.   Various cell structures.

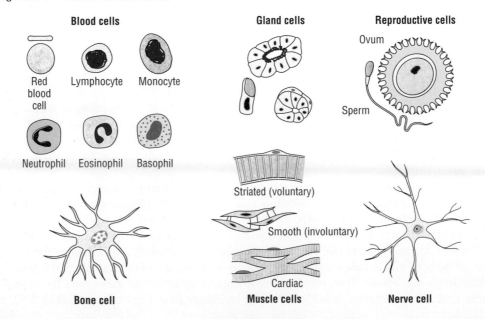

Figure 2-5. Homeostasis. The human body stays in balance by compensating with changes. When the body needs fluid, a person becomes thirsty and drinks water, which is then absorbed in the intestines. Conversely, if the body retains too much fluid, it reacts by excreting water from the kidneys (urine), skin (perspiration), intestines (feces), and lungs (water droplets as we exhale).

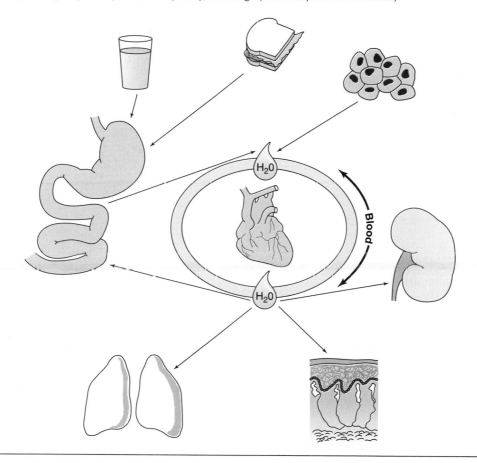

healthy body maintains constancy of its chemical components and processes in order to survive. Each organ system and body structure plays a part in maintaining homeostasis.

Another important function of the human body is **metabolism.** This process involves making necessary substances or breaking down chemical substances in order to use energy. **Catabolism** is a series of chemical reactions produced in cells to change complex substances into simpler ones while simultaneously releasing energy. This process provides energy for all body functions, whether for moving a chair or for allowing a heart to beat. Conversely, **anabolism** is a process by which cells use energy to make complex compounds from simpler ones. It allows synthesis of body fluids, such as sweat, tears, saliva, and chemical constituents (enzymes, hormones, and antibodies). Both phases are required to maintain metabolic functions in a healthy individual.

As mentioned previously, in a normal, healthy body, structural and functional aspects work together. Organization of all the body structures, such as cells, tissues, organs, and systems, together with proper functioning, such as digestion, respiration, circulation, nerve sensitivity, movement, and secretion, provide for a healthy individual. Systems working together can keep a body metabolizing properly and in homeostasis, which is the basis of survival.

Laboratory testing can provide a wealth of information about the individual organ systems and the integrated processes. Specimens, such as blood, bone marrow, urine, cerebrospinal fluid (CSF), pleural fluid, biopsy tissue, seminal fluid, and others, can be microscopically analyzed, assayed, and cultured to determine pathogenesis.[1,2]

■ MAJOR ORGAN SYSTEMS

This section summarizes the functions of the 11 major organ systems (Table 2–2). For each body system, a corresponding box provides a brief summary of the structure, function, disorders, and common diagnostic tests for that system.

INTEGUMENTARY SYSTEM

The **integumentary system** consists of the skin, hair, sweat and oil glands, teeth, and fingernails (Box 2–1). It is primarily involved in protective and regulatory functions. Intact skin protects the deeper tissues by providing a barrier to entering microorganisms and foreign bodies and by protecting such tissues from heat, cold, and other hazardous exposures. The skin also prevents water loss or allows for perspiration as needed by the body during exercise, fever, or weather conditions. Sebaceous glands in the skin produce oils for hair and skin protection, and sweat glands produce perspiration, which helps cool the body as needed and eliminates some waste. **Melanin** in the skin provides skin color and protects

Table 2-2. Normal Body Functions Controlled by Organ Systems

NORMAL BODY FUNCTIONS	ORGAN SYSTEMS
Protection	Integumentary
Support	Skeletal
Movement	Muscular
Control	Nervous
Regulation	Endocrine
Fluid Regulation	Cardiovascular
Transport	Lymphatic
Environmental Control and Exchange	Respiratory
	Digestive
	Urinary
Birth	Reproductive

BOX 2–1.   INTEGUMENTARY SYSTEM

Components:

- Skin, sweat and oil glands
- Hair
- Fingernails
- Teeth

Functions:

- Protects underlying tissues
- Regulates body temperature
- Eliminates some wastes
- Receives sensory stimuli, such as touch, pressure, temperature, pain
- Prevents water loss

Disorders:

- Acne
- Burns
- Carcinoma and other skin cancers
- Fungal infections
- Herpes
- Impetigo
- Keloid
- Pediculosis
- Pruritus
- Psoriasis

Diagnostic Tests:

- Biopsies
- KOH preparations for skin scrapings
- Tissue cultures
- Microbiological cultures

---

underlying tissues from absorbing ultraviolet rays. Ultraviolet light stimulates production of inactive vitamin D in the skin. The liver and kidneys then activate vitamin D so that it is beneficial to the body. Other functions of the skin are to store fat in the layers next to the underlying tissues and to allow an individual to experience sensations, such as touch, temperature, pain, and pressure. Hair on the head provides protection by acting as a heat insulator, eyebrows keep perspiration out of the eyes, eyelashes protect eyes from foreign objects, and hairs in the nasal passages filter out dust and harmful microorganisms. Likewise, fingernails protect the tips of the hands. Teeth aide in breaking up food to begin the digestive process.

Integumentary system disorders include bacterial infections, such as acne, impetigo (caused by *Staphylococcus aureus*), and decubitis ulcers; viral infections, such as fever blisters or cold sores, rubeola, rubella, chickenpox, and herpes zoster (shingles); fungal infections, such as ringworm and athlete's foot; allergic reactions, such as dermatitis and eczema; psoriasis; and skin cancers, such as malignant melanoma. Diagnostic tests for many of these conditions involve skin scrapings; bacteriologic, viral, or fungal tissue cultures; potassium hydroxide (KOH) preparations; or biopsy staining procedures.

SKELETAL SYSTEM

The **skeletal system** refers to all bones and joints of the body. This system comprises primarily two types of tissue: bone and cartilage. Bone is composed of cells surrounded by calcified intercellular substances that allow for a rigid structure. **Cartilage** is composed of similar cells, but these cells are surrounded by a gelatinous material, instead of calcified substances, that allows for more flexibility. Likewise, tendons and ligaments provide flexibility and leverage. The skeletal system serves the body in five major ways: support, protection for softer tissues (brain and lungs), movement and leverage, **hematopoiesis** (blood cell formation) in the bone marrow, and mineral storage (Box 2–2).

More than 200 bones are contained in the human body, and they are classified into four groups on the basis of their shapes. Long bones include leg bones (e.g., femur, tibia, fibula) and arm and hand bones (e.g., humerus, radius, ulna, phalanges). Short bones include carpals and tarsals, or wrist and ankle bones, respectively. Among flat bones are several cranial bones, the ribs, and the scapulae (or shoulder blades). Finally, irregular bones include cranial bones (e.g., sphenoid, ethmoid) and bones of the vertebral column (e.g., vertebrae, sacrum, coccyx).

Bones are connected to each other by a variety of joints that permit flexion, extension, abduction (away from median), adduction (toward median), rotation, and combinations of these movements (Fig. 2–6). Bone structure differs between male and female skeletons. Besides being somewhat larger and heavier, the male has a pelvis that is deeper with a narrow pubic arch. In contrast, the female pelvis is shallow and broad and has a wider pubic arch to facilitate childbirth.

In general, bones consist of several layers covered by a membrane, the periosteum. The periosteum contains blood vessels that bring blood from inside to the outer layer. The outer layer, compact bone, is more rigid and heavier than the inner layer, which is like a honeycomb. This inner layer is called *spongy bone* but is just as strong as compact bone. In the center of a bone is the marrow, which produces most blood cells. Approximately 5 billion RBCs are produced daily by about $\frac{1}{2}$ lb (227 g) of bone marrow. Marrow is located in all the bones of an infant, but in adults it is in the skull, sternum (or breastbone), vertebrae, hipbones, and ends of the long bones.[1]

Minerals stored in bones include calcium and phosphorus. When these minerals are needed in other parts of the body, they are released from bone through the bloodstream.

BOX 2–2.   SKELETAL SYSTEM

Components:

- Bones
- Cartilage
- Tendons
- Ligaments
- Joints

Functions:

- Provides support
- Protects organs
- Allows leverage and movement
- Produces blood cells
- Stores minerals

Disorders:

- Arthritis
- Bursitis
- Gout
- Osteomyelitis
- Osteoporosis
- Rickets
- Tumors

Diagnostic Tests:

- Alkaline phosphatase (ALP)
- Calcium
- Complete blood cell (CBC) count
- Erythrocyte sedimentation rate (ESR)
- Phosphorus
- Synovial fluid analysis
- Uric acid
- Vitamin D

Plate 1. Superficial anatomy of the heart. (Top) Anterior (sternocostal) view of the heart showing major anatomic features. (Bottom) Posterior (diaphragmatic) surface of the heart. (Coronary arteries are shown in red, coronary veins in blue.)

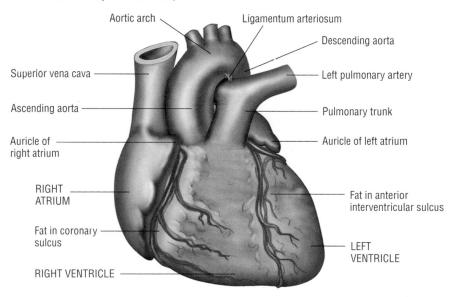

Aortic arch

Ligamentum arteriosum

Descending aorta

Superior vena cava

Left pulmonary artery

Ascending aorta

Pulmonary trunk

Auricle of right atrium

Auricle of left atrium

RIGHT ATRIUM

Fat in anterior interventricular sulcus

Fat in coronary sulcus

LEFT VENTRICLE

RIGHT VENTRICLE

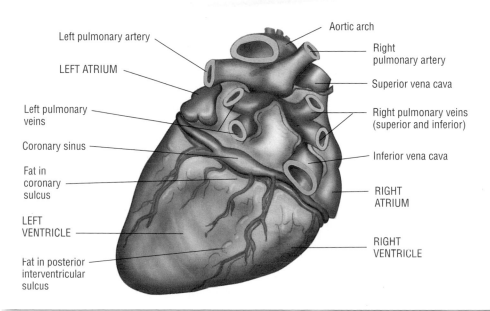

Left pulmonary artery

Aortic arch

Right pulmonary artery

LEFT ATRIUM

Superior vena cava

Left pulmonary veins

Right pulmonary veins (superior and inferior)

Coronary sinus

Inferior vena cava

Fat in coronary sulcus

RIGHT ATRIUM

LEFT VENTRICLE

RIGHT VENTRICLE

Fat in posterior interventricular sulcus

Plate 2. Sectional anatomy of the heart. A diagrammatic frontal section through the heart showing major landmarks and the path of blood flow through the atria and ventricles.

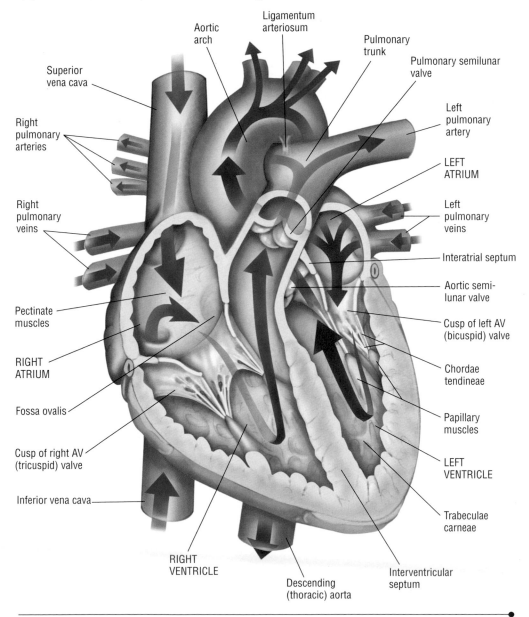

Plate 3. The pulmonary circuit. The right ventricle of the heart pumps blood into the pulmonary artery (pulmonary trunk) which divides into the right and left pulmonary arteries that go to each lung. In the lungs the arteries branch extensively into small arteries and arterioles, then to capillaries. The capillaries surround the alveoli so that exchange of oxygen and carbon dioxide can take place. The capillaries flow into veins and finally into the two pulmonary veins that return blood to the heart through the left atrium This oxygenated blood will then travel to the rest of the body. (Note that the pulmonary veins contain oxygenated blood. They are the only veins that carry blood with a high oxygen content. All other veins of the body carry blood with a low oxygen content.)

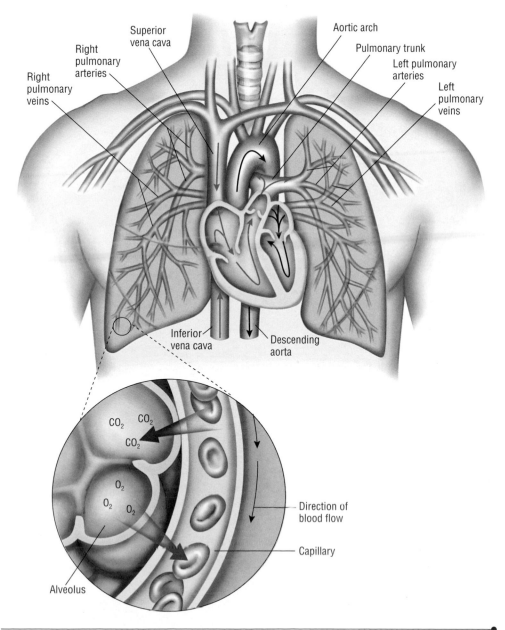

Plate 4. Exchange of gases in systemic and pulmonary capillaries. Oxygen (O_2) and carbon dioxide (CO_2) molecules are carried in red blood cells by hemoglobin (Hb) molecules. In the systemic or tissue capillaries, O_2 is released and CO_2 is picked up. When the red cell returns to the pulmonary capillaries in the lungs, CO_2 is released and O_2 is picked up.

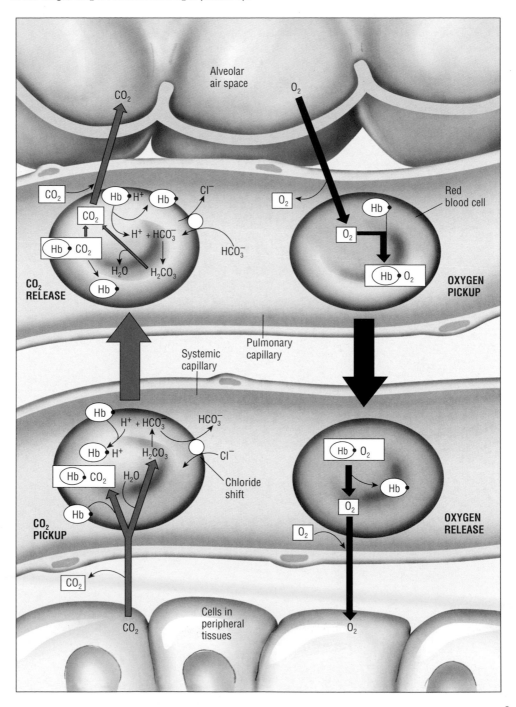

Plate 5. The arterial system.

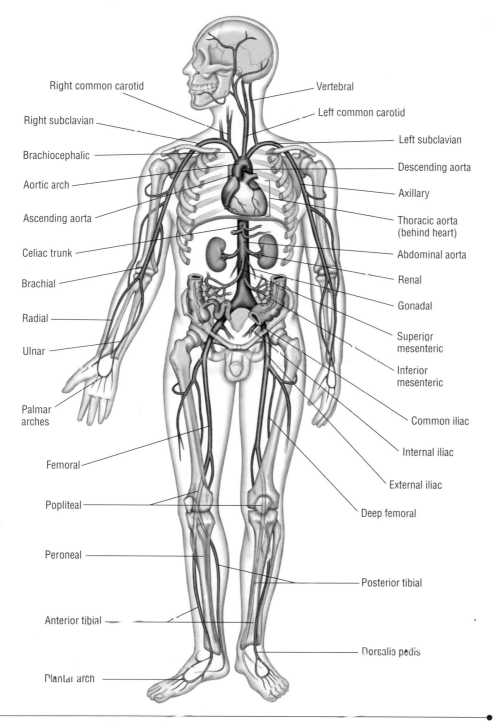

Right common carotid

Right subclavian

Brachiocephalic

Aortic arch

Ascending aorta

Celiac trunk

Brachial

Radial

Ulnar

Palmar arches

Femoral

Popliteal

Peroneal

Anterior tibial

Plantar arch

Vertebral

Left common carotid

Left subclavian

Descending aorta

Axillary

Thoracic aorta (behind heart)

Abdominal aorta

Renal

Gonadal

Superior mesenteric

Inferior mesenteric

Common iliac

Internal iliac

External iliac

Deep femoral

Posterior tibial

Dorsalis pedis

Plate 6. An overview of the venous system.

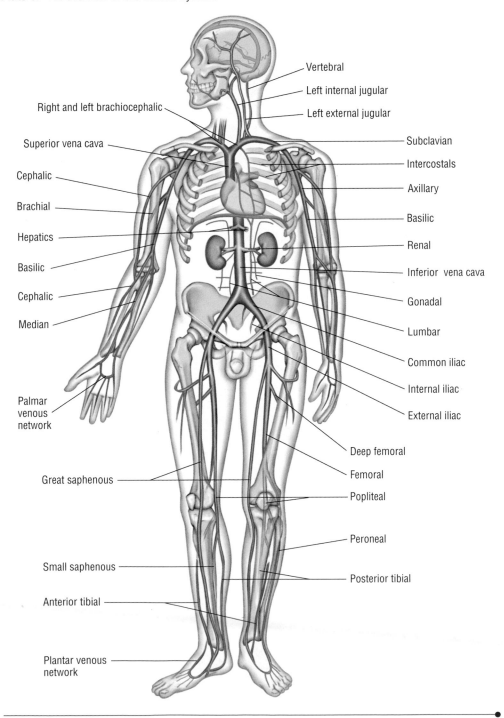

Vertebral

Left internal jugular

Left external jugular

Right and left brachiocephalic

Superior vena cava

Subclavian

Intercostals

Cephalic

Axillary

Brachial

Basilic

Hepatics

Renal

Basilic

Inferior vena cava

Cephalic

Gonadal

Median

Lumbar

Common iliac

Internal iliac

Palmar
venous
network

External iliac

Deep femoral

Great saphenous

Femoral

Popliteal

Peroneal

Small saphenous

Posterior tibial

Anterior tibial

Plantar venous
network

Plate 7. Venous drainage of the abdomen and chest.

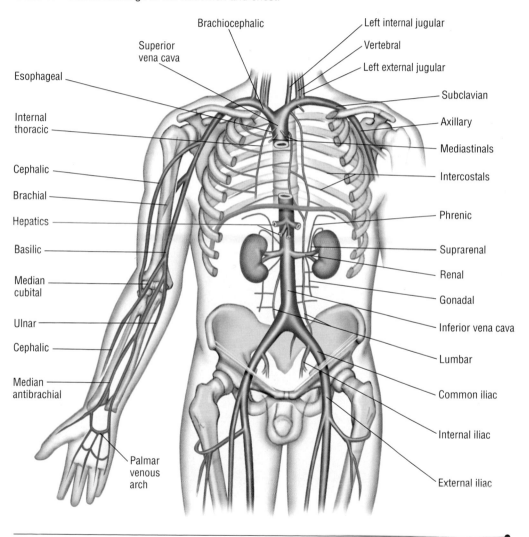

Brachiocephalic

Left internal jugular

Superior
vena cava

Vertebral

Left external jugular

Esophageal

Subclavian

Internal
thoracic

Axillary

Mediastinals

Cephalic

Intercostals

Brachial

Hepatics

Phrenic

Basilic

Suprarenal

Median
cubital

Renal

Gonadal

Ulnar

Inferior vena cava

Cephalic

Lumbar

Median
antibrachial

Common iliac

Internal iliac

Palmar
venous
arch

External iliac

Plate 8. Circulation through vessels of the forearm in warm and cold environments. **A.** Circulation through the blood vessels of the forearm in a warm environment. Blood enters the limb in a deep artery and returns to the trunk in a network of superficial veins. These veins radiate heat into the environment through the overlying skin. **B.** Circulation through the blood vessels of the forearm in a cold environment. Blood now returns to the trunk via a network of deep veins that flow around the artery. The amount of heat loss is reduced, as is indicated in C. **C.** Countercurrent heat exchange occurs as heat radiates from the warm arterial blood to the cool venous blood flowing in the opposite direction. By the time the arterial blood reaches the distal capillaries, where most of the heat loss to the environment occurs, it is substantially cooler than it was when it left the trunk. This mechanism reduces the rate of heat loss while conserving body heat. In effect, the countercurrent exchange traps heat near the trunk.

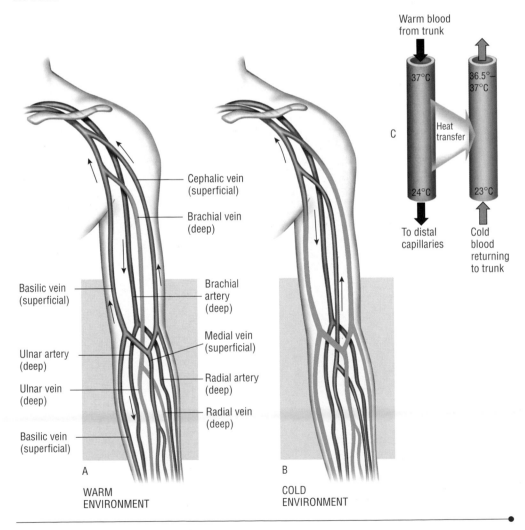

Warm blood
from trunk

37°C 36.5°–37°C

C Heat
transfer

24°C 23°C

To distal
capillaries

Cold
blood
returning
to trunk

Cephalic vein
(superficial)

Brachial vein
(deep)

Basilic vein
(superficial)

Brachial
artery
(deep)

Ulnar artery
(deep)

Medial vein
(superficial)

Ulnar vein
(deep)

Radial artery
(deep)

Basilic vein
(superficial)

Radial vein
(deep)

A

B

WARM
ENVIRONMENT

COLD
ENVIRONMENT

Figure 2-6.   Skeleton.

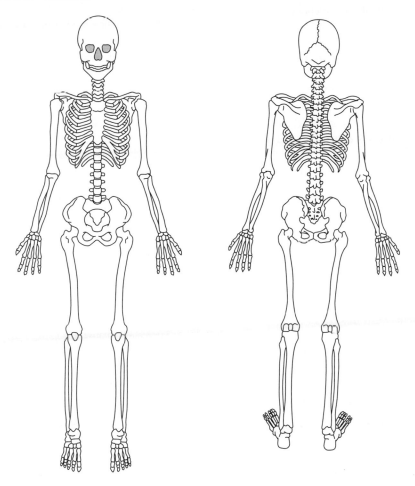

Skeletal system disorders include inflammatory conditions, such as arthritis and bursitis; gout; bacterial infections, such as osteomyelitis; porous bone conditions, such as osteoporosis; developmental conditions, such as gigantism, dwarfism, and rickets; and bone tumors. Laboratory assessment of skeletal system disorders can include serum calcium and phosphate levels, serum alkaline phosphatase (ALP) levels, uric acid, vitamin D, erythrocyte sedimentation rate (ESR), complete blood cell (CBC) counts, microscopic analysis, and microbial cultures of the bone marrow and synovial fluid (fluid between joints and bones).

MUSCULAR SYSTEM

The **muscular system** refers to all muscles of the body, including those attached to bones and those along walls of internal structures, such as the heart. On the basis of location, microscopic structure, and neural control, muscles are classified as follows: (1) **skeletal (striated voluntary) muscles**—attached to bones; (2) **visceral (nonstriated [smooth] involuntary) muscles**—line the walls of internal structures, such as veins and arteries; and (3) **cardiac (striated involuntary) muscles**—make up the wall of the heart (Box 2–3). Muscles provide movement, maintain posture, and produce heat. Movement takes place not only during locomotion, but also during body movements, changes in the size of openings, and propulsion of substances (e.g., propulsion of blood through veins or passage of food through intestines). Posture is maintained during sitting and standing by continued partial contraction of specific muscles. Muscle cells that provide mechanical energy for movement also release energy in the form of heat. All three muscle types work by extending, contracting, conducting, and being easily stimulated.

Skeletal muscles (more than 400 in humans) compose approximately 40 percent of a man's body. In contrast, women have less muscle and more fat than that in men. Muscles are strongest at about age 25, but with proper nutrition and exercise, they can remain strong throughout life. Without sufficient exercise, muscles become smaller and weaker. Glycogen is the form of stored glucose in muscles. Without stores of glycogen, muscles must wait for glucose, which is transported through the bloodstream. Exercise increases the amount of glycogen available for muscles, which in turn allows them to function more easily.

Muscular system disorders include muscular dystrophy (MD), conditions that disrupt nerve stimulation (as in severe accidents or myasthenia gravis), muscle cramps and tendinitis, and viral infections, such as multiple sclerosis (MS) and polio.

Laboratory testing of muscular system disorders often involves clinical assays of specific muscle enzymes, such as creatine phosphokinase (CK) and lactate dehydrogenase (LDH), analysis of autoimmune antibodies, microscopic examination, or culturing of biopsy tissue.

BOX 2–3.   MUSCULAR SYSTEM

Components:

- Skeletal muscle
- Cardiac muscle (heart)
- Smooth muscle (walls of hollow organs)

Functions:

- Permits movement
- Produces heat
- Maintains posture

Disorders:

- Atrophy
- Muscular dystrophy (MD)
- Myalgia
- Tendinitis

Diagnostic Tests:

- Autoimmune antibodies
- Creatine phosphokinase (CPK)
- CK isoenzymes
- Lactic acid
- Lactate dehydrogenase (LDH or LD)
- Myoglobin

NERVOUS SYSTEM

The **nervous system** provides communication in the body, sensations, thoughts, emotions, and memories. Nerve impulses and chemical substances regulate, control, integrate, and organize body functions. The nervous system is composed of specialized nerve cells (**neurons**), the brain, the spinal cord, brain and cord coverings, fluid, and the nerve impulse itself. An estimated 10 billion neurons or more reside in the human body, most of which are in the brain. Sensory neurons transmit nerve impulses to the spinal cord or the brain from muscle tissues. Motor neurons transmit impulses to muscles from the spinal cord or the brain. Both the brain and the spinal cord are covered by protective membranes (**meninges**). Between these protective membrane layers are CSF-filled spaces that provide a cushion for the brain and the spinal cord. The brain has many vitally important areas. Along with the cranial nerves, its functions include all mental processes and many essential motor, sensory, and visceral responses. The spinal cord and the spinal nerves control sensory (touch), motor (voluntary movement), and reflex (knee-jerk) functions. Reflexes are responses to stimuli that do not require communication with the brain. A simple reflex, such as moving a finger from something hot, occurs even before the brain realizes the pain. Specific cranial and spinal nerves control all complex or simple action processes in the body. In summary, the nervous system is the primary communication and regulatory system in the body (Box 2–4).

Nervous system disorders include infectious conditions, such as encephalitis, meningitis, tetanus, herpes, and poliomyelitis, and conditions such as amyotrophic lateral sclerosis (ALS), MS, Parkinson's disease, cerebral palsy (CP), tumors, epilepsy, hydrocephaly, neuralgia, and headaches. Laboratory diagnosis of nervous system disorders is not very spe-

---

BOX 2–4. NERVOUS SYSTEM

Components:

- Brain
- Spinal cord
- Nerves
- Sense organs: eyes, ears, tongue, and sensory receptor in the skin

Functions:

- Allows communication throughout the body and regulates body functions
- Detects sensations
- Controls movements and physiological functions
- Controls intellectual processes

Disorders:

- Amyotrophic lateral sclerosis (ALS)
- Encephalitis

- Epilepsy
- Hydrocephaly
- Meningitis
- Multiple sclerosis (MS)
- Neuralgia
- Parkinson's disease
- Shingles

Diagnostic Tests:

- Acetylcholine receptor antibody
- Cerebrospinal fluid (CSF) analysis
- Cholinesterase
- Drug levels

cific. Chemical assays can reveal drug interactions, as well as hormonal, protein, and enzyme alterations. Infections can be detected by bacterial, viral, or fungal cultures or by the presence of specific antibodies in the CSF.

RESPIRATORY SYSTEM

Respiration allows for the exchange of gases between blood and air. Once gases enter the blood, the circulatory system transports them between lungs and tissues. Together, the respiratory and circulatory systems carry O_2 to the cells and remove CO_2 from the tissue cells. Oxygen allows the body to burn its fuel from the nutrients eaten. It makes up about one fifth of the air around us. The average person inhales and exhales about 15 times per minute or approximately 20,000 times per day. As a person breathes in, the O_2 travels through air passages to the lungs. In the lungs, the exchange of gases occurs. Oxygen is exchanged for CO_2, which is then breathed out as the person exhales.

The main components of the **respiratory system** are in the head, the neck, and the thoracic cavity and include the nose, the pharynx, the larynx, the trachea, the bronchi, and the lungs (Box 2–5).

Receptors in the nose provide the sense of smell and allow for changes in voice. The nose also functions as the primary filter for air entering the body. It catches impurities and chemical substances that may irritate the respiratory system. In the nose, the throat, and the bronchial tree, mucus is continuously produced to trap unwanted particles and prevent

---

BOX 2–5.   RESPIRATORY SYSTEM

Components:

- Nasal cavity
- Pharynx
- Larynx
- Trachea
- Bronchi
- Lungs

Functions:

- Filters air, exchanges gases
- Supplies oxygen and removes carbon dioxide
- Helps regulate blood pH
- Protects vocal cords

Disorders:

- Respiratory tract infections
- Tonsillitis
- Asthma
- Bronchitis
- Cystic fibrosis
- Emphysema
- Pleurisy
- Pneumonia
- Tuberculosis
- Respiratory distress syndrome
- Respiratory syncytial virus
- Rhinitis

Diagnostic Tests:

- Alkaline phosphatase (ALP)
- Arterial blood gases
- Complete blood cell (CBC) count
- Bronchial washings
- Drug levels
- Electrolytes
- Microbiological cultures
- Pleuracentesis
- Sputum cultures
- Tuberculin skin test

them from entering the lungs or vocal cords. Tiny hairlike cilia line the passageways and sweep the mucus to the nose and mouth so that it can be coughed up, sneezed, or swallowed. The pharynx is a tubelike passageway for both food and air. Along with the larynx (voice box), it determines the quality of voice. The trachea and the bronchial passages provide openings for outside air to reach the lungs. Within the bronchi are grapelike **alveolar sacs** that are enveloped by capillaries and allow diffusion between air and blood. The lungs are structured into millions of branches of alveoli with surrounding capillaries and therefore can quickly take in large amounts of O_2 and release large amounts of CO_2 if they are functioning properly. (Refer to Plate 4 in the Color Atlas.) The lungs are soft and spongy and reach from just above the collarbone down to the diaphragm. They have no muscles; consequently, the diaphragm and other surrounding muscles help enlarge and contract the chest cavity as respiration occurs. Humans have two lungs; the right lung has three lobes, and the left lung has only two, to allow room for the heart. An adult's lungs hold 3 to 4 qt (approximately 3 to 4 L) of air, depending on how vigorously the person is moving or exercising. In patients with pneumonia, the alveolar sacs become inflamed, and fluid or waste products block the minute air spaces, thus normal O_2 and CO_2 exchange is difficult.

Red blood cells transport O_2 and CO_2 as part of a molecule called *hemoglobin*. After O_2 crosses the respiratory membranes (in the lung) into the blood, about 97 percent of the O_2 combines with the iron-containing heme portion of hemoglobin. The remaining 3 percent dissolves in plasma. Hemoglobin carries O_2 from the alveolar capillaries through the blood vessels to the tissue capillaries. Oxygen and CO_2 rapidly combine with hemoglobin to form oxyhemoglobin and carbaminohemoglobin, respectively (Fig. 2–7). (Refer to Plate 5 in the Color Atlas.)

Association (chemical combination) and dissociation (chemical release) with hemoglobin depends on the gaseous pressure. In lung capillaries, O_2 pressure (partial pressure of oxygen [P_{O_2}]) increases and CO_2 (partial pressure of carbon dioxide [P_{CO_2}]) decreases, which

Figure 2-7. Oxygen (O_2) and carbon dioxide (CO_2) are transported by hemoglobin inside red blood cells. Red blood cells move from the lungs (where they pick up O_2) to the tissues (where O_2 is needed). When the hemoglobin releases the O_2 in the tissues, it picks up CO_2, and the red blood cells transport it back to the lungs. CO_2 is released in the lungs and is replaced by more O_2. Thus, the cycle continues, and the body has enough oxygen to function normally.

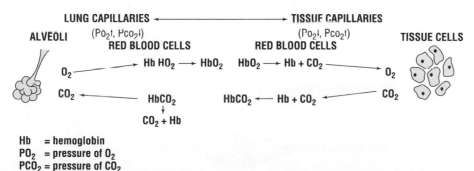

allows O_2 to rapidly associate, or combine chemically, with hemoglobin, and CO_2 to disso-ciate, or be released, from carbaminohemoglobin. Thus, humans inhale O_2 into the lungs and exhale CO_2 from the lungs. In tissue capillaries, the opposite occurs: O_2 pressure de-creases and CO_2 pressure increases, which allows O_2 to dissociate from oxyhemoglobin and CO_2 to combine with hemoglobin. Thus, O_2 is released into tissues and muscles, and CO_2 is picked up, taken to the lungs, and exhaled (Fig. 2–8).

Carbon dioxide has an important effect on the pH (acidity) of the blood. Normal body pH has a narrow range of between 7.35 and 7.45. Deviations from the normal or reference range can be dangerous and deadly. As CO_2 levels increase, the blood pH decreases (becomes more acidic). As the CO_2 level in the blood increases, chemoreceptors in the brain cause a faster and deeper rate of respiration (**hyperventilation**) in order to blow off excess CO_2 from the body. (The urinary system also plays a role in maintaining body pH, as described later in this chapter.) Gas pressure and blood pH levels can be measured in the clinical lab-oratory from appropriate blood samples.

Respiratory system disorders include infectious conditions, such as tuberculosis, laryn-gitis, bronchitis, whooping cough, pneumonia, and influenza; conditions such as asthma, emphysema, and cystic fibrosis; and tumors. Laboratory blood tests for chemical con-stituents (sodium, chloride, bicarbonate, ALP, and potassium) often indicate respiratory ab-

Figure 2-8. Enclosed circulatory system. Oxygenated blood (red) comes from the lungs and is pumped by the heart to the organs and tissues. After O_2 is released, the blood becomes deoxygenated (blue) and is pumped through the heart back to the lungs.

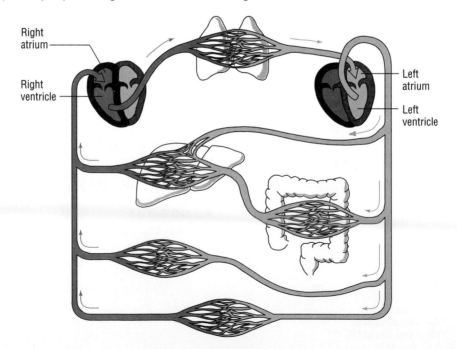

Right atrium

Right ventricle

Left atrium

Left ventricle

normalities. Lung biopsies, throat swabs, sputum cultures, and bronchial washings can be examined microscopically or cultured for pathogenic microorganisms, such as fungi; bacteria, such as acid-fast bacilli; and parasites. Pathogenic microorganisms can cause respiratory infections, such as the common cold, sore throats, tonsillitis, rhinitis, coughs, sneezing, runny noses, bronchitis, and more serious diseases, such as tuberculosis, *Pneumocystis carinii* pneumonia, Legionnaires' disease, pleurisy, respiratory distress syndrome, respiratory syncytial virus, and other types of pneumonia. Tuberculosis (TB) is caused by acid-fast bacilli that destroy lung tissue. It can be caught early using a TB skin test. In cases of pneumonia, the air sacs in the lungs fill with fluid, and gaseous exchanges cannot occur. *Pneumocystis* infections are considered opportunistic infections (i.e., they become pathogenic when the patient is immunosuppressed) and are associated with acquired immunodeficiency syndrome (AIDS).

DIGESTIVE SYSTEM

The **digestive system** functions, first, to break down food chemically and physically into nutrients that can be absorbed and used by body cells, and, second, to eliminate the waste products of digestion. The gastrointestinal (GI) tract is made up of the following components: mouth, pharynx, esophagus, stomach, intestines, and some vital accessory organs, such as salivary glands, teeth, liver, gallbladder, pancreas, and appendix (Box 2–6). Many proteins, enzymes, and juices are released by these components to facilitate digestion, absorption, and movement through the GI tract. The passageway of the GI tract through which food travels is known as the *alimentary canal.* It begins at the mouth and ends at the anus. In an adult, the average length of the alimentary canal is 27 feet. Circular muscles that surround the intestines contract to assist the movement of food through the body. These

---

BOX 2–6.   DIGESTIVE SYSTEM

Components:

- Mouth
- Salivary glands
- Esophagus
- Stomach
- Intestines
- Liver and gallbladder
- Pancreas
- Teeth
- Appendix
- Pharynx

Functions:

- Breaks down food physically and chemically
- Absorbs nutrients
- Removes solid waste

Disorders:

- Cancer
- Ulcers
- Polyps
- Parasitic infections

Diagnostic Tests:

- Occult blood test
- Ova and parasite analysis

wavelike contractions are called **peristalsis.** One meal can take 15 hours to 2 days to pass through the alimentary canal. Peristalsis is such an effective process that a person can even swallow upside down. If the process is reversed, vomiting enables the body to reject food. Saliva moistens food and contains an enzyme that helps begin the breakdown of carbohydrates into simple sugars, such as glucose. (If a salt cracker is chewed a long time, saliva begins the breakdown process so it may taste sweet.) Also, the liver secretes bile, which aids in fat digestion and absorption. In addition, it is involved in carbohydrate metabolism, protein and fat catabolism, and synthesis of many vital blood proteins for clotting and regulatory purposes. Each component functions either mechanically or chemically to keep the body in homeostasis.

The digestive system helps regulate the intake and output of essential proteins, carbohydrates, fats, minerals, vitamins, and water. The body can then use these substances by catabolizing them for stored energy or by anabolizing them to build other complex compounds, such as hormones, other tissue proteins, and enzymes. Levels of these constituents can be clinically measured in the laboratory from blood specimens and other body fluids. Materials that are not digested in the alimentary canal are eliminated from the body as fecal material or urine.

Disorders of the oral cavity can consist of dental caries or tooth decay, and periodontal disease, which is an inflammation and degeneration of the gums, ligaments, and bone around the teeth. Stomach disorders can include hiatial hernias (protrusion through the diaphragm), vomiting, and ulcers. Intestinal disorders (affecting small and large intestines) include polyps, maldigestion, malabsorption, cancer, appendicitis, constipation, diarrhea, dysentery, and hemorrhoids. Liver inflammation is referred to as *hepatitis* and can be caused by various agents, such as excessive alcohol consumption and viral hepatitis. A common disorder of the gallbladder is gallstones, which can cause blockage of the bile duct, pain, and inflammation. Numerous bacterial and parasitic infections can also affect the digestive tract. Examples include staphylococcal food poisoning, salmonellosis, typhoid fever, cholera, giardiasis, tapeworms, pinworms, hookworms, and ascariasis (roundworm). Specific diagnostic tests may include tissue biopsies, an occult blood test, bacterial cultures, and analysis for ova and parasites.

URINARY SYSTEM

 The primary purpose of the **urinary system** is to produce and eliminate urine. This system consists of two kidneys, two ureters, one bladder, and one urethra (Box 2–7). The kidneys' main function is to regulate the amount of water, electrolytes (sodium, potassium, chloride, calcium, phosphate, magnesium), and nitrogenous waste products (urea) from protein metabolism. The proper concentration of these blood constituents is vital to life. Electrolytes function to maintain the body's acid–base balance. The normal ratio of acid (carbonic acid) to base (bicarbonate) is 1:20. Blood pH and blood gas determinations provide useful information about acid–base balance in the body. Normal blood pH is within a range of 7.35 to 7.45. As blood passes through the specialized kidney cells, called *glomeruli,* water and solutes are filtered out. Only the necessary amounts of these substances are reabsorbed into the blood. The rest are excreted as waste products in the urine. Ureters collect urine as it forms and transport it to the bladder, which serves as a reservoir until the urine can be voided. The urethra is the terminal component of the urinary system. In women, it is merely a passageway from the bladder, whereas in men, it eliminates both urine and semen from the body.

BOX 2–7.   URINARY SYSTEM

Components:

- Kidneys
- Ureters
- Bladder
- Urethra

Functions:

- Filters blood to eliminate waste
- Helps maintain blood pH
- Regulates water balance

Disorders:

- Nephritis
- Renal failure

- Kidney stones
- Cystitis
- Uremia
- Urinary tract infection (UTI)

Diagnostic Tests:

- Albumin
- Ammonia
- Blood urea nitrogen (BUN)
- Creatinine clearance
- Electrolytes
- Osmolality
- Urinalysis
- Urine cultures

Two thirds of human body weight is water. About 60 percent of the body's water is inside cells, and the rest is in the bloodstream or tissue fluids. The salt content of the body's water is extremely important for survival. When excess salt is in the tissues, the kidneys eliminate it; if there is excess water, the kidneys eliminate it. If the kidneys are not functioning properly, a mechanical filtering process (dialysis) must be used or one of the kidneys must be replaced with a transplant.

Acidosis occurs when the blood pH decreases to less than 7.35. If the condition worsens, the individual can become comatose. **Respiratory acidosis** results when the respiratory system is unable to eliminate adequate amounts of CO_2 (in conditions such as a collapsed lung or blockage of respiratory passages). **Metabolic acidosis** occurs when the kidneys cannot eliminate acidic substances (in conditions such as diabetes mellitus). Such acidosis can result in kidney (renal) failure and death.

Alkalosis results when the blood pH increases to more than 7.45. **Respiratory alkalosis** results from hyperventilation or the loss of too much CO_2 from the lungs. **Metabolic alkalosis** usually results from excessive vomiting or an abnormal secretion of certain hormones that cause excess elimination of hydrogen ions (from CO_2). The kidneys are vitally important in compensating for *respiratory* acidosis or alkalosis. Conversely, the respiratory system is vitally important in compensating for *metabolic* acidosis or alkalosis.

Laboratory assessment of urinary function includes the detection of osmolality, chemical constituents, such as proteins, blood, microorganisms, and cells in the urine, as well as chemical analysis of albumin, ammonia, blood urea nitrogen, blood pH, blood gases, and electrolytes in the blood. Various urine collection techniques and preservatives are available. The creatinine clearance test evaluates the degree to which kidneys are filtering out waste products of metabolism.

REPRODUCTIVE SYSTEM

Male reproductive structures include the testes, the seminal vesicles, the prostate gland, the epididymis, the seminal ducts, the urethra, the scrotum, the penis, and the spermatic cords. The primary functions of this system are spermatogenesis (sperm production); storage, maintenance, and excretion of seminal fluid; and secretion of hormones (the most important of which is testosterone). Female reproductive structures include the ovaries, the fallopian tubes, the uterus, the vagina, the vulva, and the mammary glands. These structures play a role in ovulation, fertilization, menstruation, pregnancy, labor, lactation, and secretion of hormones (estrogens and progesterone) (Box 2–8.)

A sperm is one of the smallest cells in the body, whereas the mature egg is the largest. Each of these cells contains a nucleus with 23 chromosomes. Because a mother's egg and a father's sperm contain different sets of DNA, various genetic characteristics are paired. One of the pairs of chromosomes determines the sex of the fetus. The egg contains only an X chromosomes; however, the sperm may contain an X or a Y chromosome. Therefore, if an X sperm fertilizes the egg, an XX pair of chromosomes forms, and the neonate will be a girl. If a Y sperm fertilizes the egg, an XY pair forms, and the neonate will be a boy. The 46 combined chromosomes contain the DNA-coded blueprint for the newborn. The DNA controls not only the sex, but all characteristics, such as height; eye, hair, and skin color; immunity to diseases; allergies; and many other factors.

Disorders of the **reproductive system** include cancers, infertility, cysts, and **sexually transmitted diseases (STDs),** such as gonorrhea, genital herpes, syphilis, and **human immunodeficiency virus (HIV).** Diagnostic tests for such disorders include semen and cytogenetic analysis, as well as biopsies, Pap smears, and microbiological and viral cultures of infected areas. Blood tests include hormonal analysis (e.g., estrogen, follicle-stimulating hormone [FSH], luteinizing hormone [LH], human chorionic gonadotropin [HCG], testos-

---

BOX 2–8. REPRODUCTIVE SYSTEM

Components:

- Male: testes, penis, duct system, glands
- Female: ovaries, uterine tubes, uterus, vagina, external genitalia
  Accessory organs: mammary glands

Functions:

- Secretes hormones
- Produces germ cells for reproduction (sperm and ova)
- In the female, maintains fetus and produces milk for nourishment of neonate

Disorders:

- Cervical, ovarian, uterine cancer
- Infertility
- Ovarian cyst
- Prostate, testicular cancer
- Sexually transmitted diseases (STDs)

Diagnostic Tests:

- Acid phosphatase
- Estrogen
- Follicle-stimulating hormone (FSH)
- Human chorionic gonadotropin (HCG)
- Luteinizing hormone (LH)
- Microbiological cultures
- Pap smear
- Rapid plasma reagin (RPR)
- Testosterone
- Tissue analysis

terone) the rapid plasma reagin [RPR] test for syphilis, and acid phosphatase and prostatic specific antigen (PSA) for diagnosing and monitoring of prostate cancer.

ENDOCRINE SYSTEM

The human body has two types of glands. **Exocrine glands** secrete fluids, such as sweat, saliva, mucus, and digestive juices, which are transported through channels or ducts. **Endocrine glands,** or ductless glands, release their secretions (hormones) directly into the bloodstream. This glandular system has the same functions as those of the nervous system: communication, control, and integration. **Hormones** play an important role in metabolic regulation that influences growth and development, in fluid and electrolyte balance, in energy balance, and in acid–base balance. Hormonal imbalances can lead to severe disorders, such as dwarfism, gigantism, and sterility.

Endocrine glands include pituitary, thyroid, parathyroid, thymus, and adrenal glands, as well as ovaries and testes (Box 2–9). The **pituitary gland,** or *master gland,* as it is sometimes called, stimulates the other glands to produce hormones as needed. It controls and regulates hormone production through chemical feedback. The pituitary hormones also regulate retention of water by the kidneys, cause uterine contractions during childbirth, stimulate breast milk production, and produce growth hormone (GH). This hormone con-

---

BOX 2–9.   ENDOCRINE SYSTEM

Components:

- Hormone-producing structures: pituitary, pineal, thyroid, parathyroid, thymus, and adrenal glands
- Ovaries, testes, and pancreas

Functions:

- Composes a communications system that uses hormones as chemical messengers
- Helps maintain homeostasis
- Regulates body activities, such as metabolism and reproduction

Disorders:

- Addison's disease
- Cushing's syndrome
- Dwarfism
- Acromegaly
- Gigantism
- Diabetes insipidus
- Diabetes mellitus
- Hypo- and hyperthyroidism
- Hyperinsulinism
- Hypoglycemia
- Goiter
- Cretinism

Diagnostic Tests:

- Adrenocorticotropic hormone (ACTH)
- Aldosterone
- Antidiuretic hormone (ADH)
- Cortisol
- Erythropoietin
- Glucagon
- Glucose tolerance tests (GTTs)
- Growth hormone (GH)
- Insulin
- Renin
- Serotonin
- Thyroid function: triiodothyronine (T_3), thyroxine (T_4), thyroid-stimulating hormone (TSH)

trols growth by regulating the nutrients that are taken into cells. It also works with insulin to control blood sugar levels. If blood sugar is not controlled, diabetes mellitus, the most common disorder of the endocrine system, can result. The thyroid gland produces a hormone that affects cell metabolism and growth rate. Parathyroid glands regulate calcium and phosphorus in the blood and the bones. The thymus gland affects the lymphoid system. The **adrenals** (two glands) produce hormones as a result of emotions like fright or anger. This hormone production causes an increase in blood pressure, widened pupils, and heart stimulation. The adrenals also produce hormones that regulate carbohydrate metabolism and electrolyte balance.[1] As mentioned earlier, ovaries and testes produce estrogens and progesterone, and testosterone, respectively. The pineal gland secretes melatonin, a regulatory hormone. The pancreas contains exocrine tissue, which secrets pancreatic juice to aid in digestion and endocrine tissue to secrete hormones, such as insulin and glucagon.

Disorders are frequently inherited and result in excessive or insufficient hormone production. Diseases of this system include Addison's disease, Cushing's syndrome, dwarfism, acromegaly, giantism, diabetes insipidus, diabetes mellitus, hypo- or hyperthyroidism, hyperinsulinism, hypoglycemia, goiter, and creatinism.

Because hormones are transported by the bloodstream, abnormalities are easily detected by analyzing blood samples. Chemical assays are available for all types of hormones and provide very specific and sensitive results. In addition, specific thyroid function tests (triiodothyronine [T_3], thyroxine [T_4], and thyroid-stimulating hormone [TSH]) are available.

LYMPHATIC SYSTEM

The **lymphatic system** consists of lymph, lymphocytes, lymph vessels, lymph nodes, tonsils, the spleen, bone marrow, and the thymus gland (Box 2–10). Three main functions of the system are to maintain fluid balance in the tissues by filtering blood and lymph fluid, to provide a defense against disease, and to absorb fats and other substances from the digestive tract. About 30 L of fluid passes from the blood to the tissue spaces each day. If more

---

BOX 2–10.   LYMPHATIC SYSTEM

Components:

- Lymph vessels and nodes
- Spleen
- Thymus gland
- Tonsils
- Bone marrow

Functions:

- Maintains tissue fluid balance
- Filters blood and lymph
- Produces white blood cells to protect the body from disease
- Absorbs fats

Disorders:

- Tumors
- Immune disorders
- Infectious processes

Diagnostic Tests:

- Bone marrow analysis
- Cell surface markers

than 3 L were retained in the tissue, edema (swelling) would result. The lymph nodes filter lymph fluid, and the spleen filters blood, removing microorganisms or other foreign substances. Enlarged or swollen lymph nodes are common after infections. Lymphatic organs contain lymphocytes, macrophages, and other cells that provide immunity and protection against infections from microorganisms.

Disorders involving the lymphatic system are tumors (such as lymphoma and Hodgkin's disease), immune disorders, and infectious processes. Some immune disorders can be analyzed from blood samples, bone marrow, or both. Lymph nodes, however, are often surgically removed or aspirated so that cells can be analyzed or cultures performed. Analysis of markers on the surface of the cellular material is also diagnostically valuable.

CARDIOVASCULAR SYSTEM

For study purposes and to complete the overview of all organ systems, the **circulatory system** is briefly summarized in Box 2–11. This system is reviewed in greater depth and scope in Chapter 3.

BOX 2–11.   CIRCULATORY OR CARDIOVASCULAR SYSTEM

Components:

- Heart
- Blood vessels
- Blood

Functions:

- Transports oxygen and nutrients to the cells and transports carbon dioxide and wastes away
- Transports hormones and other substances throughout the body
- Regulates body temperature
- Helps defend against diseases

Disorders:

- Anemia
- Angina pectoris
- Hemophilia
- Embolus
- Leukemia
- Phlebitis
- Polycythemia
- Thrombocytopenia
- Thrombus
- Aortic stenosis
- Bacterial endocarditis

- Congestive heart failure
- Myocardial infarction (MI)
- Pericarditis
- Thrombophlebitis
- Varicose veins

Diagnostic Tests:

- Arterial blood gases
- Bone marrow analysis
- Complete blood cell (CBC) count and differential
- Erythrocyte sedimentation rate (ESR)
- Ferritin
- Hemoglobin and hematocrit (H&H)
- Indices (MCH, MCV, MCHC)
- Iron
- AST
- Cholesterol
- Creatine phosphokinase (CPK)
- Total iron-building capacity (TIBC)
- Coagulation studies: bleeding time, prothrombin time (PT), partial thromboplastin time (PTT), fibrin degradation product
- Triglycerides
- Potassium
- Lactic dehydrogenase (LDH)

SELF STUDY

KEY TERMS

Acidosis
Adrenals
Alkalosis
Alveolar Sacs
Anabolism
Anatomy
Anterior
Body Planes
Cardiac (Striated Involuntary) Muscles
Cartilage
Catabolism
Centriole
Circulatory System
Cytoplasm
Deoxyribonucleic Acid (DNA)
Digestive System
Dorsal
Endocrine Glands
Endoplasmic Reticulum
Exocrine Glands
Frontal Plane
Genes
Golgi Apparatus
Hematopoiesis
Homeostasis
Hormones
Human Immunodeficiency Virus (HIV)
Hyperventilation
Integumentary System
Lateral
Lymphatic System
Lysosomes

Medial
Melanin
Meninges
Metabolic Acidosis
Metabolic Alkalosis
Metabolism
Mitochondria
Muscular System
Nervous System
Neurons
Nucleolus
Nucleus
Peristalsis
Physiology
Pituitary Gland
Posterior
Reproductive System
Respiratory Acidosis
Respiratory Alkalosis
Respiratory System
Ribosomes
Sagittal Plane
Sexually Transmitted Diseases (STDs)
Skeletal (Striated Voluntary) Muscles
Skeletal System
Steady State
Transverse Plane
Urinary System
Ventral
Visceral (Nonstriated, Smooth, Involuntary) Muscles

STUDY QUESTIONS

The following may have *one* or *more* answers:

1. Which of the following body systems provide protection and support, and allow the body to move?

   a. integumentary
   b. skeletal
   c. muscular
   d. lymphatic
   e. digestive

2. Which of the following body systems provides for CO_2 and O_2 exchange?

   a. nervous
   b. muscular
   c. respiratory
   d. reproductive
   e. endocrine

3. Which of the following body systems is the primary regulator of hormones?

   a. digestive
   b. endocrine
   c. urinary
   d. integumentary
   e. nervous

4. The skeletal system provides which of the body's functions?

   a. support
   b. protection of tissues
   c. calcium storage
   d. blood cell formation
   e. leverage and movement

5. Germ cells are defined as

   a. sperm
   b. ova
   c. mammary glands
   d. neurons
   e. hair follicles

6. Which of the following pairs of words describe opposite regions or planes of the body?

   a. anterior/posterior
   b. distal/proximal
   c. anterior/ventral
   d. lateral/medial

7. The pituitary gland is often referred to as which of the following?

   a. respiratory control gland
   b. master gland
   c. lymph tissue
   d. germ cells

8. How many chromosomes are contained in human cells?

   a. 25
   b. 50
   c. 46
   d. 100
   e. 1000

9. What portion of human body weight is water?

   a. ninety percent
   b. one half
   c. one fourth
   d. two thirds

10. Homeostasis refers to which of the following?
    a. chemical imbalance
    b. steady-state condition
    c. balanced chemistry
    d. thousands of genes
    e. anabolism

References

1. Guy JF: *Learning Human Anatomy: A Laboratory Text and Workbook.* Norwalk, CT; Appleton & Lange: 1992.
2. Martini F: *Fundamentals of Anatomy and Physiology.* 3rd ed. Englewood Cliffs, NJ; Prentice Hall: 1995.

3

THREE

■

The Circulatory System

CHAPTER OUTLINE

CHAPTER OBJECTIVES

Upon completion of Chapter 3, the learner is responsible for the following:

1. Identify and describe the structures and functions of the heart.

2. Trace the flow of blood through the cardiovascular system.

3. Identify and describe the structures and functions of different types of blood vessels.

4. Identify and describe the cellular and noncellular components of blood

5. Locate and name the veins most commonly used for phlebotomy procedures.

6. Describe the phases of hemostasis.

7. Describe how to take a person's blood pressure and pulse rate.

All body systems are linked by the **cardiovascular system,** a transport network that can affect every cell, tissue, and organ within seconds. To maintain homeostasis, the cardiovascular system must provide for the rapid transport of water, nutrients, electrolytes, hormones, enzymes, antibodies, cells, and gases to all cells. In addition, it contributes to body defenses and the coagulation process and controls body temperature, much like the cooling system in a car. The primary components of the cardiovascular system include circulating fluid (**blood**), a pump (the **heart**), and numerous connected tubes (the **circulatory system,** or **blood vessels**). This chapter discusses these three main components of the cardiovascular system and the processes by which they function.

An important point to remember is that the lymphatic system, which was covered in Chapter 2, is closely integrated with the cardiovascular system. Both systems share transport vessels and empty their cells and contents into the bloodstream; however, the main purpose of the lymphatic system is to circulate lymph fluid to and from the tissues and to produce blood cells that aid in body defenses. Lymph tissue is found in lymph nodes, the thymus, the spleen, the intestine, the bone marrow, the liver, and the tonsils.

■ THE BLOOD

Circulating blood provides nutrients, oxygen, chemical substances, and waste removal for each of the billions of individual cells in the body. These functions, which are summarized in Box 3–1, are essential to homeostasis and life. Any region of the body that is deprived of blood may die within minutes.

Whole blood is composed of water, solutes, and cells. In general, humans have approximately 5 qt (4.73 L) of whole blood. The volume varies according to body weight, however. For instance, adult men usually have 5 to 6 L of whole blood, whereas adult women usually have 4 to 5 L. Abnormally low or high blood volumes can seriously affect other parts of the cardiovascular system. For example, a high blood volume (hypervolemia) can place stress on the heart because the heart must push extra fluids around the body.[1,2]

Whole blood is composed of approximately 3 qt (2.84 L, or about 60 percent) of plasma and 2 qt (1.89 L, or about 40 percent) of cells. Plasma contains 92 percent water and 8 percent solutes. Solutes include proteins, such as albumin, globulins, and fibrinogen; metabo-

BOX 3–1.   FUNCTIONS OF THE BLOOD

Transportation	Carry gases
	Carry oxygen from the lungs to the tissues
	Carry carbon dioxide from the tissues to the lungs
	Transport waste products to sites such as the kidneys for excretion
	Transport antibodies and white blood cells to defend against pathogenic microbes and viruses
Disburse nutrients	Distribute nutrients absorbed in the digestive tract to all organs of the body
	Take nutrients released from fat, muscle, or tissues for use in other parts of the body
Regulation	Regulate the blood pH in all parts of the body
	Regulate electrolyte balance to maintain a "steady state" condition
Hemostasis	Restrict fluid loss when blood vessels are damaged
	Formation of blood clots to prevent bleeding
Regulation	Control body temperature by redistribution of heat

lites, such as lipids, glucose, nitrogen wastes, and amino acids; and ions, such as sodium (Na), potassium (K), calcium (Ca), magnesium (Mg), and chloride (Cl).

Circulating blood cells are classified as **red blood cells (RBCs, or erythrocytes), white blood cells (WBCs, or leukocytes),** and **platelets (thrombocytes).** Approximately 99 percent of the circulating cells are RBCs. White blood cells are divided further into cell lines called **granulocytes (basophils, neutrophils, eosinophils), lymphocytes,** and **monocytes.** (Refer to Table 3–1.)

All blood cells develop from undifferentiated stem cells in the **hematopoietic** (blood-forming) tissues, such as the bone marrow. Stem cells are considered immature cells because they have not developed into their functional state. As the stem cells mature, they differentiate into the different cell lines mentioned in the preceding paragraph. The maturing cells are given specific names on the basis of the cell type that they will produce. The cells undergo changes in the nucleus and cytoplasm so that when they reach the circulating blood, they become fully mature and functional. These changes are clearly visible when staining techniques and light microscopy are used, or they can be distinguished by specialized hematology instruments.

ERYTHROCYTES

Red blood cells measure about 7 μm in diameter. Normally, when in the circulating blood, RBCs have no nuclei. Prior to reaching maturity in the bone marrow, RBCs lose their nuclei and simultaneously become biconcaved disks. Within each mature RBC are millions of hemoglobin molecules; each molecule is capable of carrying four oxygen (O_2) molecules. As mentioned in Chapter 2, hemoglobin can also carry carbon dioxide (CO_2).

Red blood cells are formed in the bone marrow from nucleated stem cells. Once the stem cell becomes committed to being an RBC, it matures through several stages, all of which are morphologically different if viewed under a microscope. The process occurs during several days, and the stages are called *rubriblast, prorubricyte, rubricyte, metarubricyte, reticulocyte,* and *mature RBC.* Because nomenclature differs among laboratories, however, the

Table 3–1. Blood Cells

CELLS	NUMBER/ SIZE	FUNCTION	FORMATION	DESTRUCTION
Erythrocytes (RBCs)	4.5–5.5 million/ mm³; size 6–7 μm	Transport O_2 and CO_2	Bone marrow	Fragmentation and removal in spleen, liver, and bone marrow; life span, ≅ 120 days
Leukocytes (WBCs)	5000–9000/mm³; size 9–16 μm	Defense	Granulocytes in bone marrow; nongranular WBCs in all lymphatic tissue	Removed in spleen, liver, bone marrow; life span–1 day to years
Thrombocytes (platelets)	250,000–450,000/ mm³; size 1–4 μm	Clotting	Bone marrow	Removed in spleen; life span–9 to 12 days

Abbreviations: RBCs, red blood cells; WBCs, white blood cells.

terms *pronormoblast, basophilic normoblast, polychromatic normoblast,* and *orthochromatic normoblast* can also be used for the first four stages.

The life span of RBCs is approximately 120 days in the circulating bloodstream. After this time, they begin to fragment and rupture. Cells in the liver, spleen, and bone marrow phagocytize the destroyed RBCs and begin to break down the hemoglobin into iron-containing pigments (hemosiderin) and bile pigments (bilirubin and biliverdin). The bone marrow reuses the iron for new RBCs, and the liver excretes the bile pigments into the intestines.[2]

Millions of RBCs are continuously being formed and destroyed daily. So that it can maintain a normal supply of these cells, the bone marrow must have an adequate supply of several substances, including amino acids, vitamin B complexes, and minerals, such as iron. Deficiencies of any of these substances or failure of the bone marrow to function properly may result in anemia.

The surface membranes of RBCs contain antigens that designate the individual's blood type. Red blood cells with A antigen are type A, cells with B antigen are type B, RBCs containing both A and B antigens are type AB, and RBCs with neither A nor B antigens are type O. These antigens constitute the **ABO blood group system.** ABO antibodies (also called *agglutinins*) are present in plasma and provide protection and cross-reactions with opposing antigens. For example, type A blood contains anti-B, which will attack type B RBCs. Conversely, type B blood contains anti-A, which will cross-react with type A blood cells. Type O whole blood contains anti-A and anti-B, and type AB does not contain A or B antibodies. Type O is the most common blood type (46 percent of the U.S. population), followed by types A (40 percent), B (10 percent), and AB (4 percent).

Another commonly recognized blood group system contains the **Rh factor.** If the RBCs contain the antigen for Rh factor, the individual is considered Rh positive. Rh-negative people do not have the Rh-factor antigen on their RBCs. In contrast to the ABO system, in the Rh system, the plasma of Rh-negative people does not have anti-Rh agglutinins. Rh antibodies are present only if the body has been exposed to Rh-positive RBCs. This situation may occur accidentally by transfusion or during pregnancy. When an Rh-negative mother is carrying an Rh-positive fetus (the Rh-positive gene comes from the father), she becomes sensitized to the Rh-positive blood during delivery when the placental connection breaks down and when bleeding occurs. The mother then develops Rh antibodies. If she becomes pregnant again, the Rh antibodies will cross-react with the Rh-positive blood of the fetus. This condition can result in hemolytic disease of the newborn (HDN). It is preventable by administration of RhoGam (anti-Rh agglutinins) during and after the first pregnancy.[2]

! Clinical Alert

Blood transfused into a patient must never contain antibodies to the patient's blood group antigens on the red cells because such antibodies can cross-react with specific RBC antigens and destroy the red cells. When this type of cross-reaction occurs, the RBCs clump together (or agglutinate) and may rupture (hemolyze). Red blood cell clumps and fragments can clog small blood vessels and cause damage to the kidneys, lungs, heart, or brain. One situation in which a cross-reaction may occur is when a patient is transfused with blood that has been accidentally mistyped or confused with another patient's. Such a reaction can be rapidly fatal to the inappropriately transfused patient. (See Table 3–2 for a list of antibodies present in various blood types.)

Table 3–2. ABO Blood Types

BLOOD TYPE	ANTIGENS ON RBC	ANTIBODIES IN SERUM/PLASMA
A	A	Anti-B
B	B	Anti-A
AB	AB	Neither anti-A nor anti-B
O	None	Anti-A and anti-B

Abbreviations: RBC, red blood cell.

To prevent a cross-reaction, physicians often request **cross-match testing,** which involves exposing a blood donor's blood to the patient's (recipient) blood. This procedure detects cross-reactivity. In addition to ABO and Rh, at least 48 possible cross-reactions can occur because of numerous antigens on the blood cells and antibodies in sera.

Type O individuals are called *universal donors.* Their RBCs can be transfused into a person with any ABO type because their RBCs do not contain A or B antigens to react with either the anti-A or the anti-B present in type B or type A blood, respectively.

LEUKOCYTES

White blood cells (leukocytes) differ in color, size, shape, and nuclear formation, and they are divided into two major groups: granular (with granules in the cytoplasm) and agranular (without cytoplasmic granules). **Neutrophils, eosinophils,** and **basophils** are **granulocytes.** Neutrophilic granules stain bluish with neutral dyes, and their nuclei generally have two or more lobes. These granulocytes are often referred to as *polymorphonuclear (PMN) leukocytes.* Eosinophilic granules stain orange-red with acidic dyes. Their nuclei normally have two lobes. Basophilic granules stain dark purple or black with basic dyes, and their nuclei are often S-shaped. Agranular leukocytes, lymphocytes, and monocytes have relatively large nuclei (see Fig. 3–1 and the Color Atlas).

Leukocytes function primarily as part of the body's defense mechanism. The cells phagocytize or ingest pathogenic microorganisms. Consequently, lymphocytes play a role in immunity and in the production of antibodies.

White blood cells are formed in bone marrow and lymphatic tissues. The exact life span of a cell varies with cell type from 1 day to several years. Normally, blood contains 5000 to 9000 leukocytes/mm^3, with designated percentages for each cell line. The morphological characteristics of leukocytes and erythrocytes are routinely analyzed by using special staining techniques and visualizing the cells under the microscope. Categorization of cells and abnormalities are noted on the test report called a **differential,** which can be performed manually or by using specialized instrumentation. Hematology instruments are able to produce automated differentials at a high speed in a cost-effective manner, whereas manual readings require significant expertise and time to interpret microscopic analysis.

Leukocytes contain specific cell surface antigens that are expressed at certain times during the development of the various WBC types. These antigens can be characterized with sophisticated techniques, such as flow cytometry and monoclonal antibodies, in the clinical laboratory. Using these laboratory techniques, clinicians can tell more precisely how mature or immature the WBCs are in the bone marrow, peripheral blood, or both.

Figure 3–1. Human blood cells.

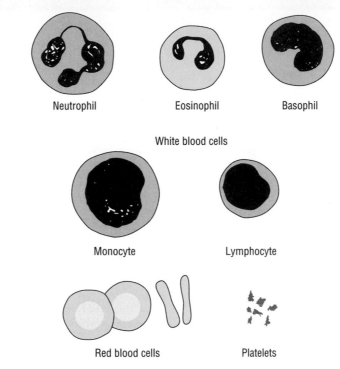

White blood cells

Neutrophil   Eosinophil   Basophil

Monocyte   Lymphocyte

Red blood cells   Platelets

THROMBOCYTES

Platelets are much smaller than other blood cells. They are fragments of **megakaryocytes** (*mega* means big), which are located in the bone. Normally, there are 250,000 to 450,000 platelets/mm^3. Platelets help in the clotting process by transporting needed chemicals for clotting, forming a temporary patch or plug to slow blood loss, and contracting after the blood clot has formed. Their life span is 9 to 12 days.

PLASMA

The liquid portion of the blood, without cells, is called **plasma**. If a chemical agent called an **anticoagulant** is added to prevent clotting, a blood sample can be separated by centrifugation into the cells and the plasma (Fig. 3–2).

Plasma is composed of 90 percent water and 10 percent solutes, which include nutrients, such as glucose, amino acids, fats, metabolic wastes (urea, uric acid, creatinine, and lactic acid), respiratory gases (O_2 and CO_2), regulatory substances (hormones, enzymes, and electrolytes), and protective substances (antibodies). The cellular portion of the specimen contains WBCs, platelets, and RBCs. If the specimen is centrifuged or allowed to settle, the

Figure 3–2. Blood specimens with and without anticoagulant, respectively.

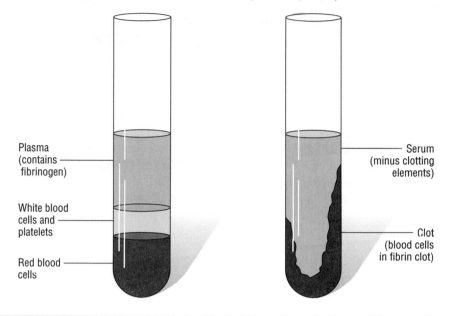

Plasma (contains fibrinogen)

Serum (minus clotting elements)

White blood cells and platelets

Red blood cells

Clot (blood cells in fibrin clot)

RBCs (the heaviest) will sink to the bottom of the tube. The WBCs and platelets form a thin white layer above the RBCs called the **buffy coat.** The fluid plasma portion remains on the top.

SERUM

If a blood specimen is allowed to clot, the result is **serum** plus blood cells meshed in a fibrin clot. Serum contains essentially the same chemical constituents as plasma, except the clotting factors and the blood cells are contained within the fibrin clot (Fig. 3–2).

■ THE HEART

The human heart is a muscular organ about the size of a man's closed fist. (Refer to the color atlas for detailed representations of the structural and anatomic components of the heart.) The heart contains four chambers and is located slightly left of the midline in the thoracic cavity. The two **atria** are separated by the interatrial septum (wall), and the interventricular septum divides the two **ventricles.** Each atrium shares a valve with the ventricle on the same side. Heart valves are positioned for blood to flow in one direction only and to prevent backflow.

The right atrium of the heart receives blood from two large veins, the **superior vena cava** and the **inferior vena cava.** The superior vena cava brings blood from the head, neck, arms, and chest; the inferior vena cava carries O_2-poor blood from the rest of the trunk and the legs. Once the blood enters the right atrium, it passes through the heart valve (right atrioventricular, or tricuspid, valve) into the right ventricle. When blood exits the right ventricle, it begins the **pulmonary circuit,** where it enters the right and left pulmonary arteries. Arteries of the pulmonary circuit differ from those of the systemic circuit because they carry deoxygenated blood. Like veins, they are usually shown in blue on color-coded charts. These vessels branch into smaller arterioles and capillaries within the lungs, where gaseous exchange occurs (O_2 is picked up, and CO_2 is released). (Refer to Chapter 2 for more information about respiratory gas exchange.) From the respiratory capillaries, blood flows into the left and right pulmonary veins and then into the left atrium. The left atrium also has a valve (left atrioventricular, or bicuspid, or mitral, valve). Blood flows through the mitral valve into the left ventricle. When blood exits the left ventricle, it passes through the aortic semilunar valve and into the **systemic circuit** by means of the ascending aorta. The systemic circuit carries blood to the tissues of the body. If a valve malfunctions, blood flows backward and a heart murmur results. The right side of the heart pumps O_2-poor blood to the lungs to pick up more O_2; the left side pumps O_2-rich blood toward the legs, head, and organs.

Figure 3–3. Sphygmomanometer.

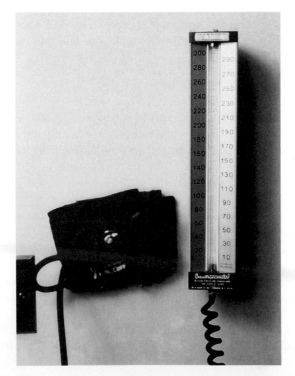

The heart's function is to pump sufficient amounts of blood to all cells of the body by contraction (systole) and relaxation (diastole). Because the lungs are close to the heart, and the pulmonary arteries and veins are short and wide, the right ventricle does not need to pump very hard to propel blood through the pulmonary circuit. Thus, the heart wall of the right ventricle is relatively thin. On the other hand, the left ventricle must push blood around the systemic circuit, which covers the entire body. As a result, the left ventricle has a thick, muscular wall and a powerful contraction.

Blood pressure increases during ventricular systole and decreases during ventricular diastole. Blood pressure not only forces blood through vessels, but also pushes it against the walls of the vessels like air in a balloon. Therefore, it can be measured by how forcefully it presses against vascular walls. The instrument used for such measurements is called a *sphygmomanometer,* or a *blood pressure cuff* (Fig. 3–3). When blood pressure is reported, **systolic pressure** and **diastolic pressure** are written with a slash between the two numbers (e.g., 120/80) (Figs. 3–4 and 3–5, and Box 3–2).

The average heart beats 60 to 80 times per minute. Children have faster heart rates than adults, and athletes have slower rates because more blood can be pumped with each beat. During exercise, the heart beats faster to supply muscles with more blood; during and after meals, it also beats faster to pump blood to the digestive system; and during fever, the heart pumps more blood to the skin surface to release heat. The heart rate (pulse rate) is measured by feeling for a pulse and counting the pulses per minute (Fig. 3–4 and Box 3–2).

■ THE VESSELS AND CIRCULATION

Three kinds of blood vessels exist in the human body: **arteries, veins,** and **capillaries.** The largest artery **(aorta)** and veins **(venae cavae)** are approximately 1-in. wide. Normally, blood vessels have smooth, flexible walls. With age, however, arterial walls may "harden" (called *hardening of the arteries* or *arteriosclerosis*). The inner walls of the vessels become rough because of cholesterol or calcium deposits. As the deposits build, blood clots may form that clog the artery further, and the blood supply to tissues is reduced. In serious cases, this lack of blood results in a stroke (if the blood supply in the brain is reduced) or a heart attack (if the blood supply in the coronary, or heart, vessels is reduced).

ARTERIES

Arteries are highly oxygenated vessels that carry blood away from the heart (efferent vessels). They branch into smaller vessels called **arterioles** and into capillaries. The principal arteries of the body are indicated in the Color Atlas. Arteries are normally bright red in color, have thicker elastic walls than veins do, and have a pulse.

VEINS

Blood is carried toward the heart by the veins (afferent vessels). Because the blood in veins flows against gravity in many areas of the body, these vessels have one-way valves and rely on weak muscular action to move blood cells. The one-way valves prevent backflow of blood.

Figure 3–4. The pressure points indicated may be used to check a patient's pulse. Blood pressure is commonly measured using a sphygmomanometer at the site of the brachial artery.

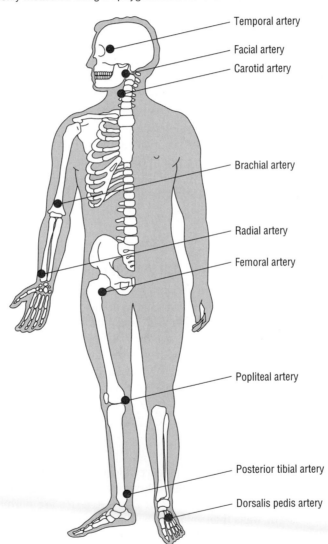

Figure 3–5. Major arm veins. Note that the *cephalic vein* extends almost the entire length of the arm. The superficial *median cubital vein* serves as a connection between the cephalic and basilic veins. The subclavian, brachial, and axillary veins are deeper veins.

1. **Subclavian vein**
2. **Brachial vein**
3. **Axillary vein**
4. **Cephalic vein**
5. **Basilic vein**
6. **Median cubital vein**

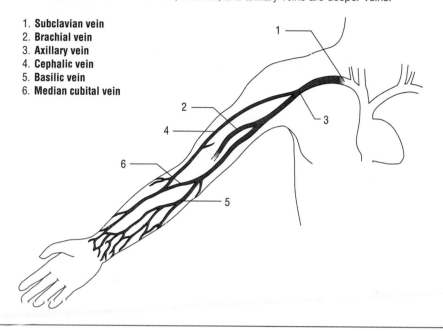

All veins except the pulmonary veins contain deoxygenated blood, are normally dark red in color, and have thinner walls than arteries. The principal veins of the body are also indicated in the Color Atlas.

Phlebotomists should be familiar with the principal veins of the arms and legs (Figs. 3–5 to 3–8). The forearm vein most commonly used for venipuncture is the **median cubital vein** because it is generally the largest and best anchored vein. Others that are acceptable are the **basilic vein** and the **cephalic vein.**

CAPILLARIES

Microscopic vessels that carry blood and link arterioles to **venules** (minute veins) are called *capillaries.* Capillaries may be so small in diameter as to allow only one blood cell to pass through at any given time. Gas exchange occurs in the capillaries of tissues.

■ HEMOSTASIS AND COAGULATION

Hemostasis (not to be confused with homeostasis) is the maintenance of circulating blood in the liquid state and retention of blood in the vascular system by preventing blood loss. When a small blood vessel is injured, the hemostatic process repairs the break and stops

> ## BOX 3–2.   PULSE RATE AND BLOOD PRESSURE MEASUREMENT
>
> ### Pulse Rate
>
> 1. To take a pulse measurement, begin by pressing two fingertips (usually the second and third fingers, not the thumb) on an artery. Choose an artery that lies against a solid mass, such as a bone; the most common site is the radial artery of the wrist (at the base of the thumb). Other possible sites include the temporal, facial, carotid, brachial, femoral, popliteal, posterior tibial, and dorsalis pedis arteries. The pulse is felt as a pressure against the fingertips.
>
> 2. Measure the pulse rate by counting the pulses for 60 seconds. The normal adult pulse rate is about 75 per minute.
>
> ### Blood Pressure
>
> Blood pressure is measured by an instrument called a *sphygmomanometer,* or *blood pressure cuff.* Values on the instrument relate to millimeters of mercury (mm Hg) in a tube at certain points. Systolic pressure, the highest, is measured when the artery receives blood. Diastolic pressure, the lowest, is measured when the heart's ventricles relax. Blood pressure is reported with two numbers, one for the systolic pressure and one for the diastolic pressure (e.g., the normal average adult reading of 120/80 means that the systolic pressure measures 120 mm Hg and the diastolic pressure measures 80 mm Hg).
>
> 1. Place the inflatable cuff around the patient's upper arm so that the cuff squeezes the brachial artery.
>
> 2. Place a stethoscope over the artery distal to the cuff, then inflate the cuff until the pressure reads approximately 30 mm Hg. At this point, the brachial artery collapses, the flow of blood stops, and the sound of the pulse disappears.
>
> 3. Slowly let the air out of the cuff. At first, blood enters only at peak systolic pressure, and the stethoscope picks up the sound of blood pulsing through the artery. As air is removed from the cuff, the sounds change because the artery is remaining more open. When the cuff pressure decreases to less than diastolic pressure, blood flow becomes continuous, and the sound of the pulse becomes muffled or disappears completely. The pressure reading when the pulse appears corresponds to the peak systolic pressure (the first number reported). When the pulse fades, the pressure reading (the second number reported) has reached diastolic levels.
>
> *Note:* Blood pressure changes frequently. For this reason, ambulatory pressure-monitoring devices are available that provide a continual printout of the patient's blood pressure. Normal blood pressure fluctuates from lows around 2:00 AM to peak values during the day.

the hemorrhage. The first (vascular) phase in this process is **vasoconstriction,** which decreases the blood flow to the injured vessel and the surrounding vascular bed. In the second (platelet) phase, platelets degranulate, clump together, and adhere to the injured vessel in order to form a plug and inhibit bleeding. In phase three (**coagulation**), many specific coagulation factors are released and interact to form a **fibrin** meshwork or blood clot. This clot seals off the damaged portion of the vessel. Phase four (clot retraction) occurs when the bleeding has stopped. The entire clot retracts to bring torn edges closer together. In phase five (**fibrinolysis**), final repair and regeneration of the injured vessel occurs, and the clot slowly begins to dissolve as other cells carry out further repair.

The coagulation process (phase three) is a result of numerous coagulation factors. For simplicity, it is divided into two systems: intrinsic and extrinsic. All coagulation factors required for the **intrinsic system** are contained in the blood, whereas the **extrinsic factors**

Figure 3–6. Major arm veins. Since all individuals are unique, the exact location of veins may vary from one to another. This figure depicts variations in venous patterns in the arms of two individuals.

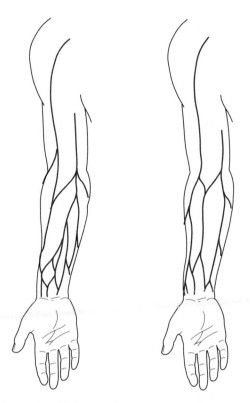

are stimulated when tissue damage occurs. For example, blood vessels are lined with a single layer of flat endothelial cells and are supported by subendothelial cells and collagen fibers. Normally, endothelial cells do not react or attract platelets; however, they do produce and store some clotting factors. When the clotting sequence is initiated by vessel injury, endothelial cells react with degranulated platelets in forming the fibrin plug (Fig. 3–9).[2]

Large- or medium-sized veins and arteries require rapid surgical intervention to prevent bleeding. Bleeding of small arteries and veins can, however, be controlled by the hemostatic process.

Disorders of the hemostatic process are serious. Overactive clotting can cause clots within the body, such as an embolus or a thrombus, or disseminated intravascular coagulation (DIC) disease. Drugs such as heparin and Coumadin (warfarin), which suppress clotting factors, can be used to prevent such problems. On the other hand, if clotting factors are not produced by the body, excessive bleeding may occur, as in hemophilia.

Figure 3–7. Major leg veins. The *femoral vein* is a deep vein. Note that the *greater saphenous vein* is the longest vein in the body. It ascends up the medial side of the leg and the medial thigh and empties into the femoral vein in the groin area. The *lesser saphenous vein* comes up the lateral side of the ankle and enters the deeper *popliteal vein* behind the knee.

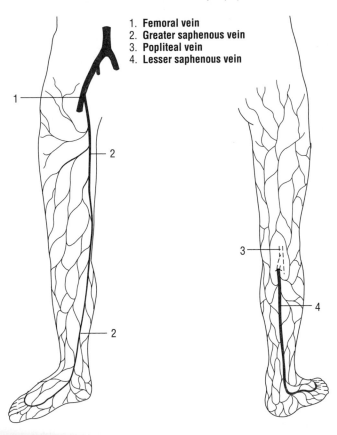

1. **Femoral vein**
2. **Greater saphenous vein**
3. **Popliteal vein**
4. **Lesser saphenous vein**

Figure 3–8. Overview of the pattern of circulation. Venous blood flow is on the left side of the diagram, and arterial flow is on the right side. RA, right atrium; RV, right ventricle; LA, left atrium; LV, left ventricle.

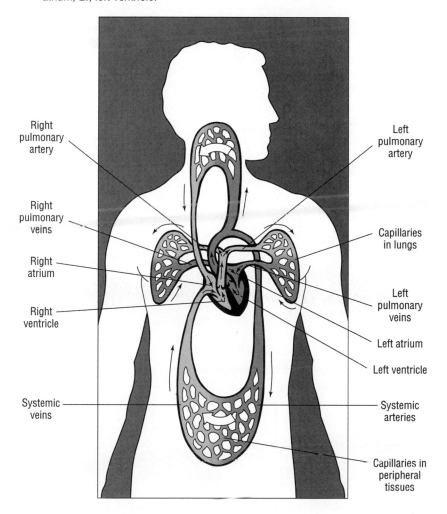

Right pulmonary artery

Right pulmonary veins

Right atrium

Right ventricle

Systemic veins

Left pulmonary artery

Capillaries in lungs

Left pulmonary veins

Left atrium

Left ventricle

Systemic arteries

Capillaries in peripheral tissues

Figure 3–9. Clotting response.

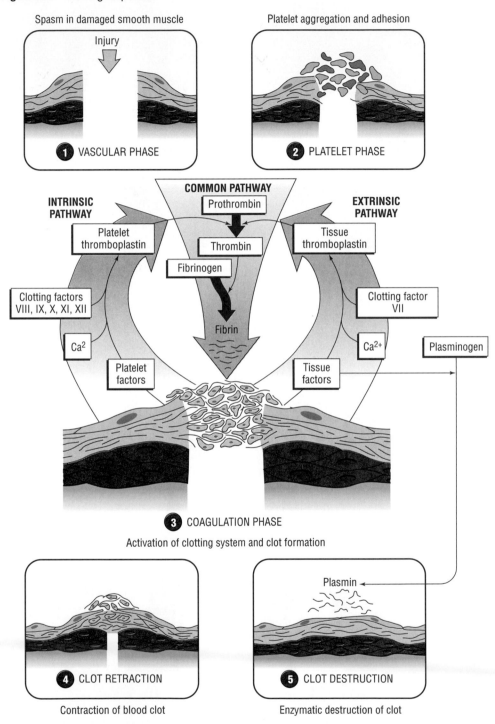

Spasm in damaged smooth muscle

Injury

1 VASCULAR PHASE

Platelet aggregation and adhesion

2 PLATELET PHASE

COMMON PATHWAY

Prothrombin

INTRINSIC PATHWAY

Platelet thromboplastin

Thrombin

Fibrinogen

EXTRINSIC PATHWAY

Tissue thromboplastin

Clotting factors VIII, IX, X, XI, XII

Ca^2

Fibrin

Clotting factor VII

Ca^{2+}

Plasminogen

Platelet factors

Tissue factors

3 COAGULATION PHASE

Activation of clotting system and clot formation

4 CLOT RETRACTION

Contraction of blood clot

Plasmin

5 CLOT DESTRUCTION

Enzymatic destruction of clot

■ DIAGNOSTIC ASSESSMENT

The number of RBCs, their morphological traits, and their hemoglobin content can be determined from an anticoagulated blood specimen in the clinical hematology laboratory. Platelets and WBCs can be assessed on the basis of number and morphological features. The results of a WBC differential count enumerate specific cell lines in percentages. Platelet function, as well as each coagulation factor, can be measured from anticoagulated blood specimens in the coagulation section of the clinical hematology laboratory. In addition, bone marrow, which is removed by a physician from the iliac crest of the hip, can be stained and studied microscopically in the hematology laboratory for the detection of abnormal numbers and morphological characteristics of blood cells.

Tests for blood types and cross-matches for donor blood are done in an immunohematology, a transfusion, or a blood banking laboratory. Serum and plasma constituents, including nutrients, metabolic wastes, respiratory gases, regulatory substances, and protective substances, can all be evaluated in the clinical chemistry laboratory.

Blood pressure and **pulse rate** measurements are performed as part of routine physi- cal assessments (Figs. 3–3 to 3–6). High blood pressure can cause a stroke when a vessel ruptures in the brain. Having slightly low blood pressure is generally considered to be a healthier state than having high blood pressure; however, if a person's pressure is too low, blood will not flow to the head, and a faint feeling may result. In these cases, the best response is to lower the head to restore and increase blood flow to the head.

SELF STUDY

KEY TERMS

ABO Blood Group System
Anticoagulant
Aorta
Arteries
Arterioles
Atria
Basilic Vein
Blood
Blood Pressure
Blood Vessels
Buffy Coat
Capillaries
Cardiovascular System
Cephalic Vein
Circulatory System
Coagulation
Cross-Match Testing
Diastolic Pressure
Differential
Extrinsic Factors
Fibrin
Fibrinolysis
Granulocytes (Basophils,
    Neutrophils, Eosinophils)
Heart
Hematopoietic

Hemostasis
Inferior Vena Cava
Intrinsic System
Lymphocytes
Median Cubital Vein
Megakaryocytes
Monocytes
Plasma
Platelets (Thrombocytes)
Pulmonary Circuit
Pulse Rate
Red Blood Cells (RBCs or
    Erythrocytes)
Rh Factor
Serum
Superior Vena Cava
Systemic Circuit
Systolic Pressure
Vasoconstriction
Veins
Venae Cavae
Ventricles
Venules
White Blood Cells (WBCs
    or Leukocytes)

STUDY QUESTIONS

The following questions may have *one* or *more* answers.

1. Whole blood consists of which of the following?

   a. water
   b. solutes

   c. cells
   d. tissue

2. Which type of blood cell is most numerous in the circulating blood?

   a. red blood cell
   b. white blood cell

   c. platelet
   d. macrophage

3. Identify the four chambers of the heart.

   a. right atrium, right
      ventricle
   b. superior vena cava,
      inferior vena cava

   c. left atrium, left ventricle
   d. ascending aorta, descending
      aorta

4. The liquid portion of an anticoagulated blood specimen is called

   a. plasma
   b. serum

   c. cellular components
   d. oxygenated blood

5. Which of the following veins are most commonly used for venipuncture procedures?

   a. popliteal
   b. brachial
   c. median cubital

   d. cephalic
   e. basilic

6. Functions of the blood include which of the following?

   a. transportation of gases,
      enzymes, and hormones
   b. regulation of pH and
      electrolytes

   c. regulation of body temperature
   d. transportation of waste
      products

7. Blood pressure is reported in which of the following ways?

   a. diastolic pressure only
   b. diastolic pressure/systolic
      pressure

   c. systolic pressure/diastolic
      pressure
   d. systolic pressure only

8. Which of the listed circulating blood cells have no nuclei?

   a. neutrophils
   b. erythrocytes

   c. basophils
   d. eosinophils

9. The most common blood type is

   a. A
   b. B

   c. AB
   d. O

10. The coagulation process occurs in phases that include the

   a. vascular phase
   b. platelet phase

   c. coagulation phase
   d. clot-retraction phase

References

1. Guy JF. *Learning Human Anatomy: A Laboratory Text and Workbook.* Norwalk, CT: Appleton & Lange; 1992.

2. Martini F. *Fundamentals of Anatomy and Physiology.* 3rd ed. Englewood Cliffs, NJ: Prentice
   Hall; 1995.

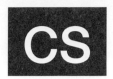

PHLEBOTOMY CASE STUDY

■

Changing Roles in Phlebotomy Practice

Ms. Sanborn had been working in the hospital clinical laboratory for 4 years as a phlebotomist. She was highly regarded by her laboratory colleagues because of her efficiency in blood collection on three different units of the hospital, her assistance with specimen processing, and overall attention to details. She was recognized by her department as outstanding in her ability to communicate effectively with patients. Outside of work she routinely socialized with her co-workers on weekends. As part of the hospital restructuring plan, she was reassigned to report to a nursing director on a surgical unit of the hospital. Her new work duties included phlebotomy, glucose bedside testing, clerical functions on the unit, and occasional patient transportation from the unit to other parts of the hospital as needed. She was very reluctant to leave her friends and old job duties in the laboratory to be relocated to the surgical unit. Ms. Sanborn knew that all the phlebotomists' positions in the hospital were being reassigned, and she did not want to work anywhere else because she felt loyal to the hospital. She was too proud to complain about her unhappiness with the situation.

QUESTIONS:

1. Name three trends in the health care industry that might be contributing to the hospital's changes. How could Ms. Sanborn learn more about these changes?
2. List four character traits that Ms. Sanborn should remember about working with health care teams.
3. Describe the positive professional character traits exhibited by Ms. Sanborn and how they may be beneficial in her new job assignment.

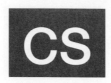

PHLEBOTOMY CASE STUDY

■

Collection From the Dorsal Side of the Hand

Mr. Whitefield, a phlebotomist who recently completed his training program at Amber Community College, acquired a position at Oakhaven Hospital on the early morning shift. One morning, he was informed by the nurse on the orthopedic floor that any blood collections from Patient Davis should be taken while Mr. Davis is in the supine position and that all collections should be taken from the left dorsal hand.

QUESTIONS:

1. Is the dorsal area the same as the proximal area? Explain the similarities or differences.

2. Should Mr. Davis sit up or lie down during the blood collection?

3. *Orthopedic* refers to what type of specialty?

SAFETY PROCEDURES

PART II PROVIDES A MORE DETAILED LOOK at safety and regulatory factors that affect the health care professional in practicing phlebotomy and associated procedures. The chapters cover methods for protecting patients and providers from the risks of infections and hazardous situations, ways to document information about phlebotomy practices, and procedures for proper transportation of specimens and documentation essentials.

Chapter 4, Infection Control, describes the essentials of infection control, which include surveillance, knowledge of the chain of infection, and isolation protocol. Detailed procedures are presented that are designed to protect the patient from infections and to protect the employee from being exposed. Infection control programs designed for various hospital units are also described.

Chapter 5, Safety and First Aid, provides basic procedures for safe handling of specimens, equipment, and reagents in the work setting. Topics covered include fire, electrical, radiation, mechanical, and chemical safety and emergency care procedures and exposure control issues.

Chapter 6, Specimen Documentation and Transportation, provides the essentials of documentation for the clinical or medical record. Special components that relate to phlebotomy practice are highlighted, such as specimen requisition forms, labels, and reports. Specimen transportation and delivery procedures are also described for settings within a hospital and ambulatory sites. Manual and computerized processes are also discussed.

FOUR

■

Infection Control

CHAPTER OUTLINE

CHAPTER OBJECTIVES

Upon completion of Chapter 4, the learner is responsible for the following:

1. Define the term *nosocomial infection.*
2. Identify the basic programs for infection control.
3. Explain the proper techniques for hand washing, gowning, gloving, masking, double bagging, and entering and exiting the various isolation areas.
4. Identify the potential routes of infection and methods for preventing transmission of microorganisms through these routes.
5. Describe the various isolation procedures and reasons for their use.

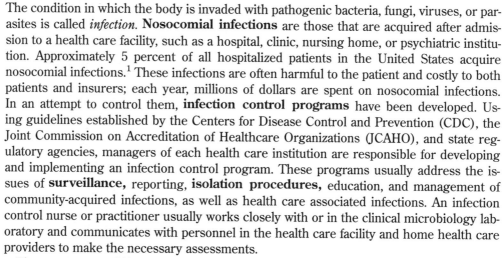

The condition in which the body is invaded with pathogenic bacteria, fungi, viruses, or parasites is called *infection.* **Nosocomial infections** are those that are acquired after admission to a health care facility, such as a hospital, clinic, nursing home, or psychiatric institution. Approximately 5 percent of all hospitalized patients in the United States acquire nosocomial infections.[1] These infections are often harmful to the patient and costly to both patients and insurers; each year, millions of dollars are spent on nosocomial infections. In an attempt to control them, **infection control programs** have been developed. Using guidelines established by the Centers for Disease Control and Prevention (CDC), the Joint Commission on Accreditation of Healthcare Organizations (JCAHO), and state regulatory agencies, managers of each health care institution are responsible for developing and implementing an infection control program. These programs usually address the issues of **surveillance,** reporting, **isolation procedures,** education, and management of community-acquired infections, as well as health care associated infections. An infection control nurse or practitioner usually works closely with or in the clinical microbiology laboratory and communicates with personnel in the health care facility and home health care providers to make the necessary assessments.

There are many different guidelines for the isolation of patients and the protection of health care workers (e.g., category-specific isolation, blood and body fluid precautions, body substance isolation, and/or standard or universal and transmission-based precautions) that are discussed in this chapter. Whatever the system in place, the main issues for health care workers are to understand what pathogens can infect them, how such pathogens are transmitted, and how to protect themselves in the workplace.

The cornerstones for infection protection of the health care worker, particularly phlebotomists are as follows:

- Frequent handwashing.
- Use of barrier garments and personal protective equipment.
- Waste management of contaminated materials.

These protective procedures must become part of a phlebotomist's routine procedures and standards for practice. These practices are also discussed in Chapters 7 and 8.

■ SURVEILLANCE

In most health care institutions, the infection control program involves monitoring and collecting data on several specific populations, such as (1) patients at a high risk of infection;

(2) patients with previously acquired infections; (3) personnel or patients accidentally exposed to a communicable disease, contaminated equipment, or hazardous reagents; (4) patients in certain areas of the hospital or in certain rooms; and (5) patients in ambulatory settings, such as home or long-term care facilities. The health care worker should be aware of these special circumstances for two reasons. First, the phlebotomist can take the necessary precautions to prevent infecting him- or herself or the patient. Second, he or she can mentally prepare to deal with these special patients in a professional and humanistic manner. Because each health care facility has its own infection control program and policy manual, the health care worker should read and be familiar with both.

Infection control surveillance also involves the classification of infections according to prevalence rates. The prevalence rates of commonly identified nosocomial infections are represented in Figure 4–1. Each of the infections cited in this figure can be transmitted in a variety of ways, and each health care worker should realize that he or she can be a potential recipient or transmitter of infectious agents. Table 4–1 lists causative agents for nosocomial infections.

Figure 4–1. Prevalence of nosocomial infections. CSF, cerebrospinal fluid.

(From Castle M, Ajemian E. *Hospital Infection Control*. New York: John Wiley & Sons: 1987, with permission.)

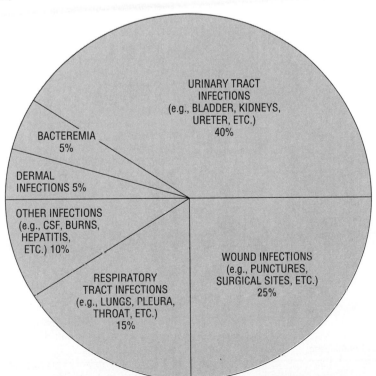

Table 4–1. Pathogenic Agents Causing Nosocomial Infections

BODY AREAS OR HOSPITAL AREAS	COMMONLY IDENTIFIED PATHOGENIC AGENTS
Blood and cerebrospinal fluid	Any microorganisms
Burn unit	All Gram-negative bacilli Gram-positive rods Fungi
Dialysis unit	Hepatitis and other viruses Bacteria Fungi
Ear	*Pseudomonas aeruginosa* *Streptococcus pneumoniae* Gram-negative bacilli
Eye	*Staphylococcus aureus* *Neisseria gonorrhoeae* Gram-negative bacilli *Moraxella lacunata* *Haemophilus influenzae* *S. pneumoniae* *P. aeruginosa*
Gastrointestinal tract	*Salmonella* sp. *Shigella* sp. *Yersinia enterocolitica* Enteropathogenic *Escherichia coli* *Vibrio cholerae* *Campylobacter* sp. Parasitic protozoans *Candida albicans* Some viruses
Genital tract	*N. gonorrhoeae* *Haemophilus vaginalis* *C. albicans* (yeast)
Intensive care or postoperative care unit	Any microorganisms
Nursery unit	*S. aureus* Group B *Streptococcus* *E. coli* *S. pneumoniae* Other Gram-negative bacilli Viruses
Respiratory tract	*Streptococcus pyogenes* *Corynebacterium diphtheriae* *Bordatella pertussis* *Staphylococcus epidermidis* *S. aureus* *S. pneumoniae* *H. influenzae* Any Gram-negative bacilli Fungi Certain viruses
Skin	*S. aureus* *S. pyogenes* *C. albicans* Smallpox Herpes virus Enterovirus Measles
Urinary tract	Any microorganism in sufficient numbers
Wounds and abscesses	Any microorganisms

Infection control programs also monitor employee health programs. The primary objective is to minimize the risk of infection or hazardous circumstances for employees and patients. Most employees are screened for the following diseases prior to employment: measles, mumps, tuberculosis, hepatitis, diarrheal disease, syphilis, and skin diseases. Immunization for a variety of diseases is often made available initially and throughout employment, free of charge. Often, the hospital stipulates policies for employees with specific infections or employees who have been exposed to certain infections, such as those listed in Table 4–2.

For the employee's protection, many types of warning labels are used. Among these are color-coded isolation signs and radiation hazard signs. Radiation signs may be posted on the hospital doors of patients treated with radioactive isotopes. In general, a short period of contact with these patients is not significant; however, the National Committee for Clinical Laboratory Standards (NCCLS) recommends that pregnant employees avoid contact with these patients.[2]

Table 4–2. Employee Infections or Special Circumstances*

DISEASE	WORK STATUS	DURATION OF WORK OR WORK LIMITATIONS
Conjunctivitis, infectious	Off	Until discharge ceases
Draining abscess, boils, and so forth	Off	Until drainage stops, if employee has patient contact
Chicken pox (varicella)	Off	For 7 days after eruption first appears in normal host, provided lesions are dry and crusted when he or she returns
Diarrhea *Shigella* *Salmonella*	Variable	Individual, depending on extent of symptoms, cultures, and evaluation by Personnel Health Services
Gonorrhea	May Work	
Hepatitis A	Off	Until 7 days after onset of jaundice (must bring note from private physician upon return)
Hepatitis B	Off	Must bring note from private physician upon return
Hepatitis C	May Work	Period of infectivity has not been determined
Herpes simplex	May Work	Evaluation by Personnel Health Services, depending on work area
Herpes zoster (shingles)	No patient contact	If able to work, may do so
Human immunodeficiency virus	May work with restriction	Evaluated by Employee Health Physician
Influenza and upper respiratory infections	Variable	Until acute symptoms resolve
Impetigo	Off	No patient contact until crusts are gone

(continued)

Table 4–2. *(continued)*

DISEASE	WORK STATUS	DURATION OF WORK OR WORK LIMITATIONS
German measles (rubella)	Off	Until rash clears (minimum of 5 days)
Measles	Off	Until rash clears (minimum of 4 days)
Mononucleosis	Off	At discretion of private physician
Positive PPD Conversion	May Work	Evaluation by chest x-ray and follow-up by Personnel Health Services
Pregnancy (first or second trimester)	May Work	Avoid contact with patients having viral or rickettsial infections, tuberculosis, or those being treated with radioactive material
Pregnancy (third trimester)	May Work	Avoid contact with patients in any type of isolation
Active TB	Off	Until under treatment and smears are negative for 2 weeks
Scabies	Off until treated	
Strep throat (Group A)	Off	May work 24 hours after being placed on appropriate antibiotic therapy and symptom free
Weeping dermatitis	No patient contact	No patient contact until acute symptoms resolve

Abbreviations: PPD, purified protein derivative; TB, tuberculosis.

*Sample guideline for employees with infection; their work status and when they can return to work.

(References: Castle M, Ajemian E. *Hospital Infection Control.* New York: John Wiley & Sons; 1987, and Bennett J, Brachman P. *Hospital Infections.* 3rd ed. Boston: Little, Brown & Co.; 1992)

■ CHAIN OF INFECTION

Nosocomial infections result when the **chain of infection** is complete. The three components that make up the chain are the **source, mode of transmission,** and **susceptible host.**[3]

SOURCE

In a normal environment, relatively few things are sterile; therefore, potential sources of infection cover a wide range. Inanimate objects, as well as people, are colonized with various microorganisms, many of which help carry out normal body functions. Some of these microorganisms, however, are more pathogenic than others. For example, relatively few *Shigella* organisms need to be ingested before a diarrheal infection occurs. With *Salmonella,* however, large numbers of the organisms must be ingested before symptoms appear. Conversely, numerous anaerobic and aerobic bacteria must be present in the gastrointestinal (GI) tract for normal metabolism to occur.

Regarding the sources of nosocomial infections, infection control practitioners must consider the amount of contamination, viability of the infectious agent, virulence of the agent, length of time from contamination to contact, and the manner in which the agent is transmitted from the source. Sources of nosocomial infection are numerous in the health care environment (Table 4–3). For instance, human hands provide a warm, moist environment for microorganisms. Therefore, a physician, phlebotomist, or nurse can transmit organisms from themselves or an infected patient to another potential host. Uniforms or other clothing that comes in contact with infectious agents and is then worn around other patients is another potential source of infection. Likewise, medical instruments that come into contact with open wounds, mucous membranes, or organs can transmit microorganisms. For example, an instrument, such as a fiber-optic bronchoscope, may be used repeatedly only if thoroughly decontaminated after each use. Otherwise, it may be implicated in transmitting bacterial pneumonia. Although many other pieces of invasive equipment are also potential transmitters unless adequately sterilized, some pieces of equipment that can become contaminated with bacteria are less likely to cause infection. As an example, tourniquets come in contact with intact skin but are less likely to be sources of infection. They should, however, also be decontaminated after each use.

MODE OF TRANSMISSION

The second link in the chain of infection involves transmission from the source to the next host. **Pathogenic agents** may be transmitted by five modes: (1) direct contact, (2) air, (3) medical instruments, (4) other objects, and (5) other vectors. Direct contact involves close or intimate contact with an infected person. For example, some patients acquire staphylococcal infections, chickenpox, hepatitis, or diarrhea after touching other infected individuals. During contact, the infective microorganism rubs off one person onto another. Hand washing is the best means of preventing infections transmitted by this route.

Microscopic airborne droplets may carry infectious agents, such as the causative agent of tuberculosis and Legionnaire's disease. Droplets may become airborne in the following instances: when an individual coughs or sneezes, when linens are shaken, when dust is stirred by sweeping, or when ventilation is inadequate. Preventive measures include wearing a mask, isolating specific patients, and ensuring good ventilation.

As mentioned previously, invasive medical instruments may expose a susceptible patient to pathogenic agents. To prevent instrument-induced infections, health care personnel should change or decontaminate instruments, such as tourniquets and catheters, after each use. Needles should be used only once, then disposed of in appropriate containers.

Other inanimate objects, such as toys in the pediatric areas, common toilets and sinks, linens, and water fountains are all potential modes of transmission. Objects that can harbor

Table 4–3.   Considerations for Sources of Nosocomial Infections

Health care personnel (e.g., lack of hand washing between patients)
Visitors
Medical instruments (e.g., contaminated needles, intravenous [IV] catheters, Foley catheters,
    bronchoscopes, respiratory therapy equipment)
Medical reagents (e.g., IV fluid)
Other patients (e.g., those having severe wound drainage)

infectious agents and transmit infection are called **fomites.** Fomites that are found in health care settings are listed in Table 4–4. Preventing transmission by fomites can be accomplished by following isolation techniques, using **sterile technique** for injections or venipuncture, wearing gloves during equipment handling, and restricting the use of common toys or facilities.

Many insects (mosquitoes, ticks, fleas, mites) and rodents act as vectors in transmitting infectious diseases, such as plague, rabies, and malaria. Patients may be exposed to these vectors in unsanitary conditions in a home setting or in areas where the diseases are prevalent.

SUSCEPTIBLE HOST

The third link in the chain of infection is the susceptible host. Factors that affect a host's susceptibility are age, drug use, the degree and nature of the illness, and the status of the immune system. The patient's progress in the hospital significantly affects his or her chances of acquiring an infection. Underlying diseases, such as diabetes, acquired immune deficiency syndrome (AIDS), and cancer, as well as therapeutic measures (chemotherapy, radiation therapy, antibiotics), all change the status of the body and make it a potential host for infection.

BREAKING THE CHAIN

Infection control programs aim at breaking the infection chain at one or more links, as shown in Figure 4–2. Hand-washing procedures for sterile technique, proper waste disposal, appropriate laundry services, and housekeeping are ways of controlling the sources. Isolation techniques, control of insects and rodents, and use of disposable equipment and supplies help interrupt the modes of transmission. Host susceptibility is controlled by speeding the patient's recovery. Immunizations, transfusions, proper nutrition, medication, and adequate exercise all help the patient to regain health.

Table 4–4.   Fomites Found in Health Care Facilities

Computer keyboards
Door knobs
Telephones
Countertops
Scrub suits
Phlebotomy trays
Eyeglasses
Pens and pencils
Water-faucet handles
Laboratory coats
Manuals and books
Phlebotomy supplies and equipment
IV equipment

Figure 4–2. The chain of nosocomial infection can be interrupted by infection control procedures.

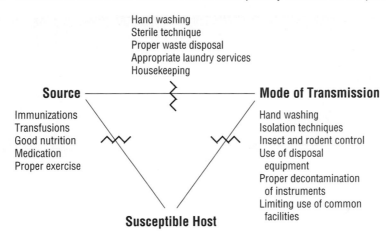

Hand washing
Sterile technique
Proper waste disposal
Appropriate laundry services
Housekeeping

Source ———————— **Mode of Transmission**

Immunizations
Transfusions
Good nutrition
Medication
Proper exercise

Hand washing
Isolation techniques
Insect and rodent control
Use of disposal
  equipment
Proper decontamination
  of instruments
Limiting use of common
  facilities

Susceptible Host

■ ISOLATION PROCEDURES

Isolation procedures, methods of removing diseased individuals from society, date to antiquity. Although the supplies for and methods of isolation have been updated, the fear of being contaminated and the stigma associated with a patient in isolation are still present. The psychological effects of being a patient in isolation are profound. Therefore, the health care provider should make an effort to reduce the patient's anxiety by communicating in a calm, professional, and reassuring manner.

NEW CDC ISOLATION GUIDELINE

In the past, isolation procedures were established in varying degrees. They ranged from sterile rooms or wards to isolation procedures for one disease only. Isolation techniques were formally divided into two types by the CDC: category-specific precautions and disease-specific precautions.[3] The new federal guideline on hospital isolation precautions may clarify the instances in which specific infection control actions should be taken.[4,5] The change should avoid the inconsistent use of universal precautions and **body substance isolation (BSI)** practices (both described later in this chapter) among health care facilities.

Under the new guideline: (1) **standard precautions** are combined with isolation practices for moist and potentially infectious body substances (BSI practices) into a single set of safeguards, which are to be used for the care of all patients; (2) the old categories of isolation and disease-specific precautions have been collapsed into three sets of precautions based on the route of transmission: airborne, droplet, and contact; and (3) specific syndromes in both adult and pediatric patients that are highly suggestive of infection are listed.

Hospitals have the option to continue with alternative isolation procedures; therefore, they may continue with previously used procedures. The most common types of procedures in use have been the category-specific isolation precautions, shown in Figure 4–3 and discussed later in this chapter and in Box 4–1.

Figure 4–3.   Isolation signs and warning signs.

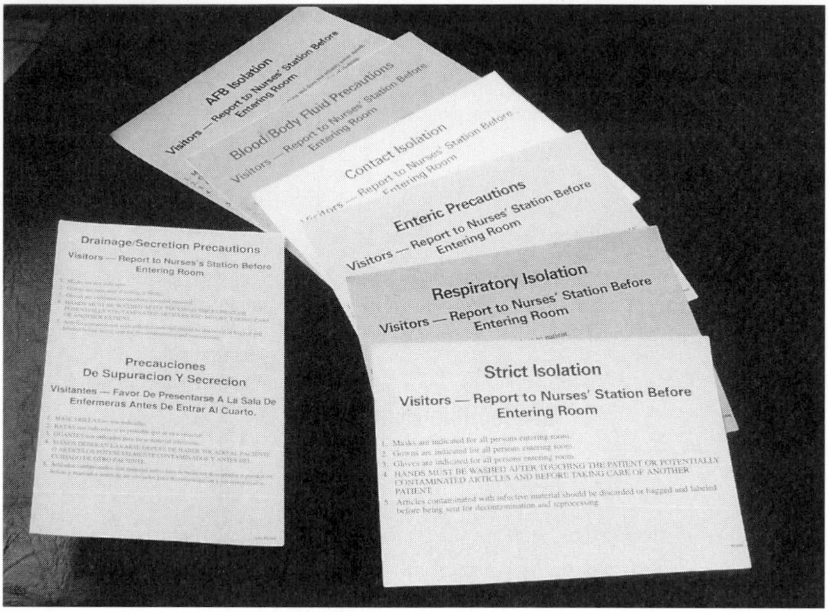

STANDARD PRECAUTIONS

Standard precautions are a combination of the universal precautions and the BSI practices. These precautions apply to blood, *all* body fluids, nonintact skin, and mucous membranes. Standard precautions are designed to reduce the risk of transmission of microorganisms from both recognized and unrecognized sources of infection in health care facilities. All the steps of the universal precautions apply to the standard precautions for health care workers involved in blood collection.

CATEGORY-SPECIFIC ISOLATION PRECAUTIONS

Strict or Complete Isolation

Strict (complete) isolation has been required for patients with contagious diseases—that is, diseases that may be transmitted by direct contact and by air. Examples include anthrax, rabies, smallpox, measles, chicken pox, plague, diphtheria, and streptococcal and staphylococcal pneumonia. The patients are housed in private rooms with closed doors, and all articles in the room should be handled as if they are contaminated. Patients are usually restricted to their rooms. If they must be moved, they should be covered appropriately. Personnel entering these rooms must wear gowns, masks, and gloves. Hand washing is critically important. All items taken into the room must be left there in the appropriate location (Box 4–1).

BOX 4–1.   ISOLATION TECHNIQUE FOR PHLEBOTOMISTS

Principle:

Health care personnel must practice isolation techniques when collecting specimens from infectious patients. Doing so helps prevent transmission of the disease to the health care provider and to other patients and other health care providers.

Procedure:

1. Check the sign posted on the door of an isolation room. It will tell you the type of isolation and to what extent the isolation procedures must be followed. The types of isolation are as follows:
   a. *Complete (strict):* anthrax, rabies, smallpox, measles, chickenpox
   b. *Respiratory:* whooping cough, meningococcal meningitis, mumps, rubella
   c. *Protective (reverse):* immunosuppressed or burn patient
   d. *Drainage/secretion:* postoperative, skin infections
   e. *Enteric: Salmonella, shigella,* typhoid fever, hepatitis A
   f. *Contact:* group A strep, pneumonia, rubella
   g. *Tuberculosis (or AFB):* tuberculosis

2. Check with the nursing station to find out the patient's diagnosis. Female personnel who are pregnant or think they might be should avoid all patients isolated for viral or rickettsial infections. Pregnant women in their last trimester should not go into *any* isolation rooms.

3. Except for protective isolation, any equipment taken into the room must be left there. Make sure that a needle–tube assembly, a tourniquet and a pen are in the room before entering. Protective isolation rooms should have the needle–tube assembly and a tourniquet already in the room. Isolation rooms will have either an anteroom in which isolation equipment is kept or a cart outside the door for the same purpose.

4. Put on a sterile gown, touching only the inside. Make sure that your back is completely covered, and tie the belt. Pull the sleeves all the way down.

5. Place a mask over your nose and mouth. Tie both ties comfortably around your head. For AFB isolation, an air-purifying particulate respirator must be worn.

6. Put on disposable gloves, trying not to touch the palms with your hands. When entering a protective isolation room, wash your hands thoroughly before you put on *sterile* disposable gloves. Pull the gloves up over the sleeves of the gown.

7. Invert the isolation bag halfway inside out and leave it near the door outside the room. Take only the equipment that you will need into the room. Leave the requisition slip on the cart outside the room.

8. Check the patient's armband and collect your specimen. Label the specimen with the information on the patient's armband, leaving the pen in the room.

9. Dispose of the needle in the sharps biohazardous box in the room. Throw the cotton swab and any gauze flats into the biohazardous container in the room.

10. Before placing the tubes in the isolation bag, wipe the outside of the tubes with a paper towel moistened with cold water to remove any blood that may be on the outside of the tubes. Touching only the inside of the biohazardous bag, place the tubes inside the bag, standing in the doorway of the room. Touch only the inside of the bag; avoid touching other items or areas outside the room with gloved hands.

11. Wash your gloved hands in the patient's room. Dry your hands and turn off the faucet with a paper towel.

12. Remove your gown by breaking the paper tie and touching only the inside. Fold it with the contaminated side on the inside and discard it.

(continued)

BOX 4–1. *(continued)*

13. Remove the first glove.
14. Remove your other glove by sliding the index finger of the opposite hand between the glove and your hand. Discard the gloves.
15. Wash your hands again, using a paper towel to turn off the faucet.
16. Leave the unit: Place a clean paper towel over the door knob and open the door. Hold the door open with one foot and discard the paper towel in the wastebasket beside the door. Place the tubes of blood in the isolation container for return to the laboratory.
17. Check the labeled tubes against the requisition slip to be sure that the patient from whom blood was collected was the patient for whom the tests were ordered.
18. Wash your hands at the nursing station before going to the next patient's room.

Quality Control:

The only means of quality control is strict adherence to the procedure.

(From Hermann Hospital Clinical Laboratories, Houston, TX, with permission.)

Respiratory Isolation

Respiratory isolation has been required for patients with infections that may be transmitted over short distances through the air (droplet transmission). Examples include whooping cough, meningococcal meningitis, mumps, and measles. Patients are housed in private rooms with closed doors. Anyone entering the room must wear a mask, as should the patient if he or she is moved. All contaminated supplies should be disposed of in the patient's room.

Enteric Isolation

Enteric isolation has been required for patients with infections that are transmitted by ingestion of the pathogen. Examples include diarrheal diseases—such as *Salmonella, Shigella, Escherichia coli, Clostridium difficile, Yersinia, Staphylococcus, Campylobacter, Vibrio,* and amebic dysentery—and other parasitic infections. Ideally, patients should be housed in private rooms. Their bathroom facilities should *not* be used by hospital personnel, other patients, or visitors. People entering these rooms should wear gowns and gloves. All contaminated materials should be disposed of in the patient's room, including the tourniquet.

Drainage/Secretion Isolation

Drainage/secretion isolation has been required after surgery or if a patient is admitted with a skin infection. Postoperative wounds, catheters, and intravenous (IV) devices may become infected, and microorganisms can be transmitted to other patients by direct or indirect contact. Patients are generally restricted to their rooms, and all entering people should wear gowns and gloves. When these patients are moved, procedures to prevent transmission should be implemented (e.g., covering the infected site).

Contact Isolation

Contact isolation was designed to prevent the spread of highly transmissible infections that do not warrant strict isolation but are conveyed primarily by direct contact. This type of isolation is necessary for pediatric patients having acute respiratory infections (e.g., influenza, pneumonia), patients with major skin infections that are draining severely, and patients with antibiotic-resistant microorganisms. Masks are required for health care workers who must go near the patient. Gowns are indicated if soiling is likely, and gloves are always indicated for performing the phlebotomy. Hands must be washed before and after the use of gloves. The gown, mask, and gloves must be discarded or bagged and labeled before they are sent for decontamination and reprocessing.

Tuberculosis Isolation

Tuberculosis isolation has been indicated for patients with infectious tuberculosis. This type of isolation is sometimes referred to as *AFB* (acid-fast bacilli) to protect the patient's confidentiality. Because multiple cases of drug-resistant tuberculosis have been reported, guidelines were developed for health care workers who come in contact with these patients. The guidelines emphasize the importance of and necessity for wearing an air-purifying, particulate respirator when the health care worker must share air space with the patient having infectious tuberculosis.[6]

DISEASE-SPECIFIC ISOLATION PRECAUTIONS

Another type of isolation precautions has been designed to prevent the transmission of most of the common infectious diseases in the United States. This type of isolation protocol has been used less often than the category-specific precautions because **disease-specific isolation** precautions include specific procedures for dealing with more than 150 diseases. These diseases are listed in the older version of the CDC isolation guideline.[7]

BSI PRACTICES

Body substance isolation (BSI) is a newer, alternative isolation system. This type of isolation focuses on the isolation of potentially infectious moist body substances (blood, urine, saliva, feces, sputum, wound drainage, and other body fluids).[8] This isolation technique is based on the presumption that all body substances may carry infectious agents and thus, precautions should be used whenever health care personnel are working with any of these substances.

The BSI technique focuses on isolation of moist body substances through the use of barrier precautions, primarily gloves, and diagnosis of patients who have some of the diseases that are transmitted by air. A stop-sign alert (Fig. 4–4) must be placed on the door of any room inhabited by a patient with one of these diseases. Before entering a room with a stop-sign alert, the health care worker must consult the floor nurse who will determine whether he or she should wear a mask to collect the blood specimens.

Body substance isolation includes the following:[8]

1. Gloves must be worn for contact with blood, body fluids, secretions, mucous membranes, nonintact skin, and all moist substances from the body. Gloves *must* be changed between patients. Hand washing must also occur after and before each patient's blood collection. If running water is not available (e.g., home health care setting), the health care provider should use the decontaminating rinses or foams available through various vendors for hand washing.
2. A fluid-resistant gown, mask, and goggles should be worn when secretions, blood, or body fluids are likely to spill or splash onto the clothing of the health care worker.

Figure 4–4.   Stop-sign alert for body substance isolation.

**REPORT TO FLOOR NURSE
BEFORE ENTERING**

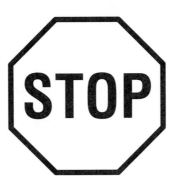

**FAVOR DE ANUNCIARSE A LA ENFERMERA DE PISO
ANTES DE ENTRAR AL CUARTO**

3. Soiled articles must be placed in a biohazardous container or bag. If the container or bag is contaminated on the outside, it should be placed in a double bag, as discussed subsequently in this chapter.
4. Needles should never be recapped. They, and other sharp items (e.g., lancets), should be placed in rigid, puncture-resistant, biohazardous containers that display the required labels. Before going to off-site settings (e.g., home health care visits), the health care worker must remember to take a biohazardous container along for sharps disposal.
5. Private rooms and additional precautions are necessary for patients with certain diseases (e.g., pulmonary tuberculosis, contagious diseases requiring strict isolation, cancer patients requiring reverse isolation).
6. Health care workers must be immunized against infectious agents transmitted by airborne or droplet routes (e.g., measles, mumps, rubella) before entering the rooms of patients with these infections.

■ UNIVERSAL STANDARD PRECAUTIONS FOR HEPATITIS AND HIV

Patients who are infected with blood-borne pathogens, such as hepatitis or HIV, cannot always be readily detected. Therefore, the CDC states that "under universal precautions, all patients should be assumed to be infectious for HIV and other blood-borne pathogens."[9] These universal precautions eliminate the need for a separate isolation category of "blood and body-fluid precautions." Universal and standard precautions have been combined as universal standard precautions to include BSI practices. The following six points summarize the necessary precautions for preventing the transmission of blood-borne pathogens.[9,10]

Clinical Alert

1. All health care workers should routinely use appropriate barrier precautions to prevent skin and mucous membrane exposure when contact with blood or other body fluids of any patient is anticipated. Barriers (e.g., gloves, facial masks, respirators, gowns, shields) are also referred to as *personal protective equipment (PPE)*. Gloves should be worn (a) for touching blood and body fluids, mucous membranes, or nonintact skin of all patients; (b) for handling items or surfaces soiled with blood or body fluids; and (c) for performing venipunctures and other vascular access procedures. Gloves should be changed after contact with each patient. Masks and protective eyewear or face shields should be worn to prevent exposure of mucous membranes of the mouth, nose, and eyes during procedures that are likely to generate droplets of blood or other body fluids. Fluid-resistant gowns or aprons should be worn during procedures that are likely to generate splashes of blood or other body fluids. As explained in the section of this chapter entitled "Tuberculosis Isolation," a personal respirator should be used if the risk of aerosolized *Mycobacterium tuberculosis* is present.

2. Hands and other skin surfaces should be washed immediately and thoroughly if contaminated with blood or other body fluids. Hands should be washed immediately after gloves are removed.

3. All health care workers should take precautions to prevent injuries caused by needles, scalpels, and other sharp instruments or devices (a) during procedures, (b) when cleaning used instruments, (c) during disposal of used needles, and (d) when handling sharp instruments after procedures. To prevent needlestick injuries, health care workers should not recap needles, purposely bend or break them by hand, remove them from disposable syringes, or otherwise manipulate them by hand. After they are used, disposable syringes and needles, scalpel blades, and other sharp items should be placed in puncture-resistant containers for transport to the reprocessing area.

4. Although saliva has not been implicated in HIV transmission, to minimize the need for emergency mouth-to-mouth resuscitation, health care workers should ensure that mouthpieces, resuscitation bags, or other ventilation devices are available for use in areas in which the need for resuscitation is predictable.

5. Health care workers who have exudation lesions or weeping dermatitis should refrain from all direct patient care and from handling patient care equipment until the condition resolves.

6. Pregnant health care workers are not known to be at greater risk of contracting HIV infection than health care workers who are not pregnant; however, if a health care worker develops HIV infection during pregnancy, the infant is at risk of infection resulting from perinatal transmission. Because of this risk, pregnant health care workers should be especially familiar with and strictly adhere to precautions to minimize the risk of HIV transmission.

■ OSHA STANDARDS FOR OCCUPATIONAL EXPOSURE TO BLOOD-BORNE PATHOGENS

Occupational Safety and Health Administration (OSHA), an agency of the US Department of Labor, requires employers to provide measures that will protect workers exposed to biological hazards. On December 6, 1991, OSHA standards for occupational exposure to blood-borne pathogens, based mainly on the use of the hepatitis B vaccine and the previously described CDC recommendations regarding universal precautions, were published.[10]

BLOOD-BORNE EXPOSURE PROCEDURES

OSHA requires managers at health care facilities to provide a confidential medical evaluation, treatment, and follow-up for any employee who has had a blood-borne exposure incident (e.g., needle stick).

Immediately after an exposure incident, the employee must (1) decontaminate the needle-stick site with an appropriate antiseptic (e.g., iodine) for 30 seconds or (2) flush the exposed mucous membrane site (e.g., eyes) with water for 10 minutes. Then, he or she should report the incident to his or her supervisor, who will direct the employee to the appropriate clinic for medical evaluation, treatment, and counseling.

The medical evaluation involves the following five steps[9]:

1. The exposed health care worker's blood is tested for HIV in an accredited laboratory.
2. The source individual is identified and tested for HIV and HBV, if the person gives permission. For possible exposure to hepatitis C, it is recommended to test the source for anti-HCV.[11]
3. If the source individual tests positive for HIV, the exposed health care worker is given counseling and evaluated for HIV infection immediately, 6 weeks, 12 weeks, and 6 months later. Also, azidothymidine (AZT) therapy is provided to the exposed employee as soon as possible, preferably within 1 hour of exposure.

The health care worker exposed to HCV should have baseline and 6-month follow-up testing for anti-HCV and ALT (alanine aminotransferase) activity.[11]

4. If the source individual does not consent to testing and is in a high-risk category, the exposed health care worker is given immune globulin or an HBV vaccination; however, no prophylaxis is available for HCV exposure.[11]
5. The exposed health care worker is counseled to be alert for acute viral symptoms within 12 weeks of exposure.

This entire medical evaluation must be completely confidential.

■ ISOLATION FOR HOSPITAL OUTBREAKS

Occasionally, outbreaks of particular infections occur in one or more hospital areas. For example, infection control surveillance may reveal that the nursery unit is having an excessive

Clinical Alert

OSHA standards require the employer to provide the following:

1. An implementation and compliance program requiring all employers and employees to observe universal standard precautions.
2. PPE devices to minimize the risk of infection from blood-borne pathogens (e.g., fluid-resistant gowns, goggles, respirators).
3. Engineering practice controls that isolate or remove the blood-borne pathogen hazard from the health care facility (e.g., sharps disposal containers, self-sheathing needles).
4. Work practice controls that change the manner in which a blood collection task is performed to reduce the likelihood of exposure (e.g., prohibiting needle recapping; prohibiting eating, drinking, or smoking in the clinical laboratory).
5. Appropriate cleaning methods in blood and other body fluid collection areas to prevent exposure to infectious agents (e.g., use of 10 percent solution of household bleach as a disinfectant for the area).
6. The hepatitis B virus (HBV) vaccine available at no cost to employees. The HBV vaccine protects against HBV, as well as delta hepatitis. The hepatitis virus is the most frequently occurring laboratory-associated infectious agent. It attacks the liver and is a life-threatening blood-borne pathogen.
7. Postexposure follow-up for employees exposed to HBV, HIV, or other blood-borne pathogens. The follow-up must involve an immediate confidential medical evaluation of the employee with continued evaluation and counseling at periodic intervals. The employee's medical record must include the employee's name, social security number, and HBV vaccination dates. Health care workers are concerned about HIV and hepatitis C virus (HCV) because they are blood-borne pathogens that lead to a poor prognosis if workers are exposed by needle stick or another method. Although the incidence of HIV and/or hepatitis C viral infections occurring as a result of on-the-job exposure is relatively low, caution must be used because no vaccine is available for protection.
8. Training and educational information on blood-borne pathogens (e.g., HIV, HCV, and HBV) available for employees at no cost and accessible during the employees' working hours. These training sessions must occur at the beginning of task assignments involving occupational exposure to blood-borne pathogens. Each employee must have annual training on this topic, and each employer must maintain an accessible copy of OSHA's blood-borne pathogen standards with statementsthat relate these standards to the specific health care facility's environment.
9. Labels and signs that warn of biological hazards and contaminated waste. These labels and signs must be affixed to appropriate refrigerators, freezers, waste containers, and storage cabinets containing infectious materials. The labels must be fluorescent orange or orange-red, bearing the word *biohazard* in English and other predominant languages spoken in the region (e.g., *peligro biologico* in Spanish). In addition, the biohazard symbol shown in Chapter 5. Figure 5–5 should be on the label. Alternatively, red or orange bags may be substituted for labels.

number of cases of staphylococcal infection. To control the outbreak, the infection control staff may dictate the need for special precautions, isolation procedures, or employee screening for staphylococcal carriers. Any health care worker entering or exiting these areas should be made aware of the special circumstances.

■ PROTECTIVE, OR REVERSE, ISOLATION

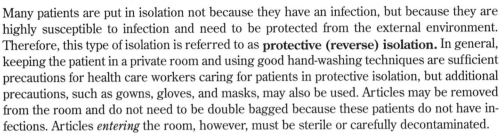

Many patients are put in isolation not because they have an infection, but because they are highly susceptible to infection and need to be protected from the external environment. Therefore, this type of isolation is referred to as **protective (reverse) isolation.** In general, keeping the patient in a private room and using good hand-washing techniques are sufficient precautions for health care workers caring for patients in protective isolation, but additional precautions, such as gowns, gloves, and masks, may also be used. Articles may be removed from the room and do not need to be double bagged because these patients do not have infections. Articles *entering* the room, however, must be sterile or carefully decontaminated.

A few hospitals in the United States have large protective isolation facilities for patients with combined immunodeficiencies who must live in an environment that is completely sterile. All food and articles are sterilized before they are taken into the patient's room. Some patients must live their entire lives in such a protected environment.

■ INFECTION CONTROL IN HOSPITAL UNITS

Other areas where patients are at a high risk of infection are the nursery, the burn unit, the postoperative care unit, the intensive care unit (ICU), and the dialysis unit. The clinical laboratory plays an important role in infection control in these hospital units and is also subject to specific infection control procedures.

INFECTION CONTROL IN A NURSERY UNIT

Newborns are easy targets for infections of all sorts because their immune systems are not fully developed at birth. Neonates may pick up pathogens from their mothers, other babies, or hospital personnel. The best way to minimize infection is to use gloves and an antiseptic for hand washing. Special clothing may be worn by nursery personnel, changed daily, and limited to the unit. Bibs should be used and discarded after contact with only one baby. Often, a baby is assigned a single nurse to limit the possible sources of infection transmission. Babies whose mothers have genital herpes must be isolated from other infants. Mothers with genital herpes must also be isolated. All individuals having contact with either the mothers or the children must be gowned and gloved, and double-bagging procedures must be used for disposal of contaminated articles in the patient's room.

INFECTION CONTROL IN A BURN UNIT

Patients with burns are also highly susceptible to infection. In some institutions, infection rates for burn patients are lower because of the availability of a completely isolated environment for each patient. Each bed is surrounded by a plastic curtain with sleeves. Hospital personnel use these sleeves when having contact with the patient. All supplies and equipment are kept outside the curtain.[1]

In hospitals lacking these facilities, burn patients are housed in private rooms. Gowning, gloving, **double bagging** (as described later in this chapter), and strict hand-washing procedures should be used. All articles in the room, as well as the room itself, should be disinfected or sterilized frequently.

INFECTION CONTROL IN AN ICU OR A POSTOPERATIVE CARE UNIT

Patients in ICUs are more critically ill and, by nature, more susceptible to infections. In most hospitals, ICUs are open areas, with numerous patients in one large room so as to be more easily monitored. Patients with known infections should be isolated according to the types of infections they have, and strict hand-washing and gloving policies are necessary in all ICUs.

Postoperative patients are susceptible to infection because surgical wounds or drains enable bacteria to gain easy access to deeper tissues. Again, each patient who becomes infected should be isolated and dealt with according to the type of infection acquired.

INFECTION CONTROL IN A DIALYSIS UNIT

Patients needing dialysis are most often immunosuppressed, which makes them a high-risk group for contracting infection, especially hepatitis. Protective gowns and gloves may be worn in the unit, and strict hand-washing and gloving techniques should be adhered to.

INFECTION CONTROL IN THE CLINICAL LABORATORY

The clinical laboratory contributes to infection control programs in the following manner:

1. Maintaining laboratory records for surveillance purposes.
2. Reporting on infectious agents, drug-resistant microorganisms, and outbreaks.
3. Evaluating the effectiveness of sterilization or decontamination procedures.

Laboratory personnel must be cautious because they often handle specimens with infectious agents. Laboratorians have a higher incidence of hepatitis antigen, tuberculosis, tularemia, and Rocky Mountain spotted fever than that of other hospital personnel.[1] Many of these infections are acquired by aerosol spray, needle sticks, spills, mouth pipetting, and eating, drinking, or smoking in the laboratory. Such danger can easily be prevented or minimized by adhering to policies that prohibit mouth pipetting, eating, drinking, and smoking in the laboratory. Other useful procedures include hand washing; gloving; wearing protective clothing such as laboratory coats, scrubs, and face shields, if appropriate; surface decontamination; and careful disposal of needles.

The health care worker should remember that the quality of laboratory test results is only as good as the specimen collected. If the specimen is contaminated or improperly collected, laboratory test results reflect this fact and may be misleading. If sloppy techniques are used, the potential for mistakes and infection is greater. Table 4–5 details the infection control policies that health care workers must follow during blood collection.

Table 4–5. Infection Control Responsibilities Required in Blood Collection

Frequent handwashing

Use of personal protection equipment

Use of appropriate waste disposal practices

Maintaining good personal hygiene, including wearing clean clothes, keeping hair clean and tied
    back if necessary, keeping fingernails clean, and washing hands frequently

Maintaining good health by eating balanced meals in the designated areas, getting enough sleep,
    and getting enough exercise

Reporting personal illnesses to supervisors

Becoming familiar with and observing *all* isolation policies

Learning about the job-related aspects of infection control, and sharing this information with others

Cautioning all personnel working with known hazardous material (this can be done with proper
    warning labels)

Reporting violations of the policies

Reporting potential candidates for infection control (e.g., patients who are jaundiced)

■ SPECIFIC ISOLATION TECHNIQUES

In most hospitals, all supplies required for isolation procedures are located in an area or on
a cart just outside the patient's room. After washing their hands, health care personnel may
put on the appropriate PPE just prior to entering the room.

HAND WASHING

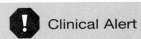 Clinical Alert

Hand washing is the most important procedure in the prevention of disease transmission
in hospitals. It should be the first and last step of any isolation procedure (Fig. 4–5 A–C).
Scrubbing for surgery requires a different procedure than washing hands for general patient care. For general purposes, hand washing usually removes potential pathogens but
does not necessarily sterilize the hands. Good technique involves soap, warm running
water, and friction.[1] Soap removes oils that may hold bacteria to the skin. Many varieties
of soap are available for general purposes; however, health care personnel who purchase
supplies should choose soaps that are mild, easy to use, and form a good lather. Rubbing
action with soap and water should continue for at least 10 seconds to create a lather over
the entire hand surface. Warm running water washes away loosened debris and lathers
the soap. Friction from rubbing the hands together loosens and removes dead skin, oil,
and microorganisms. The health care worker should thoroughly rub both sides of each
hand and between each finger. Hands should be rinsed in a downward position. After
rinsing, the faucet should be turned off by grasping the handles with paper towels to prevent reinoculation of microorganisms onto the hands. Drying of hands should be with
single-use or disposable towels or with an air dryer.

Figure 4–5. Specific isolation techniques: hand washing, gowning, masking, gloving, and double bagging. **A.** Hand-washing techniques should involve soap lather, friction between hands, and thorough washing between fingers. **B.** Washing should include the wrist areas. (*continued*)

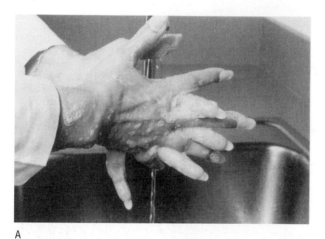

A

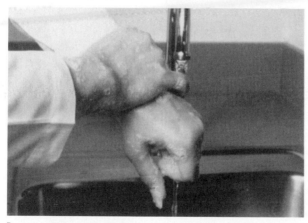

B

Figure 4–5. **C.** Lather should be rinsed. Rinsing should continue until all soap is removed. If the water must be turned off by hand, a clean paper towel should be used to grab the faucet. **D.** Gowns should be large enough to cover all clothing. Sleeves should be pulled down and the back covered. **E.** The mask should be tied in two places and should fit comfortably. **F.** Gloves should be pulled over the ends of gown sleeves. (*continued*)

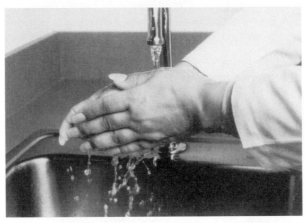

C

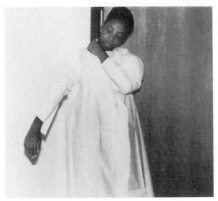

D

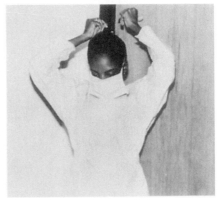

E

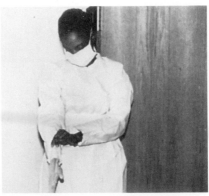

F

Figure 4–5.   **G–I.** After specimen collection, the gown should be removed from inside out. **J.** Double bagging involves two individuals, one inside the room and one outside.

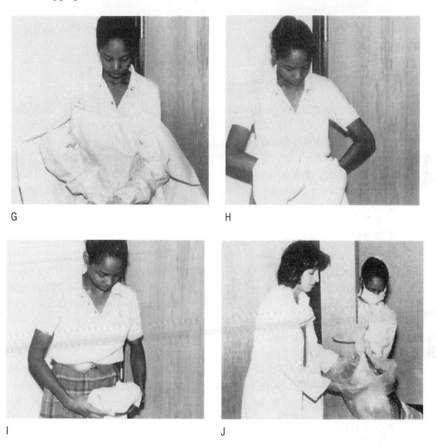

G   H

I   J

GOWNING

After hand washing, a sterile gown should be put on by touching only its inside surface. It should have long sleeves and be large and long enough to cover all clothing (Fig. 4–5D). Gowns are generally made of cloth or paper. The health care worker's back must be completely covered, the belt tied, and the sleeves pulled all the way to the wrists.

MASKING

After gowning, a mask (if necessary) may be put over the nose and mouth (Fig. 4–5E). Masks protect the health care worker from small-particle droplets that may carry infectious agents. Often, a small metal band on the mask can be shaped to fit the nose. Two ties are usually made, the first around the upper portion of the head and the second around the upper portion of the neck. Most masks become ineffective after prolonged use (20 minutes) or if they become wet.[1]

GLOVING

Chemically clean disposable gloves may be used for most isolation procedures. The exception is protective isolation procedures, for which *sterile* disposable gloves should be used. Gloves should be pulled over the ends of gown sleeves (Fig. 4–5F). Rings and other pieces of jewelry should not be worn because they may puncture a glove during patient contact. Gloves are also discussed in Chapter 8.

ENTERING AND EXITING THE ROOM

Isolation bags for transporting specimens are often available. The bag may be turned halfway inside out and left near the door outside the room, or someone may be available to hold the bag outside the door. Only the needed supplies should be taken into the room. Phlebotomy requisitions may be left outside the room on the isolation cart. If drawing a blood specimen, the health care provider may use a tourniquet in the room or leave the one brought in. The specimen should be labeled at the bedside and the pen left in the room. Used needles, swabs, and so forth should be put in appropriate containers inside the room. Any blood on the outside of the specimen container should be removed with a paper towel. While standing in the doorway, and touching only the inside of the isolation bag, the health care worker should place the specimen inside the bag. Gloved hands should be washed in the room. The faucet may be turned off with a paper towel.

The mask, if used, can be removed by carefully untying the lower tie first, then the upper one. Only the ends of the ties should be held. The mask should then be properly disposed of inside the room. In some cases, a special container for masks is placed just outside the room to prevent exposure of hospital personnel to airborne diseases while inside.

The gown is removed by first breaking the paper tie or untying the sash. It should be removed and folded with the contaminated side turned inside and with care taken not to touch the uniform (Fig. 4–5 G–I). One glove may be removed, and the second one can be slipped off by sliding the index finger of the ungloved hand between the glove and the hand.

Just before leaving the room, however, hands must be washed again and a paper towel used to turn off the faucet. A clean paper towel should be used to open the door. The door should be held open with one foot and the used paper towels discarded in the wastebasket directly inside the patient's room.

Once outside the room, the requisition forms may be checked again, placed carefully in the isolation bag, and sealed. Care must be taken to avoid touching the inside of the bag holding the specimen. Personnel should wash their hands again before proceeding with other duties.

DISPOSING OF CONTAMINATED ITEMS

Trash, linens, and other articles in an isolation room may be removed by using one sturdy biohazardous bag or the double-bagging procedure. Double bagging involves putting contaminated material in one bag and sealing it inside the room. A different person should stand outside the doorway with another opened, clean, impermeable bag (Fig. 4–5J). The person standing outside the room should have the ends of the bag folded over the hands to shield them from possible contamination. The sealed bag from the room may then be placed inside the clean bag. The person outside the room can then fold over the edges, expel the air, and seal the outer bag. The bag must be labeled with biohazard warnings.

PREVENTION OF LABORATORY-ACQUIRED INFECTIONS

As mentioned previously, health care workers must be extremely cautious with biohazardous specimens. Policies and procedures for handling such specimens should be defined in the laboratory policy manual and should be reviewed periodically by health care workers who collect and transport specimens. Infections from these specimens may be spread during collection and handling by means of several routes. The actual occurrence of an infection from a biohazardous specimen depends on the virulence of the infecting agent and the host's susceptibility.

CLINICAL ALERT

The following are possible routes of infection from collected specimens and therefore should be considered when health care personnel must collect or process specimens for laboratory assays:

1. *Skin contact.* Virulent organisms can enter through skin abrasions and cuts or through the conjunctiva of the eye. Thus, scratches from needles and broken glass must be avoided. If the health care worker has a cut or an abrasion, he or she should always wear a laboratory coat, gloves, and protective adhesive tape over the cut or abrasion to prevent possible inoculation from infectious specimens. He or she must also avoid rubbing the eyes.
2. *Ingestion.* Failure to wash contaminated hands and subsequent handling of cigarettes, gum, food, or drinks can result in an infection from a biohazardous specimen. Each employee must comply with the safety rules of the laboratory to prevent transmission of infections.
3. *Airborne.* As discussed in other sections, aerosol spray created from patient's specimens by careless splashing or centrifugation must be prevented. Dangerous, infectious aerosol spray can be caused from popping tops off blood specimen vacuum tubes and centrifugating the blood specimens. To protect against blood exposure during this hazardous step, manufacturers recently developed different types of items that minimize airborne transmissions (see Chapter 7, Blood Collection Equipment). Prior to centrifugation, vacuum tubes should be inspected for cracks, and tubes with wet rims should be wiped dry. The centrifuge brake should not be applied to save time because braking can cause infectious aerosol formation. Centrifuged infectious specimens must not be poured because of the potential hazards from aerosol formation. Instead, the contents should be transferred by using a disposable pipette with a rubber bulb or its equivalent and gently transferring the contents down the wall of the aliquot tube or tubes.

STERILE TECHNIQUE FOR HEALTH CARE WORKERS

All health care personnel should realize that bacteria and other microorganisms can be found everywhere. For example, human skin is covered with bacteria. Because of this fact, all health care personnel should be responsible for cleanliness and maintaining sterility when handling instruments, catheters, IV supplies, or other devices that come into contact with patients.

The health care worker is responsible for using sterile supplies for skin punctures and venipunctures and antiseptics for patient preparation. Alcohol pads are often used to cleanse skin sites for venipuncture. Although rubbing with alcohol pads destroys most of the bacteria, it does not destroy all microorganisms. A special decontamination procedure is required to obtain a sterile site. Venipuncture for blood cultures requires this type of preparation, as discussed thoroughly in Chapter 12.

New needles and most blood collection tubes are sterilized by the manufacturers. Once the covering of a needle or a lancet is removed, the needle or lancet should not touch anything until it punctures the skin. If it accidentally touches *anything* prior to contact with the skin site, it must be discarded appropriately and replaced with a new one. If a needle is used for an unsuccessful venipuncture, it too *must* be discarded and replaced with a new one before another puncture is attempted.

Sterile technique and isolation procedures may require sterile gloves. If this is the case, the health care worker must make sure that the package of gloves indicates that they are sterile. Some manufacturers produce gloves that are *chemically clean* but not necessarily *sterile.* Most sterile gloves are available in various hand sizes. If the gloves do not fit properly, they may interfere with the procedure. Use of gloves is also discussed in Chapter 7 on Blood Collection Equipment.

DISINFECTANTS AND ANTISEPTICS

Disinfectants are chemical compounds used to remove or kill pathogenic microorganisms.[12] Chemical disinfectants are regulated by the Environmental Protection Agency (EPA). **Antiseptics** are chemicals used to inhibit the growth and development of microorganisms but do not necessarily kill them. Antiseptics may be used on human skin, whereas disinfectants are generally used on surfaces and instruments because they are too corrosive for direct use on skin. An intermediate-level disinfectant with a product label claiming that the disinfectant is HIVcidal or tuberculocidal, or a disinfectant having a chlorine bleach dilution of 1:10, should be used to disinfect tourniquets and items contaminated with blood or other body fluids. A more diluted solution of chlorine bleach (1:32) is used for routine cleaning of surfaces.[13] Table 4–6 lists some of the more common hospital disinfectants and antiseptics used.

Table 4–6.   Common Antiseptics and Disinfectants for the Health Care Setting

COMPOUND	USES AND RESTRICTIONS
Alcohols	
Ethyl (70%)	Antiseptic for skin
Isopropyl (70%)	Antiseptic for skin
Chlorine	
Chloramine	Disinfectant for wounds
Hypochlorite solutions	Disinfectant
Ethylene oxide	Disinfectant (toxic)
Formaldehyde	Disinfectant (noxious fumes)
Glutaraldehyde	Disinfectant (toxic)
Hydrogen peroxide	Antiseptic for skin
Iodine	
Tincture	Antiseptic for skin (can be irritating)
Iodophors	Antiseptic for skin (less stable)
Phenolic compounds	
1–2% phenols	Disinfectant
Chlorophenol	Disinfectant (toxic)
Hexachlorophene	Antiseptic for skin (used in surgery)
Chlorhexidine	Antiseptic for skin
Hexylresorcinol	Antiseptic for skin
Quaternary ammonium compounds	Antiseptic for skin (ingredient in many soaps)

SELF STUDY

KEY TERMS

Antiseptics

Body Substance Isolation (BSI)

Chain of Infection

Contact Isolation

Disease-Specific Isolation

Disinfectants

Double Bagging

Drainage/Secretion Isolation

Enteric Isolation

Fomites

Infection Control Programs

Isolation Procedures

Mode of Transmission

Nosocomial Infections

Occupational Safety and Health
  Administration (OSHA)

Pathogenic Agents

Protective (Reverse) Isolation

Respiratory Isolation

Source

Standard Precautions

Sterile Technique

Strict (Complete) Isolation

Surveillance

Susceptible Host

Tuberculosis Isolation

STUDY QUESTIONS

The following may have *one* or *more* answers:

1. Which of the following types of nosocomial infections are most prevalent?

   a. dermal infections

   b. wound infections

   c. respiratory tract infections

   d. urinary tract infections

2. Name the links in the chain of infection.

   a. poor isolation technique

   b. susceptible host

   c. source

   d. mode of transmission

3. What is/are the primary function(s) of isolation procedures?

   a. keep the hospital clean

   b. prevent transmission of
      communicable diseases
      environments

   c. protect the general public
      from disease

   d. provide protective

4. Nurses, physicians, and other health care workers are responsible for knowing the procedures of which type(s) of isolation?

   a. strict

   b. drainage/secretion

   c. enteric

   d. protective, or reverse

   e. respiratory

   f. universal precautions

5. Which of the following precautions prevents infectious aerosol spray?

   a. popping the cap on a vacuum collection tube rather than twisting it
   b. inspecting vacuum tubes for cracks prior to centrifugation
   c. applying the centrifuge brake to save time during centrifugation of specimens
   d. pouring the specimens into the required aliquot tubes

6. Protective isolation is generally used for

   a. an adult patient with active tuberculosis
   b. a pediatric patient who has an immunodeficiency
   c. an adult patient with meningitis
   d. a pediatric patient who has whooping cough

7. Which of the following laboratory-acquired infections is most prevalent?

   a. HIV infection
   b. Rocky Mountain spotted fever
   c. HBV infection
   d. tuberculosis

8. Enteric isolation may be required for patients with infections such as

   a. tuberculosis
   b. whooping cough
   c. *Salmonella*
   d. Rocky Mountain spotted fever

9. According to the OSHA standards for occupational exposure to blood-borne pathogens, which of the following is a PPE?

   a. 10 percent household bleach
   b. fluid-resistant gown
   c. goggles
   d. respirator

10. In Spanish, *peligro biologico* refers to the English term

    a. hepatitis
    b. biohazardous
    c. blood-borne pathogen
    d. *Salmonella*

References

1. Bennett JV, Brachman PS (eds). *Hospital Infections.* 3rd ed. Boston: Little, Brown & Co; 1992.

2. National Committee for Clinical Laboratory Standards (NCCLS). *Protection of Laboratory Workers from Infectious Disease Transmitted by Blood, Body Fluids and Tissues.* NCCLS Document M29-T2, Villanova, PA: NCCLS; 1991.

3. Castle M, Ajemian E. *Hospital Infection Control.* New York: John Wiley & Sons; 1987.

4. Department of Health and Human Services, Centers for Disease Control and Prevention (CDC): Guideline for isolation precautions in hospitals: Part I. Evolution of isolation practices and Part II. Recommendations for isolation precautions in hospitals. *Federal Register.* Fall 1995.

5. Department of Health and Human Services, Centers for Disease Control and Prevention (CDC). Part II: Recommendations for isolation precautions in hospitals (Update 2/18/97). http://www.cdc.gov/ncidod/hip/isolat/isopart2.htm

6. US Department of Health and Human Services, Centers for Disease Control and Prevention. Guidelines for preventing the transmission of *Mycobacterium tuberculosis* in health-care facilities, 1994. *Federal Register.* 1994; 59(208): 54248–54250; and Final Rule 42 CFR, Part 84, effective June 2, 1995.

7. Garner JS, Simmons BP: CDC guideline for isolation precautions in hospitals. *Am J Infect Control.* 1984; 12:103.

8. Lynch P, Cummings J, Roberts P, et al. Implementing and evaluating a system of generic infection precautions: body substance isolation. *Am J Infect Control.* 1990; 18:1–12.

9. Guidelines for prevention of transmission of human immunodeficiency virus and hepatitis B virus to health-care and public-safety workers. *MMWR.* 1989; 38(S-6).

10. US Department of Labor and Occupational Safety and Health Administration (OSHA). Occupational exposure to bloodborne pathogens; final rule (29 CFR 1910.1030). *Federal Register.* 1991; Dec 6:64004–64182.

11. Department of Health and Human Services, Centers for Disease Control and Prevention. *Hepatitis Surveillance: Issues and Answers.* Report No. 56, April, 1996.

12. Luebbert P. Choosing the appropriate disinfectant. *Lab Med.* 1992; 23(2):126.

13. Texas Department of Health (TDH). *Infection Control Manual for Public Health Clinics.* 2nd ed. Austin, TX: TDH; 1993.

5

FIVE

■

Safety and First Aid

CHAPTER OUTLINE

CHAPTER OBJECTIVES

Upon completion of Chapter 5, the learner is responsible for the following:

1. Discuss safety awareness for health care workers.

2. Explain the measures that should be taken for fire, electrical, radiation, mechanical, and chemical safety in a health care facility.

3. Describe the essential elements of a disaster emergency plan for a health care facility.

4. Explain the safety policies and procedures that must be followed in all phases of specimen collection and transportation.

5. Describe the safe use of equipment in health care facilities.

The goal of safety in the health care institution is to recognize and eliminate hazards and provide information on safety education so that employees can work in a healthy environment. Safe working conditions must be ensured by the employer and have been mandated by law under the **Occupational Safety and Health Administration (OSHA)** standards (1910.1030).[1] Knowledge of OSHA requirements and cooperation between the employer and employee concerning these requirements are necessary in all health care facilities, including home health care agencies (Box 5–1). The health care worker involved in blood collection needs to become aware of safety policies and procedures in his or her health care facility and to receive proper instruction on safety requirements.

■ SAFETY IN SPECIMEN HANDLING

Patients' specimens should be handled with caution to prevent the possibility of acquiring an infection, such as hepatitis or one associated with acquired immunodeficiency syndrome (AIDS). Health care workers who are routinely exposed to blood and body fluids must take the simple precaution of wearing gloves to protect themselves from infection. Further discussion of precautionary measures for specimen handling can be found in Chapter 4, Infection Control.

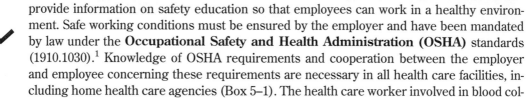

BOX 5–1.   SAFETY PRECAUTIONS FOR THE HEALTH CARE WORKER

1. Gloves must be worn during *all* phases of blood collection procedures (at inpatient and outpatient facilities). Health care workers should make every effort to avoid contact with blood, body fluids, nonintact skin, and mucous membranes.

2. Gloves must be changed between patient collections, and hands must be washed after gloves are removed.

3. A laboratory coat, a smock, or a gown must be worn during blood collection procedures and left at the laboratory or clinic when the health care worker leaves the work area. The laboratory coat must be cleaned at the health care facility.

4. A personal respirator should be used if exposure to aerosolized *Mycobacterium tuberculosis* is possible.

5. Facial protection must be provided at the health care facility and used by the health care worker if any possibility of body fluid or blood splashing exists.

6. Needles should *never* be recapped by hand.

7. All sharps, including needles and lancets, must be disposed of *carefully* in a rigid needle container.

8. Blood collection items must be disposed of according to the proper procedure for biohazardous waste disposal.

9. Blood collection devices and surfaces must be decontaminated after use.

■ EXPOSURE CONTROL

Clinical Alert

Any incident of exposure to potentially harmful or infectious substances should be reported immediately to Employee or Personnel Health, or in the absence of a separate department, to a supervisor. Each health care worker should know who to contact, where to go, and what to do if inadvertently exposed. This information is included in an **Exposure Control Plan** that is designed for that health care facility. This is important because the health care worker should seek advice about medical treatment orprophylaxis, depending on the type of exposure. Also, reporting work-related exposures is required for worker's compensation documentation. If exposures are not reported, it is difficult to prove retrospectively that an exposure was work-related.

■ PERSONAL HYGIENE

Clinical Alert

While on the job, nothing should be inserted into one's mouth (e.g., food, pencils). Hands should be washed frequently during the day; before and after contact with patients or patients' specimens; before and after eating, drinking, or smoking; and before and after using restrooms. Cosmetics should not be applied while on the job. The health care worker should avoid biting his or her fingernails and rubbing the eyes. Eating, drinking, or smoking within the specimen control section and other laboratory sections must be avoided (Fig. 5–1). No food should be placed in any laboratory refrigerator unless the refrigerator is designated "FOR FOOD ONLY." A laboratory coat should be worn completely buttoned while collecting specimens and removed prior to coffee breaks or lunch. Loose clothing, such as scarves, which might become entangled in the centrifuge, should never be worn. Long hair must be tied so that it cannot come in contact with specimens or become entangled in the centrifuge. Open-toed shoes are usually prohibited in most clinical laboratories because of potential chemical and glassware hazards.

Figure 5–1.   Required safety precautions during specimen collection and specimen processing.

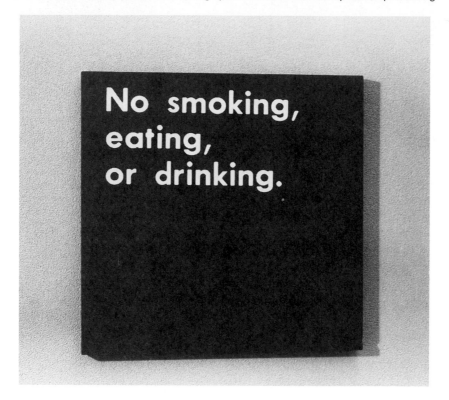

■ LABORATORY SAFETY

Laboratory safety includes a variety of policies. All health care workers, however, should remember a few key safety rules at all times.

- Patients' specimens should be covered at all times during transportation and centrifugation.
- Centrifugation of specimens should be performed within a biohazard safety hood.
- All wastes from specimen collections must be disposed of in the correct containers.
- Needles should not be recapped, bent, or broken.

Specific **Environmental Protection Agency (EPA)** and OSHA regulations, as well as state and local laws, regulate the disposal of wastes. Blood and body fluids should be disposed of through an approved biohazardous waste disposal company. Urine specimens are usually flushed down the drain with water or flushed down the toilet. These biological liquid wastes should be disposed of gently so that they do not splash onto other objects, and hand washing should not occur in sinks used for disposal of these wastes.

Needles *must not* be recapped before disposal (Fig. 5–2). Sharps, such as needles and lancets, should be disposed of in a special container that is spillproof, tamperproof, puncture resistant, and closable and that can be autoclaved. The sharps container must be labeled in red or orange, must be maintained upright, and must display the biohazard symbol (Fig. 5–3).

Figure 5–2.   Universal precautions in patient care.

(Courtesy of United Ad Label [UAL] Co., Inc., Brea, CA.)

**Includes blood
and
any body fluids**

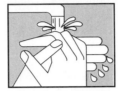

1. Wash hands BEFORE and AFTER patient care.

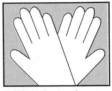

2. Wear gloves when likely to touch body substances, mucous membranes or non-intact skin.

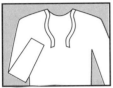

3. Wear gown when clothing is likely to become soiled.

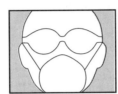

4. Wear mask and protective eyewear or a face shield when likely to be splashed with body fluids.

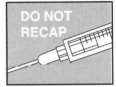

5. Place intact needle/syringe units and sharps in designated disposal container. DO NOT BREAK OR BEND NEEDLES.

Figure 5–3.   Biohazard symbol.

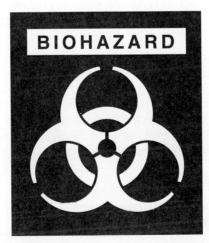

In addition, the specimen collection area should be decontaminated with a 1:10 bleach solution. Because a diluted bleach solution becomes unstable when exposed to oxygen, it must be prepared daily. Alternatively, a diluted bleach solution that is stable is available commercially. If blood or other body fluids are spilled, encapsulating powder, which is available from manufacturers of safety products (e.g., United Ad Label Direct, Brea, CA), should be used to gel the liquid for safe cleanup.

Colored biohazard labels must be affixed to all containers of regulated waste, refrigerators and freezers containing blood or other body fluids, and other containers used to store, transport, or ship these materials.

If an accident occurs, such as a needle stick, the injured health care worker should immediately cleanse the area with isopropyl alcohol and apply a Band-Aid. Then, he or she should follow the exposure control plan for that facility (i.e., notify the immediate supervisor, fill out the necessary incident and medical forms, and undergo the appropriate laboratory tests). In addition, the health care worker should be counseled and evaluated for HIV infection at periodic intervals (see "OSHA Standards for Occupational Exposure to Blood-Borne Pathogens" in Chapter 4).

■ FIRE SAFETY

Fire safety is the responsibility of all employees in the health care institution. Health care workers should be familiar with not only the use and location of the fire extinguishers, but also the procedures to follow during a fire. They should also be knowledgeable of the exact locations of fire extinguishers and fire blankets. The blankets should be available to smother burning clothes or to use as a fire shield if fire is blocking the exit. Health care institutions usually conduct periodic safety education programs in which the health care worker can participate and become skillful in and knowledgeable about the use of fire safety equipment.

CLASSIFICATION OF FIRES

The components of fire are fuel, oxygen, and heat, plus the necessary chain reaction. Four general classifications of fires have been adopted by the National Fire Protection Association (NFPA).[2] These classifications are as follows:

1. *Class A fires* occur with ordinary combustible material, such as wood, rubbish, paper, cloth, and many plastics.
2. *Class B fires* occur in a vapor–air mixture over flammable solvents, such as gasoline, oil, paint, lacquers, grease, and flammable gases.
3. *Class C fires* occur in or near electrical equipment.
4. *Class D fires* occur with combustible metals, such as magnesium, sodium, and lithium. These fires are infrequently encountered in health care institutions.

FIRE EXTINGUISHERS

Fire extinguishers are classified to correspond with each class of fire.

1. *Class A extinguishers* contain soda and acid or water and are used to cool the ordinary fire.
2. *Class B extinguishers* contain foam, dry chemicals, or carbon dioxide (CO_2) and are used to combat fires occurring in vapor–air mixtures over solvents.

3. *Class C extinguishers* contain dry chemicals, Halon (Allied Corporation, Morristown, NJ), or CO_2 (nonconducting extinguishing agents) and are used to combat electrical fires.
4. *Multipurpose (ABC) extinguishers* are frequently installed in health care institutions because they reduce the confusion associated with operating and maintaining different types of extinguishers.

As shown in Figure 5–4, the health care worker should learn how to use the various kinds of fire extinguishers in the workplace. Use of the wrong type of extinguisher may not only fail to put out the fire, but it can actually spread it.

In the event of a fire, the health care worker should *do* the following:

- Immediately pull the lever in the alarm box nearest the area he or she is in.
- Call the assigned fire number, which should be posted on or near each telephone.
- If the fire is small, attempt to extinguish it, using the proper extinguisher.
- If evacuation becomes necessary, use only the stairwells for exiting.

Figure 5–4. Proper use of fire extinguishers.

(Courtesy of Risk Analysis and Loss Control—Institutional Affairs, The University of Texas–Houston Health Science Center, Houston, TX.)

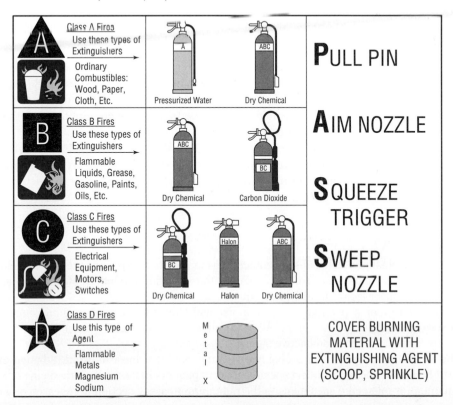

- Close all doors and windows before leaving the area.
- If clothing is on fire, drop to the ground and roll, preferably in a fire blanket.
- If caught in a fire, crawl to the exit. Because smoke rises, breathing is easier at floor level. Breathing through a wet towel is also helpful.

The health care worker should *not do* the following:

- Block entrances.
- Reenter the building.
- Panic.
- Run.

■ ELECTRICAL SAFETY

A major hazard in any area of a health care institution is the possibility of electrical current passing through a person. For example, in the clinical laboratory or physician office laboratory, the health care worker sometimes operates electrical equipment, such as a centrifuge. He or she should be aware of the location of the circuit breaker boxes in order to assure a fast response in the event of an electrical fire or an electrical shock.

The health care worker should not use electrical equipment if power cords are frayed or if control switches and thermostats are not in good working order. The centrifuge or other electrical equipment must be unplugged before maintenance is performed. Any electrical instrument that has had liquid spilled on or in it or has had liquid come in contact with the wiring should be immediately unplugged and dried prior to further use.

If an electrical accident occurs involving electrical shock to an employee or a patient, the health care worker should be aware of the following two points:

1. The electrical power source must be shut off. If this is impossible, carefully remove the electrical contact from the victim using something, such as asbestos gloves, that does not conduct electricity, or place your hand in a glass beaker and push the power supply away from the victim. The rescuer should not attempt to touch the victim without heeding these precautions.
2. Medical assistance should be called and **cardiopulmonary resuscitation (CPR)** started immediately. The victim should not be moved prior to the arrival of medical assistance. A fire blanket or other warm clothing should be put over the victim to keep him or her warm until medical help arrives.

■ RADIATION SAFETY

The three cardinal principles of self-protection from radiation exposure are time, shielding, and distance. Radiation exposure is cumulative; thus, limiting the length of exposure at any one time is a major factor in minimizing the hazard.

Areas where radioactive materials are in use and stored must have warning signs (Fig. 5–5) posted on the entrance doors. All radioactive specimens and reagents must also be properly labeled with the radioactive sign.

The health care worker will probably encounter potential hazards from radiation exposure only if he or she must collect specimens from patients in the nuclear medicine or x-ray department or must take specimens to the radioimmunoassay section in research or a clin-

Figure 5–5. Sign for possible radiation hazard.

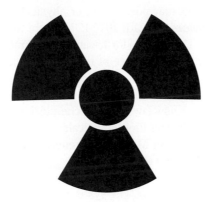

ical chemistry laboratory. Thus, the health care worker should be cautious when entering an area posted with the radiation sign and should be knowledgeable of the institution's procedures pertaining to radiation safety. Health care workers who are pregnant should be aware of the potential hazard of radiation to the fetus.

■ MECHANICAL SAFETY

The centrifuge is a frequently used instrument for blood specimen preparation and testing. Thus, a health care provider who collects and prepares blood specimens for testing should learn how to maintain this instrument and become familiar with its parts. For example, he or she should know if the carriers are in the correct position prior to use. If the carriers are not in the correct position, they can swing out of the holding disks into the side of the centrifuge. Also, the wrong head, the wrong cups, or imbalanced tubes can lead to the same dangerous problem. If this particular type of accident occurs, tubes containing patients' specimens or spinning chemicals may be propelled onto the side of the centrifuge, and broken, and a dangerous, hazardous problem created. Thus, it is of utmost importance to abide by the preventive maintenance schedule and procedures for the centrifuge.

■ CHEMICAL SAFETY

Because a health care worker must sometimes pour preservatives, such as hydrochloric acid (HCl), into containers for 24-hour urine collections and transport these specimens to the patients' floor, he or she should be knowledgeable of chemical safety. Labeling may be the single most important step in the proper handling of chemicals. Laboratorians should be able to ascertain from appropriate labels not only the contents of the container, but also the nature and extent of hazards posed by the chemicals. Carefully read the label before using any reagents.

CHEMICAL IDENTIFICATION

Various chemicals are needed in health care facilities, especially in the clinical laboratory department. Because chemicals may pose health or physical hazards, OSHA amended the *Hazard Communication Standard* (29 CFR 1910.1200, Right to Know/HCS Standard) to include health care facilities.[3,4] Thus, labels for hazardous chemicals must (1) provide a warning (e.g., corrosive), (2) explain the nature of the hazard (e.g., flammable, combustible), (3) state special precautions to eliminate risks, and (4) explain first-aid treatment in the event of a chemical leak, a chemical spill, or other exposure to the chemical. In addition to mandating labels, the Right to Know law requires chemical manufacturers to supply **material safety data sheets (MSDSs)** for their chemicals. The MSDS is required for any chemical with a hazard warning label. An MSDS lists general information, precautionary measures, and emergency information.

The NFPA developed a labeling system for hazardous chemicals that is frequently used in health care facilities (Fig. 5–6). The system uses a diamond-shaped symbol, four colored quadrants, and a hazard rating scale of 0 to 4. The health hazard is shown in the blue quadrant, the flammability hazard is shown in the red quadrant, the instability hazard is indicated in the yellow quadrant, and the specific hazard is shown in the white quadrant.

Figure 5–6.   National Fire Protection Association (NFPA) 0 to 4 hazard rating system.

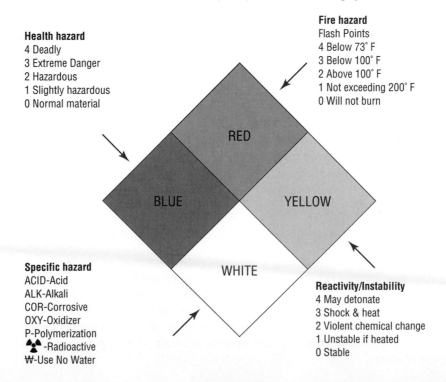

Health hazard
4 Deadly
3 Extreme Danger
2 Hazardous
1 Slightly hazardous
0 Normal material

Fire hazard
Flash Points
4 Below 73° F
3 Below 100° F
2 Above 100° F
1 Not exceeding 200° F
0 Will not burn

Specific hazard
ACID-Acid
ALK-Alkali
COR-Corrosive
OXY-Oxidizer
P-Polymerization
☢-Radioactive
W̵-Use No Water

Reactivity/Instability
4 May detonate
3 Shock & heat
2 Violent chemical change
1 Unstable if heated
0 Stable

PROTECTIVE MEASURES

The proper clothing must be worn when a health care worker is working with chemicals. A buttoned laboratory coat, safety glasses, and gloves provide protection and prevent skin contact. When transporting acids or alkalis, an *acid carrier* should be used. It is a specially designed container for carrying large quantities of hazardous solutions.

The entrance of any room in which hazardous chemicals are in use or in storage must be posted with a caution sign specifying the types of chemicals present. No chemicals should be stored above eye level because of the danger of breakage or spillage involved in reaching. All explosives should be stored in an explosionproof or a fireproof room that is separate from the flammables.

SAFETY SHOWERS AND THE EYEWASH STATION

Safety showers should be nearby for use if an accidental chemical spill occurs. Because permanent damage to the skin can result from chemical burns, the victim of a chemical accident must immediately rinse for at least 15 minutes after removing contaminated clothing.

In case of a chemical spill in the eye, the victim should rinse his or her eyes at the eyewash station for a minimum of 15 minutes. Contact lenses must be removed prior to the rinsing in order to thoroughly cleanse the eyes. The victim should not rub the eyes because doing so may cause further injury. If someone is hurt in a chemical spill, it is preferable to take the victim to the emergency department for treatment after his or her eyes have been rinsed for 15 minutes.

CHEMICAL SPILL CLEANUP

If a chemical spill occurs, the health care worker should obtain a spill cleanup kit from the clinical chemistry section. The kit includes absorbents and neutralizers to clean up acid, alkali, mercury, and other spills. The absorbent and neutralizer used depend on the type of chemical spill and have an indicator system that identifies when the spill has been neutralized and can be considered safe for sweepup and disposal. The health care worker should become familiar with the procedures for cleaning up chemical spills in his or her place of employment.

DISPOSAL OF CHEMICALS

Chemical wastes that are water soluble, such as acids and alkalis, can be flushed down the sink with cold water; however, acids and alkalis should be poured into a large amount of water before flushing them down the sink. The acid *must* be added to the water and not vice versa to prevent a violent chemical reaction.

■ EQUIPMENT AND SAFETY IN PATIENTS' ROOMS

Each member of the health care team is responsible for the safety of the patient. All health care professionals are responsible for patient safety from the time the patient enters the health care setting until his or her departure. As a matter of general patient safety, the phlebotomist should do the following when in the patient's room:

1. Make certain that all specimen collection supplies, needles, and equipment are either properly disposed of or returned to the specimen collection tray after blood collection.
2. Check to see whether the bed rails are up or down. Always place bed rails up before leaving the patient if they were up when you entered the room.
3. Report unusual odors to the nursing station because a pipe may be broken and be leaking gas or liquid.
4. Check for food or liquid spilled on the floor, urine spills, or intravenous (IV) line leakage. Areas on which the patient and health care professionals walk must be dry. They should be free of obstacles and slipping hazards. Thus, in cases of spills, make certain that the area is cleaned and dried for the safety of the patient and hospital personnel.
5. During blood collection, be very cautious not to touch any electrical instrument located adjacent to the patient's bed because if the instrument malfunctions, the health care worker may ground the patient and, as a result, a microshock could pass through the health care worker and into the patient. A serious problem could result from such a shock if the patient has an electrolyte imbalance or is wet with perspiration or other fluid. Furthermore, the needle inserted in the patient's arm could produce ventricular fibrillation and death if the patient has a pacemaker or an unstable heart ailment.
6. Report the following problem immediately to the nursing station: If the patient has an IV line and the site is swollen and red, the IV needle is probably no longer in the vein and the IV solution is infiltrating into the surrounding tissues. Some chemicals in IV solutions are toxic to body tissue, so gangrene could result from such infiltration. Also, if blood is backing up the IV line from the needle insertion to the IV drip container, the IV solution container is empty. Report this problem immediately.
7. If the patient's alarm for the IV drip is sounding, report this problem to the nursing station immediately.
8. If the patient is in unusual pain or is unresponsive, notify the nursing station immediately.

◼ PATIENT SAFETY OUTSIDE THE ROOM

Health care workers should be aware of possible hazards to patients outside the patients' rooms. As a matter of general safety practice, the following guidelines should be followed:

1. Because trays, carts, and ladders may be placed around a hallway corner, the health care worker should be careful not to travel too quickly from one room to another and around corners.
2. Items lying on the floor, such as flower petals, may cause someone to slip and should be reported for cleanup.
3. Avoid running in a health care facility because patients and visitors may become alarmed and begin to run as well. Also, someone may be hurt if the health care worker runs into him or her (e.g., a cardiac patient walking in the hall with an inserted IV stand or another health care worker carrying a specimen collection tray).

■ DISASTER EMERGENCY PLAN

Many health care institutions have developed procedures to be followed in case of a hurricane, flooding, earthquake, bomb threat, and other disasters. The health care worker should become familiar with these procedures because he or she must be prepared to take immediate action whenever conditions warrant such action.

■ EMERGENCY PROCEDURES

The health care worker should become knowledgeable of emergency care procedures because accidents do occur even though precautionary measures are in place. He or she must be able to detach him- or herself from the emergency situation to some degree in order to perform well and deliver the best possible health care. In an emergency situation, the following objectives must be met for the victim: prevent severe bleeding, maintain breathing, prevent shock and further injury, and send for medical assistance.

BLEEDING AID

Severe bleeding from an open wound can be controlled by applying pressure directly over the wound. A clean handkerchief or other clean cloth (compress) should be placed over the wound before applying pressure by the hand. In an emergency in which a clean cloth is not available, the bare hand should be used until a cloth compress can be located. Bleeding of a limb (i.e., an arm or a leg) can be decreased by elevation. The injured portion should be raised above the level of the victim's heart unless the injured portion is broken. Even with elevation, however, pressure should be maintained on the wound until medical assistance arrives. A tourniquet should not be used to control bleeding except for an amputated, mangled, or crushed arm or leg, or for profuse bleeding that cannot be stopped otherwise.

BREATHING AID

When a victim's breathing movements stop or his or her lips, tongue, and fingernails become blue, immediate mouth-to-mouth resuscitation is needed. Any delay in using this technique may cost the victim's life. To perform mouth-to-mouth breathing, include the following:

1. See if the victim is conscious by *gently* shaking the victim and yelling, "ARE YOU OKAY?" If any possibility of a neck injury exists, do not shake the victim! If there is no response to the gentle shaking and yelling, call out for help and start aid immediately.
2. Place the victim on his or her back on a firm, flat surface. Caution must be exercised if the person has a spinal or neck injury. No twisting should occur to the victim's body.
3. Open the airway passage by checking for obstructions: tongue, chewing gum, vomitus, and so on.
4. Place one hand on the victim's forehead and, applying firm, backward pressure with the palm, tilt the head back (Fig. 5–7). Place the fingers of the other hand under the bony part of the victim's lower jaw, near the chin, and lift to bring the chin forward with the teeth almost to occlusion. The jaw should be supported as the head is tilted back. This position is called the *head-tilt/chin-lift*.

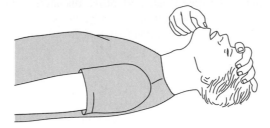

Figure 5–7.   Head-tilt/chin-lift for emergency care.

5. Listen and feel for return of air from the victim's mouth and nose for approximately 3 to 5 seconds. Also, simultaneously, look for the victim's chest to rise and fall.
6. If there is no breathing, maintain the head-tilt/chin-lift and pinch the victim's nose shut with the hand to prevent air from escaping. Open mouth widely, take a deep breath, and seal mouth over the victim's mouth (Fig. 5–8). Blow into victim's mouth. Watch for the victim's chest to rise. (If it does not, the airway is blocked and must be cleared.)
7. Give two full ventilations. If this still does not start an air exchange, reposition the head and try again. After two more ventilations, again look, listen, and feel for breathing. Improper chin and head positioning is the most common cause of difficulty with ventilation.

CIRCULATION AID

To maintain circulation in a victim, a health care provider must know the techniques of basic CPR. Thus, he or she should check with the supervisor about the availability of CPR classes

Figure 5–8.   Breathing aid in emergency situation.

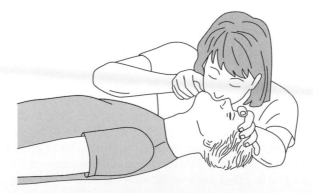

at the health care institution because this emergency technique must be demonstrated so that the employee can learn the proper skills.

SHOCK PREVENTION

Shock usually accompanies severe injury. It may result from bleeding, extensive burns, an insufficient oxygen (O_2) supply, and other traumatic events. Early signs include pale, cold, clammy skin; weakness; a rapid pulse; an increased, shallow breathing rate; and, frequently, nausea and vomiting. The main objectives in treating a shock victim are to improve circulation, to provide sufficient O_2, and to maintain normal body temperature.

The following six actions are recommended if first aid is given to a shock victim:

1. Correct the cause of shock if possible (e.g., control bleeding).
2. Keep the victim lying down.
3. Keep the victim's airway open. If he or she vomits, turn head to the side so that the neck is arched.
4. In the absence of broken bones, elevate the victim's legs so that the head is lower than the trunk of the body.
5. Keep the victim warm.
6. Call for emergency assistance.

Actions that are *not* recommended include the following:

1. Giving fluids to a victim who has an abdominal injury (the person is likely to require surgery or a general anesthetic).
2. Giving fluids to an unconscious or a semiconscious person.

SELF STUDY

KEY TERMS

Cardiopulmonary Resuscitation
(CPR)

Environmental Protection Agency
(EPA)

Exposure Control Plan

Material Safety Data Sheets
(MSDSs)

Occupational Safety and
Health Administration
(OSHA)

STUDY QUESTIONS

The following may have *one* or *more* answers:

1. If a fire occurs in or near electrical equipment, which of the following fire extinguishers should be used?

    a. class A extinguisher

    b. class B extinguisher

    c. class C extinguisher

    d. ABC extinguisher

2. What are the major principles of self-protection from radiation exposure?

    a. distance

    b. time

    c. combustibility

    d. shielding

3. Which of the following safety rules should be maintained in patients' rooms?

    a. full ashtrays should be emptied into the trash can to prevent a fire hazard

    b. unusual odors in the patient's room should be reported to the nursing station

    c. health care providers should not touch electrical instruments located adjacent to the patient's bed

    d. if the patient has an IV line and the site is swollen and reddish, this problem should be reported to the nursing station

4. The main objectives of treating a shock victim are to

    a. improve circulation

    b. provide sufficient drinking water

    c. provide sufficient oxygen

    d. maintain normal body temperature

5. In an emergency situation, which of the following is/are objective(s) that must be met for the victim?

    a. prevent severe bleeding

    b. maintain breathing

    c. prevent shock

    d. send for medical assistance

6. Which of the following should occur first if a fire breaks out in the health care facility?

   a. run from the floor where the fire is located

   b. call the assigned fire number

   c. use the fastest elevator to escape from the floor where the fire is located

   d. close all windows before leaving the area of the fire

7. The Right to Know law originated with the

   a. CDC   c. OSHA

   b. CAP   d. NFPA

8. The hazardous labeling system developed by the NFPA has the blue quadrant of the diamond to indicate:

   a. flammability hazard   c. instability hazard

   b. health hazard   d. specific hazard

9. If an electrical accident occurs involving electrical shock to an employee or a patient, the *first* thing that the health care worker should do is

   a. move the victim   c. start CPR

   b. shut off electrical power   d. place a blanket over the victim

References

1. US Department of Labor, and Occupational Safety and Health Administration (OSHA): Occupational exposure to bloodborne pathogens; final rule (29 CFR 1910.1030). *Federal Register.* 1991; Dec 6: 64004–64182.

2. National Fire Protection Association (NFPA). *National Fire Codes.* Vol. 1. Quincy, MA: NFPA; 1990.

3. Occupational Safety and Health Administration (OSHA). *Hazard Communication Standard.* 29 CFR 1910.1200. Washington, DC: OSHA; 1986.

4. Occupational Safety and Health Administration (OSHA). *Toxic and Hazardous Substances.* 29 CFR 1910.1001–1047. Washington, DC: OSHA; 1989.

■ ADDITIONAL SOURCES FOR SAFETY INFORMATION

Centers for Disease Control and Prevention (CDC)
Division of Biosafety
1600 Clifton Rd, NE
Atlanta, GA 30333
(404) 639-3883
http://www.cdc.gov

College of American Pathologists (CAP)
325 Waukegan Rd
Northfield, IL 60093-2750
(800) 323-4040 or (847) 832-7000
http://www.cap.org

Department of Transportation (DOT)
Materials, Transportation Bureau, Information Services Division
Washington, DC 20402
(202) 366-4000

Joint Commission on Accreditation of Healthcare Organizations (JCAHO)
One Renaissance
Oakbrook Terrace, IL 60181
(630) 792-5000
http://www.jcaho.org

National Committee for Clinical Laboratory Standards (NCCLS)
940 W. Valley Rd S-1400
Wayne, PA 19087-1898
(610) 525-2435
http://www.NCCLS.org

National Fire Protection Association (NFPA)
One Batterymarch Park
Quincy, MA 02269-9101
(617) 770-3000
http://www.NFPA.org

Occupational Safety and Health Administration (OSHA)
US Department of Labor
200 Constitution Ave, NW
Washington, DC 20210
(202) 523-8148
http://www.cdc.gov/niosh

6

SIX

■

Specimen Documentation and Transportation

CHAPTER OUTLINE

CHAPTER OBJECTIVES

Upon completion of Chapter 6, the learner is responsible for the following:

1. Describe the basic components of a clinical, or medical, record.
2. Identify six ways to enhance the intralaboratory communication network.
3. Describe essential elements of requisition and report forms.
4. Name three methods commonly used to transport specimens.
5. Name areas or departments that usually receive laboratory reports.

■ FUNDAMENTALS OF DOCUMENTATION

All health care organizations have methods of documenting information related to each patient and procedure that include some common elements. One document that can be found in all health care settings is the **clinical (or medical) record** for each patient. It is the definitive legal document that provides a chronological log of the patient's care. Box 6–1 describes the components most likely to be found in a medical record. In addition, numerous other documents provide a record of actions and results of the procedures that occur in the daily processes of providing health care services. Documentation in any health care setting is important for the following seven reasons[1]:

1. *Quality of care.* Documentation is used to describe what has been done and how the patient responds.
2. *Coordination of care.* Documentation is used to plan interventions, evaluate progress, and assist the health care team in making effective decisions.
3. *Accrediting and licensing.* The Joint Commission for Accreditation of Healthcare Organizations (JCAHO) and other such accrediting agencies require specific standards for documentation in each patient's clinical, or medical, record. They usually include some guidelines for containing an assessment, a plan of care, medical orders (e.g., laboratory, radiology, etc.), progress notes, and a discharge summary.
4. *Quality monitoring.* State and JCAHO regulations also mandate that ongoing quality assessment activities take place. For this purpose, the clinical record is used to collect objective, readily measurable indicators that allow these agencies to assess the structure, process, and outcomes of patient care.
5. *Peer review.* Similar to quality monitoring, peer review organizations (PROs) also use documentation in the clinical records to evaluate the quality of care for specific indicators, such as nosocomial infections, medical stability of patients, unnecessary procedures and tests, adequate discharge planning, and the occurrence of avoidable discomfort or death. PROs can impose fines, impose sanctions, or deny reimbursement for care if patient care is inappropriate.
6. *Legal protection.* Documentation in the clinical records can provide proof of the quality of care given. Documentation can serve as evidence in disability, personal injury, malpractice, and mental competency cases. Appropriate documentation is the key to winning or losing a case for individual members or employees of the health care facility.
7. *Research.* In teaching institutions, documentation can provide important data for clinical research on new therapies and procedures.

BOX 6–1.   COMPONENTS OF A CLINICAL RECORD

Each health care facility has its own method for keeping track of information in the clinical record. The amount of data and degree of documentation required vary with the particular setting and the severity of each illness; thus, the clinical record in a physician's office is usually not as elaborate as one in a hospital. The following sections are commonly used in hospital clinical records:

FACE SHEET: Includes patient's name, birth date, social security number, address, and marital status; name of closest relative; list of allergies; admitting diagnosis; assigned diagnosis-related group; and physician's name.

MEDICAL HISTORY AND PHYSICAL FORMS: Completed by the physician and the nurse; contain information about the initial assessment.

ORDER SHEET: Contains the physician's medical orders, including laboratory, radiology, pharmacy, and so forth.

NURSING CARE PLAN: Covers the nurse's plans for the patient.

GRAPHIC SHEETS: Flowcharts showing recordings of the patient's temperature, pulse rate, respiratory rate, blood pressure, weight, blood glucose levels, urinalysis results, and other assessments.

MEDICATION ADMINISTRATION RECORD: Contains information about medication dosage, route of administration, site, date, and time of administration.

PROGRESS NOTES: Cover patient's progress, intervention, and treatment; provided by the physician and the nurse.

DIAGNOSTIC TEST RESULTS: Include results from all tests performed on the patient, such as laboratory test results, radiology results, and so forth.

HEALTH CARE TEAM RECORDS: Include notes from other departments, such as physical therapy, respiratory, and the like.

CONSULTATION SHEETS: Contain evaluations by clinical specialists (e.g., rheumatologists, infectious disease specialists) who have been called in for their treatment recommendations.

DISCHARGE PLAN/SUMMARY: Reviews the patient's stay and plans for care after discharge from a hospital, including dietary, medication, and follow-up appointments.

(From Clinical Skillbuilders: *Better Documentation.* Spring House, PA, Spring House Corporation, 1992, with permission.)

General guidelines for documentation are as follows:

- *Accuracy.* Record only the facts, not opinions or assumptions; and, clinical records should never be changed or falsified to cover a mistake.
- *Completion.* Notes should be made about each event, procedure, or problem that occurs. Writing the documentation as soon as possible with the exact time of a procedure and identifying other sources of information about the process can become vitally important. For example, if a phlebotomist is unable to identify a patient because of a missing armband, the notation should include the time, the date, the name of the nurse who positively identified the patient, and the phlebotomist's name.
- *Objectivity.* Documented comments should not assign blame (e.g., "blood was not collected from Mr. Jones because nurse Daly did not complete the proper requisition.") Likewise, comments about staffing shortages or working overtime should not be recorded because it would be confusing in a courtroom in that it may or may not have a direct influence on the patient's condition.

Every notation in the patient's record should be legibly written in blue or black ink on the appropriate forms and signed. Chapter 17 addresses other legal aspects of documentation.

■ THE LABORATORY COMMUNICATION NETWORK

The major purpose of a clinical laboratory is the acquisition and determination of valid data by analytic procedures performed on patient specimens and the timely communication of those data to the physician. Specimen collection procedures are the first and most critical steps in this process. The number of persons and steps involved varies greatly depending on the size of the institution and the type of laboratory involved. Clinical laboratories may be centralized or may be decentralized, with satellites, or minilaboratories, in various locations. With each additional location or person involved, another potential source of error or delay is introduced into the system.

Sources of error in laboratory testing can be related to preanalytic variables in the following categories:

- *Patient variables.* Fasting versus nonfasting, diurnal variations, refusal to cooperate, patient is unavailable, stress or anxiety, etc.
- *Transportation variables.* Specimen leakage, tube breakage, excessive shaking, etc.
- *Specimen processing variables.* Centrifugation is inadequate, delays in processing, contamination of the specimen, exposure to heat or light, etc.
- *Specimen variables.* Hemolysis, inadequate volume in tube, inadequate mixing of anticoagulant, etc.

The individual who performs the phlebotomy is a vital link in the preanalytic phases of laboratory testing. He or she should be knowledgeable about the procedures to help prevent these sources of errors and he or she should know how to react in case of unusual circumstances. Phlebotomists should anticipate potential variables and assist in writing protocols that minimize errors.[2] Furthermore, there should be a dependable communication link among laboratory staff, physicians, patients, and other members of the health care team.

There are many ways to conceptualize the cycle of performing laboratory tests flowing from the initial test request to the specimen collection to the analytic phase to the final reporting of results. One example is shown in Figure 6–1.

The clinical laboratory must be involved not only in the activities of a central laboratory, but also of the hospital unit, of an ambulatory clinic, or other off-site locations. There is a constant overlap and interaction between internal and external functions of the laboratory. This chapter addresses the importance of this network, both inside and outside the laboratory, as well as the various nonanalytic communication components of laboratory test request specifications, test requisitioning, patient and specimen identification, specimen transport, reporting of results, and distribution of results.

In a relatively small laboratory, as in the case of a physician's office laboratory, the communication processes, both within the laboratory (intralaboratory) and with all others outside the laboratory (extralaboratory), are essentially the same. As the size of the institution increases, however, the requirements for effective and efficient intralaboratory and extralaboratory communication are expanded, and the use of computer technology is enhanced.

■ INTRALABORATORY COMMUNICATION NETWORK

Using well-written procedures in the clinical laboratory improves the communication network by ensuring continuity of methods; avoiding shortcuts; minimizing the chances of errors, specimen recollections, and reruns; preventing expensive substitutions of reagents; and enhancing quality control (QC), teaching, and safety. Overall, such procedures lead to more efficient data collection and reporting.

Figure 6–1.   A patient–physician–laboratory network can be depicted in an analytic phase (A) and a preanalytic phase (PA). (QC, quality control.)

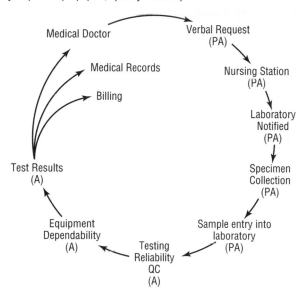

POLICY AND PROCEDURE MANUALS

Clinical laboratories have administrative or personnel policy manuals that can be consulted by all employees. The manual contains policies that are consistent with those of the larger organization (i.e., hospital or clinic). The manual is general in scope and is particularly concerned with, but not limited to, such subjects as management authorizations, organizational charts, responsibilities, personnel practices (e.g., attendance and punctuality policies, dress codes, and rules about coffee breaks), and professional protocol. Health care workers who accept positions in a clinical laboratory section should become acquainted with the laboratory policies.

Written procedures about a specific situation, event, technique, or protocol to be followed should be available to employees who will be performing the procedures or who need to know about safety procedures. One example is depicted in Box 6–2.

Technical Procedures

Technical procedures describe in detail the steps to be followed in the performance of specimen collection and each laboratory test. The College of American Pathologists (CAP) requires technical procedures to be made available on-site, at all times, to technical personnel who perform specimen collection procedures and laboratory assays.[3] The technical procedure format includes the name and title of the procedure, a description of the method, specimen requirements, procedural steps, a discussion of reagents and preparation, **reference ranges,** the clinical significance of the results, quality control instructions, calculations, re-

BOX 6–2.   SAMPLE PROCEDURES FOR DOCUMENTING SPECIFIC PHLEBOTOMY SITUATIONS

Collection Logbook Verification

1. Requests on computer-generated labels that serve as requests for phlebotomy are checked against the logbook prior to the drawing of blood. Any discrepancy should be brought to the attention of the unit secretary or nurse for resolution of orders. Any test deleted from the log by request of a unit will be circled and an explanation of the deletion, along with requester's name, will be written in the log. Any tests added to requests also should be added to the logbook. If any tests are added but not requested on computer labels, a stamped request must be made by the nursing unit personnel.

2. After the appropriate specimens have been collected, each patient's collection that is complete will be initialed by the health care worker collecting the blood and time of draw will be entered in the appropriate box in the logbook. At the bottom of the list of patients, a line is drawn and "EOR," or End of Run, is written to signify that all is complete.

Inability to Draw Specimen

1. A maximum of two laboratory employees will attempt to obtain blood from a patient.

2. Any unsuccessful attempt to obtain blood *must* be documented in the logbook and on the request slip.

Patient Unavailable

1. If you are unable to obtain blood when requested because a patient is unavailable (gone to x-ray or surgery, out of room), hold these slips until you have completed all other patients on that nursing unit. Check the patient's room again before leaving unit.

2. If the patient is still unavailable, notify the primary nurse, if available, or unit clerk. Leave the slip(s) at the desk, circle the orders, and write the following in the logbook:

    Reason patient is unavailable.

    Time and initials of collector.

    Name of nurse notified.

    The patient's blood will then be drawn on the next scheduled run.

Patient Refused

If the patient refuses to have blood drawn, notify his or her primary nurse. Often, the nurse can convince the patient to cooperate. If not, leave slips at the unit desk, with the following information written in the logbook:

    Patient refused.

    Time and initials of collector.

    Name of nurse notified.

Patient Missed

If at any time the person collecting blood is unable to obtain the blood, he or she should check to see whether another collector is available to help. If no other health care worker is available, notify the patient's nurse that the patient was missed and that another person from the laboratory will try on the next run unless the nurse requests that the attempt be made sooner. Leave the slips at the desk, with the following information written in the logbook:

    Unable to collect specimen.

    Time and initials of collector.

    Name of nurse notified.

(continued)

> ## BOX 6–2.   *(continued)*
>
> Upon returning to the laboratory, notify the supervisor. If the second person is unable to obtain the specimen, a nurse is again notified, and the previous information is again documented on the requisition form and in the logbook. At this time, request that a physician draw the blood.
>
> ### Combative Patient
>
> In cases when an adult patient is combative or verbally abusive of laboratory personnel, and nursing staff is unavailable, the health care worker should notify the supervisor. If the health care worker is instructed by the supervisor to refuse to draw blood, the primary nurse should be notified of the refusal and it must be documented in the logbook, noting:
>
> Reason for refusal.
> Name of the nurse notified.
>
> ### Unidentified Test Requested
>
> If a test is requested that cannot be found in the specimen requirement book, the nurse should be asked to consult the doctor to clarify the request. Meanwhile, the health care worker can call the laboratory for a more familiar name for the test and test requirements. If no other name can be found and no clarification is offered, he or she *must* refuse to draw a specimen for the test. The logbook should be marked "no such test," the primary nurse notified, and his or her name recorded in the logbook. The supervisor of the laboratory also should be notified.

porting requirements, approval signatures, dates, and references. Not all these sections apply to phlebotomy procedures, but they would be found when reviewing specific laboratory testing procedures.

Laboratory Administrative Procedures

The following topics are generally covered in an administrative procedure manual:

- Technical procedure format.
- Assignment of test code numbers to laboratory procedures.
- Communication with physicians and other health care professionals.
- Time cards and attendance records.
- Laboratory equipment identification and centralization of specification files.
- Handling of samples for reference laboratory work.
- Acceptable symbols, abbreviations, and units of measure.
- Handling of laboratory charges.
- Purchase and maintenance requisitions.
- Performance evaluation procedure and disciplinary policies.
- Employee folders, color-blindness records, certification records.
- Distribution of laboratory documents.
- Quality assurance procedures.
- Quality control procedures.
- Safety procedures, including fire, chemical, and radiation safety procedures and a disaster plan.
- Loan of laboratory equipment.
- Compensatory time off, annual leave, and overtime policies.
- Employee accidents.

- Laboratory library resources.
- Inventory lists of capital equipment.
- Consent to donate blood and urine specimens.
- In-service records.
- Clinical laboratory samples referred from outside sources.
- Hepatitis testing of laboratory personnel.
- Dress code.

Safety and Infection Control Procedures

Safety procedures should be distributed to all management staff and made known to all personnel. One book of safety procedures should be available in each laboratory section, including the specimen collection areas. As mentioned in Chapter 5, safety manuals should include fire safety, internal and external disaster plan, radiation safety, exposure control plan, and biological hazard, as well as a hazard communication manual indicating procedures for handling hazardous substance and infection control manuals. The infection control manual usually includes procedures for handling specimens, isolation procedures, handling precautions, disposal policies, decontamination procedures, and hand-washing procedures. Since many phlebotomy personnel are decentralized from the clinical laboratory, these policies should be accessible to them at their work stations.

QC Procedures

QC procedures pertain to the conduct of diagnostic laboratory testing. These procedures should be available in each laboratory section, including the specimen collection area, or they can be indicated in each technical procedure. QC records include information about hazards; proper use, storage, and handling; stability; expiration dates; and indications for measuring the precision and accuracy of analytic processes.

Instrument and Maintenance Manual

Other manuals or procedures that might be used in the clinical laboratory are instrument and equipment maintenance manuals. These include records of maintenance adjustments, malfunctions, and service calls regarding instruments.

CONTINUING EDUCATION

In addition to procedure manuals, ongoing in-service education programs help increase communication, safety, and efficiency in patient care. With the increasing complexity of patient care services and responsibilities, it is essential for health care workers to attend in-service education sessions within the institution and elsewhere. Certain types of continuing education, such as training about universal standard precautions, fire safety, and radiation safety, are required periodically.

STAFF MEETINGS

Intralaboratory communication is improved when regularly scheduled staff meetings are held within each laboratory section, such as the specimen collection area. They are useful for discussing problems, new policies and procedures, and for planning. Decisions made in such meetings are usually conferred to all members of the laboratory by written memoranda, minutes of meetings, or telephone contact in some cases. Minutes of these meetings should be reviewed by employees who were absent from the meeting. Employees in remote off-site locations can participate by using conference calls or videoconferencing. This saves the time and travel expense of leaving a work site to come to "headquarters" for meetings.

OTHER MODES OF INTRALABORATORY COMMUNICATION

Bulletin boards, posters, checklists, memoranda, newsletters, and clipboards are noncomputerized suggestions for disseminating current information. One person from each work area should be responsible for periodically checking and changing poster information. Computer software and hardware are also available for networking within the laboratory. **E-mail** (electronic mail), voice mail, electronic bulletin boards, product recall notices, and facsimiles (faxes) are all effective ways of communicating. Sometimes off-site laboratory facilities also have a speed-dialing telephone exchange. All individuals who practice phlebotomy must be familiar with the communications technology in their facilities.

■ EXTRALABORATORY COMMUNICATION NETWORK

PROVISION OF INFORMATION

Communication with other health care workers working outside the laboratory can be enhanced by the use of an information bulletin or a *floor book* of laboratory services, made available at least in every patient unit, both inpatient and outpatient. This information (either computerized or hard copy) contains a directory of the laboratory sections with listings of the key staff members, the location of the laboratory, telephone numbers, operating hours, reference ranges, instructions, and pertinent standard procedures of the laboratory. The methods used for collection of all specimens, as well as the proper identification, storage, preservation, and transportation mechanisms to be used, are clearly specified. In addition, an alphabetical listing of all laboratory determinations, specimen requirements, special instructions, and tables with reference ranges for each measurement are often included. (Refer to Table 6–1). A health care worker involved in specimen collection should be familiar with the floor book in order to answer questions related to the clinical laboratory specimen collections and procedures. In some hospitals, this information can be reproduced as a pocket-sized resource. This is particularly helpful to medical students, residents, fellows, and trainees.

USE OF THE TELEPHONE

The telephone is the most frequently used method of two-way communication in any setting. Health care workers must be aware of the procedures for operating it. These procedures usually include the following:

- Using effective customer service manners.
- Transferring calls.
- Placing the caller on "hold."
- Using the intercom system.
- Modifying and using voice mail messages.

Table 6–1. Sample of a Hospital's *Floor Book* of Laboratory Information

				HOSPITAL FLOOR BOOK		
TEST NO.	**PROCEDURE**	**SPECIMEN**	**AVERAGE TURN AROUND TIME**	**LABORATORY SECTION**	**COLLECTED BY**	**SPECIAL INSTRUCTION**
1220	Ionized calcium	SST tube	2 hours	Chemistry	Phlebotomist	—
1221	Serum calcium	SST tube	2 hours	Chemistry	Phlebotomist	—
1558	Complete blood count	EDTA tube	1.5 hours	Hematology	Phlebotomist	Invert tube gently to mix blood and anticoagulant

- Organizing conference calls.
- Using the speaker phone.
- Writing legible, complete messages.

Box 6–3 provides suggestions to help the health care worker communicate effectively and politely on the telephone. Additional information on effective communication is presented in Chapter 1.

CONFIDENTIALITY

Each state has statutes related to privileges between physicians and patients. Communications between a physician and a patient are generally considered privileged and must not be shared with other people without the written consent of the patient. Verbal communications and clinical documents must be kept confidential. Clinical documents include the results of testing (e.g., laboratory and radiology) and monitoring. Exceptions to this are matters for legal consultation. Health care workers who have access to patient information must be

---

BOX 6–3.   TELEPHONE TIPS

- Always speak in a polite and professional tone.
- State the department, clinic, or unit name.
- To establish a cooperative relationship, always use phrases such as the following:
    May I help you?
    Please spell your name.
    I am sorry that I cannot assist you with that matter, let me refer you to someone who can.
    Thank you.
- If speaking to patients and family members, try to use words that are easy to pronounce, concise, direct, and uncomplicated.
- Spelling a term may help you or the receiver understand or recognize what is being said.
- Restate sentences to make sure that you understand the message or instructions.
- Remain neutral in a controversy.
- Reflecting on a response before answering will help clarify your answer; however, pauses that are too long may indicate a lack of interest.
- Ask pertinent questions and have the ability to say that you do not know the answer.

careful not to disclose results or other patient information in a casual, unnecessary fashion. Discussion that does not directly relate to the health care worker's role in caring for the patient should be avoided.

ELECTRONIC TRANSMISSION (FACSIMILE) OF PRINTED MATERIALS

Each laboratory or health care institution should have clear policies related to the use of test requests or patient information that has been sent by facsimile or fax. Most laboratories find the use of a **fax machine** efficient, timely, and cost effective, especially when off-site services are offered. Precautionary measures should, however, be detailed in procedure manuals that relate to receiving an official laboratory order from the requesting physician. In addition, older fax paper copies have been known to fade with time. In cases in which the paper fades, a reproduction (photocopy) of the fax is necessary to provide a more permanent version.

■ COMPUTERIZED COMMUNICATIONS

Personal, hand-held mini-, and mainframe computers have become essential instruments in the clinical laboratory and health care setting; thus, the health care worker needs to become acquainted with computerized information systems. For example, in the clinical laboratory, the functions of a laboratory computer system include

- Entering lists of test requisitions for a patient.
- Printing patients' labels, specimen collection lists, and schedules.
- Updating the laboratory specimen accession records.
- Printing lists that identify which test procedures need to be performed on patients' specimens.
- Entering test results into the computer manually or through clinical laboratory instrumentation.
- Storing test results.
- Sending laboratory test results to the nursing stations.
- Sending patient charges to the accounting office.

Computerization of the collection process can significantly decrease errors. Without a computer, collection and specimen information must pass through several people before the sample is actually processed in the laboratory. With a computer, data are continually being checked against the computer files, and authorized individuals can add to and receive information from the accumulated data. With the combined use of hand-held computers and bar code technology, specimens can more easily and accurately be tracked through preanalytic *and* analytic phases of laboratory testing.

■ REQUISITION FORMS

Requested patient laboratory tests occur by means of the laboratory **requisition form** or a computer-generated order. Therefore, the information or instructions must be explicit, and the design and format of the request forms or computer screens to be used must be carefully considered in order to minimize handwriting, permit convenient handling, generate inexpensive and legible copies, and obtain all necessary information for laboratory testing.

Multiple-part forms, that serve as both laboratory request and report forms, represent one of the most widely used traditional formats for a manual system. These forms are also used when computer failures occur. The forms are usually of a convenient size to be easily attached to $8^{1/2} \times 11$-in. paper as is customarily used for patients' medical records. Also, these forms are easy to transport, handle, sort, and store, and they are cost effective. For example, the manual backup requisition forms designed for use at The University of Texas M.D. Anderson Cancer Center, Houston, TX, are $3^{1/4}$-in. wide by $7^{3/8}$-in. long and are usually positioned horizontally, as seen in Figure 6–2. Each form is divided into sections, one for request information and the other for results. The information in the request section (e.g., physician's name, collection time and date, clinic section) is arranged so that it always appears in the same order. This consistency allows standardization between departments and facilitates correct use. The request information must designate time specifications, or the promptness with which the test results are needed (STAT, routine, and so on); patient condition specifications or the circumstances at the time of specimen collection (preop, admission); and patient category specifications, such as inpatient or outpatient. The request side also allows room for all patient identification information, whether added by means of an Addressograph machine (Addressograph Company, Chicago, IL) or handwritten. Each form is identified by name (e.g., hematology, coagulation, chemistry) and is divided into test categories usually coinciding with the different sections of the laboratory. The forms are manufactured to provide clear copies and easy detachment (perforated edges). Color coding can be used for different request forms for ease of identification, both in the ordering of tests and in the charting of results. The name of the institution is usually included on each request form.

Certain additional specifications may be included on request slips that are to be used with a laboratory computer system or with instrumentation that generates printed results. Some request forms are used with a computerized reporting system but are designed to serve also as temporary report forms on a backup basis (Fig. 6–2A). Exact spacing specifications must be met when the request form is to be used as a printout report for certain test results.

Other variations of computerized requisitions may also be used, such as those with barcoded identification numbers. The use of barcoded labels (Fig. 6–2B) for patients' samples to reduce transcription errors and speed up sample processing, is commonplace.

Bar codes represent a series of light and dark bands of varying widths. The configuration of these bands relates to specific alphanumeric symbols (i.e., numbers and letters). In other words, each letter of the alphabet and each number has a specific code (black and white bars of varying widths). When these bands are placed together in a series, they can correspond to a name (patient or test) or a number (identification or test code). When the bar is scanned with a sensitive light or laser scanner, the series of numbers and letters is read into a computer in a precise manner. This technology is very accurate and fast. It saves time, and it keeps personnel from entering or typing information, which reduces clerical errors substantially. Bar codes not only represent patients' names and identification numbers, but also the test codes, accession numbers, billing codes, and inventory records. Many instruments used in the clinical laboratory are functioning with automatic scanners to read a barcoded label directly from the patient's sample tube as it is run through the analyzer. In addition, many laboratory supplies are packaged with bar-coded inventory labels. Figure 6–3 shows some of the many uses for bar codes in a health care facility.

Figure 6–2.   A. Multiple-part requisition forms that also serve as report forms can be stamped with Addressograph machines. These forms can be used with a computerized reporting system but are designed to serve as temporary report forms on a manual backup basis. **B.** If needed, bar-coded labels can be printed with the same information.

(Courtesy of The University of Texas M.D. Anderson Cancer Center, Division of Laboratory Medicine, Houston, TX, with permission.)

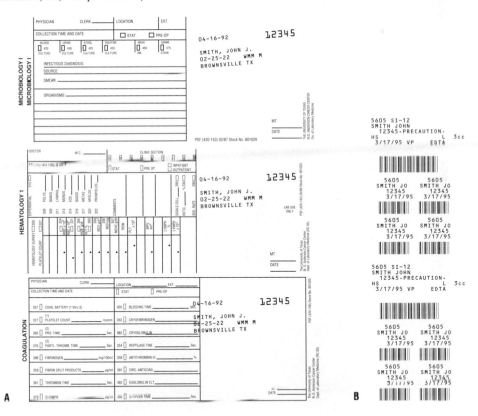

Figure 6–3. The use of bar codes can facilitate the following: **A.** Printing labels and requisition forms. **B.** Labeling specimens. **C.** Labeling blood smears. **D.** Identifying serum aliquot tubes. **E.** Processing blood samples.

(Courtesy of TimeMed Labeling Systems, Burr Ridge, IL, with permission.)

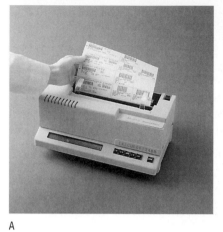

A

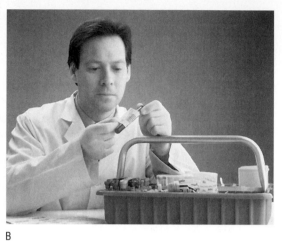

B

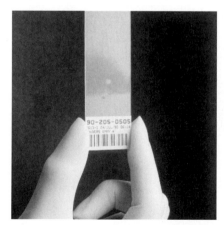

C

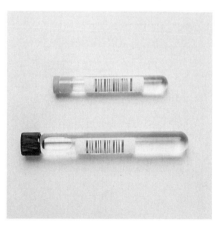

D

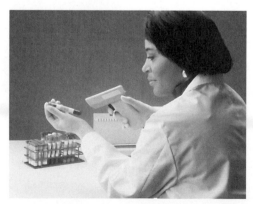

E

■ TRANSMITTAL OF THE TEST REQUEST TO THE LABORATORY

The test request mechanism formally initiates the cyclic procedure of the laboratory communication network. Two systems are commonly used for this activity. Orders for test requests can be transmitted directly to the clinical laboratory from the requesting authority through an on-line interactive computer system. In many institutions, however, manual requesting systems are still in use, sometimes using bar codes, which are then entered into the computer; other times involving a totally manual system in which the request form also serves as the final report.

On-line computer input of request information is the most error-free means of making requests. Because a computer system can perform automatic checks on the input, it does not accept a request for any test that is not in its test-information database. Likewise, it does not accept a sample of plasma or urine for a test restricted to serum. It also allows the person entering the test request to obtain accurate and up-to-date information about specific determinations, such as revised specimen collection requirements, delivery instructions, assay techniques, reference ranges, and fees. Even with hand-held computers that are used for

BOX 6–4. DAILY LOG SHEET THAT DOCUMENTS ALL SPECIMENS COLLECTED AND DELIVERED BY SPECIALIZED PHLEBOTOMY PERSONNEL CALLED *LABORATORY LIAISON TECHNICIANS (LLTS)*

DAILY WORK SHEET

UNIT _____ DATE _____ LLT _____

TOTAL PATIENT SERVICES _____ TOTAL STAT SAMPLES _____   7:00–4:00 _____
(# OF VENIPUNCTURES)
TOTAL TIMED SAMPLES _____   3:00–11:00 _____

ROOM #	PATIENT'S NAME	PATIENT #	TESTS TO BE DONE OR SPECIMENS DELIVERED	LOGGED BY	TIME TO BE COLLECTED	TIME COLLECTED	OBTAINED BY	SPECIMEN	COMMENT

(Courtesy of The University of Texas M.D. Anderson Cancer Center, Division of Laboratory Medicine, Houston, TX, with permission.)

bar code scanning, special comments may be added regarding the patient or sample (e.g., "non-fasting" or "drawn from a CVC line").

In a manual system, the multipart request forms are commonly completed at each patient unit or clinic by a member of the health care team and delivered to the laboratory. This type of system is more subject to human error. The requisition slips could be lost by the nursing service or the ward clerk prior to arriving in the clinical laboratory or by the laboratory personnel after the slips reach the laboratory. Another common source of error comes from requests that are prepared in duplicate or not at all as a result of lack of communication on the in-patient unit. These problems can be minimized by instituting a few organizational procedures, such as using a centralized location for all requisition forms, using a sorting system once the requisition slips reach the laboratory, and using a blood collection log. (Refer to Box 6–4.)

Verbal test requests are occasionally used in cases of emergency. The request should be documented on a standardized form in the laboratory prior to the specimen collection (Box 6–5). After the blood is collected, the formal laboratory request slip can be filled out and accompany the specimen to the laboratory in the routine manner.

BOX 6–5.   SAMPLE OF A DOCUMENTATION FORM USED BY THE LABORATORY IN CASES OF VERBAL TEST REQUESTS

STAT REQUESTS

Nurse:

Requesting Physician:

Location: ICU _____   ER _____   Other _____
              Room: _____

Patient:

Pick up orders on unit:
Tests Ordered: _____
_____
_____
_____

Requested by: _____

Order taken by: _____

Date _____   Time _____   AM _____   PM _____

(Adapted from a form used at The University of Texas M.D. Anderson Cancer Center, Houston, TX, with permission.)

■ SPECIMEN LABELS AND BLOOD DRAWING LISTS

Clear and accurate specimen identification is essential and must begin immediately upon collection, and it must continue through disposal of the specimen. Identification methods vary from manually copying all patient identification information onto the container to using prenumbered bar-coded labels. Manually labeling specimens can be time consuming and it can be prone to transcription errors. These problems can be prevented by using preprinted labels, which are available from many commercial sources. Some labels are gummed hospital labels that can be attached to specimens. Other labeling systems include those that can imprint a patient identification card or electronically print patient identification information onto the specimen label.

Among the most sophisticated, accurate, and efficient labels are those generated by a hospital computer system. Requisition slips for the morning blood collections can be sent to the laboratory on the previous day or entered into the computer at any time. On the basis of the laboratory orders, the computer can generate enough labels containing all the appropriate patient identification criteria for each tube required to be drawn. The labels also list the specific tests requested, the types of specimen collection tubes required for the requested tests, and the unique accession numbers or sample numbers to be used for that particular collection time. Bar codes can be used for any alphanumeric symbols. Smaller transfer labels may also be printed to label special aliquot tubes, collection tubes, cuvettes, and microscope slides. This type of system eliminates the manually written entry log used at many hospitals for recording the tests and accession number requested for each patient. Additional test requests ordered later in the day are entered into the computer, which assigns a specific time to the tests so that they can be easily separated from those requested in the morning. Labels for later collection can be computer printed or made with an Addressograph machine. Blood-drawing lists are also printed by the computer to provide a list of patients on each floor requiring blood work for the morning draw and the tests ordered, and to identify the assigned sample accession number. The health care worker initials this list after the patient's blood has been drawn, and a copy is left at the nursing unit so that caregivers attending the patient can see which specimens have already been collected. Any additional specimens collected later in the day are documented in the logbook on the floor (see Box 6-4). In this way, the personnel on the health care team has a complete list of the specimen collections taken from each patient throughout the day.

■ SPECIMEN TRANSPORTATION AND DELIVERY

Both the communication network and the quality of laboratory test results depend on the time that specimens are received for processing. Blood and other specimens must be delivered expeditiously.

BASIC HANDLING GUIDELINES

Every health care facility has a specific protocol for specimen transportation and processing. Most laboratories require the use of a leakproof plastic bag for insertion of the specimen container. This bag protects the health care worker from pathogenic (disease-producing) organisms during specimen transportation. Usually, this special transport bag has a pouch on the outside for the laboratory request slip. Thus, the potential for contamination of the request slip is eliminated. If possible, the blood in evacuated tubes and micro-collection tubes should be maintained in a vertical position to promote complete clot formation, if required, and to reduce the possibility of hemolysis. It is also imperative to handle and transport blood specimens in a gentle manner to prevent hemolyzing the specimens.

Glycolytic action from the blood cells interferes in the analysis of various chemicals (e.g., glucose, calcitonin, aldosterone, phosphorus, enzymes). Because of this, the blood samples should be transported to the clinical laboratory within 45 minutes from the time of collection so that the serum or plasma can be separated from the blood cells. The serum or plasma that is separated from the cells must be handled according to the laboratory procedure. The National Committee for Clinical Laboratory Standards (NCCLS) suggests a maximum time of 2 hours from the time of collection to the separation of sera from plasma. Once separated, sera may remain at room temperature, be refrigerated, be stored in a dark place, or be frozen, depending on the prescribed laboratory method.[4]

For transportation of specimens from remote ambulatory sites, including home health collections, the phlebotomist must still follow the handling guidelines according to Universal Standard Precautions. The phlebotomist should use the same safety equipment he or she would use in a hospital environment (e.g., closed venipuncture system, gloves, disposable laboratory coat, plastic blood collection tubes, and a biohazardous disposal container). In addition, all blood collection equipment and specimens should be transported in an enclosed or lockable container to avoid accidental spills if the automobile is in a collision. The container should have a biohazard warning label on it. Cold packs should be used in the container for transport during hot weather, or the reverse, the vehicle should be heated in cold weather. For home collections, the phlebotomist must be extra careful to dispose of waste properly and to place blood specimens in leakproof plastic bags in an upright position inside a transport container.

CHILLED SPECIMENS

For special types of specimens, chilling is required. If a health care worker is requested to transport an arterial specimen for blood gas analysis, he or she should be aware that the specimen must be transported in an airtight heparinized syringe and placed in a mixture of ice and water. The airtight container and the ice water decrease the loss of gases from the specimen. It is important to use ice water rather than solid chunks of ice; otherwise, parts of the specimen may freeze and hemolysis will result. Speed in specimen transportation is essential to prevent the loss of blood gases. Other specimens that may require chilling are those for gastrin, ammonia, lactic acid, renin, catecholamine, parathyroid hormone, prothrombin time (PT), partial thromboplastin time (PTT), and glucagon determinations.[5]

PROTECTION OF SPECIMENS FROM LIGHT

Some chemical constituents in blood, such as bilirubin, are light sensitive and decompose if exposed to light. Thus, blood collected for light sensitive chemical analysis should be protected from bright light with an aluminum foil wrapping around the tube. Other light-sensitive constituents are vitamin B_{12}, carotene, and folate, and urine specimens to be used for the detection of porphyrins.

MICROBIOLOGICAL SPECIMENS

Blood and urine specimens for microbiological culture need to be transported to the laboratory as quickly as possible so that the blood can be transferred to culture media and the urine analyzed. This enhances the likelihood of detecting pathogenic bacteria. Specimens for blood cultures can also be collected directly into culture media, which minimizes possible contamination and speeds the contact with the culture media. (Refer to Chapter 7 for additional information about blood culture collections.)

WARMED SPECIMENS

Specimens that require warming (to body temperature, 37°C) include those for testing cold agglutinins and cryofibrinogen. These special cases require a heat block for transportation and handling purposes.

LABORATORY PROCESSING OF SPECIMENS

Processing specimens may occur in one location of the clinical laboratory or in each laboratory section (e.g., hematology, clinical chemistry, clinical immunology, blood bank, coagulation), depending on the organization of the laboratory. Specimen processing can also occur in satellite laboratories. Wherever the site, it is important to know the processing requirements of the clinical laboratory so that specimens are transported and processed as quickly as possible. As discussed in Chapters 4 and 5, safety devices should be used to gain access to the blood to prevent splashing and aerosol spray from the blood sample. Efficient and safe processing of the specimens leads to better clinical laboratory test results and, thus, better patient care.

In many laboratories, the specimen collection area has a medical technologist (clinical laboratory scientist) or a medical laboratory technician who centrifuges the specimens and makes the appropriate aliquots for each section. These aliquots are then distributed to the clinical laboratory sections for testing. Some specimens must be prepared for shipping to referral laboratories. This preparation sometimes involves special packaging requirements, such as freezing the specimen to maintain stability and packaging it in a Styrofoam mailing container.

HAND DELIVERY

Many systems for specimen delivery involve hand-carried specimens and require standards for ensuring promptness. The laboratory is most often the department responsible for the collection and delivery of blood specimens. The laboratory may also be responsible for the delivery of all other patient specimens as well. Health care workers may make scheduled pickups as well as deliveries of stat specimens. The specimens should be placed in an assigned area in each hospital unit after being documented in the log book. The patient's name, hospital number, and room number; the specimens delivered; the date; the time; and the initials of the person transporting the specimen should be included on the log sheet, as shown in Box 6–6. Specimen transportation can be more easily monitored when all personnel involved use the appropriate documentation procedures and communicate openly with one another.

BOX 6–6.   SAMPLE OF A LOG SHEET USED BY LABORATORY PERSONNEL TO DOCUMENT DELIVERY OF PATIENT SPECIMENS

SPECIMEN DELIVERY

Patient Name	Location	Specimens						Date	Time	Escort Name
		CSF	Blood	Urine	Sputum	Other	Test Ordered			

Most health care workers organize blood collection trays or carts to accommodate patient specimens that need to be taken to the laboratory. A test-tube rack, slide rack, plastic holder, or cup is sufficient to hold the collected specimens. Some specimens require ice for transport, so it is wise to carry a small container with a slurry of ice water that will not leak and will fit conveniently on the tray.

TRANSPORTATION DEPARTMENT

Specimen delivery may also be performed by a transportation department within the hospital. Typically, the transportation escort or orderlies are responsible for moving patients from their nursing units to service areas, such as diagnostic radiology, physical therapy, and so forth. When a specimen and requisition form are to be delivered to the laboratory by the transportation department, the following information is usually required: type of specimen, name and hospital identification number of the patient, date and time of specimen collection, and destination of the specimen. After obtaining this information, the escort takes the specimen to the laboratory. The test request slip accompanying the specimen can also be "clocked in" at this time so that the actual delivery time can always be obtained. If any complications arise with the specimen, the escort notifies the nursing staff. Occasionally, specimens, especially stat or timed requests, may be collected and delivered to the laboratory by a nurse or a physician. Again, the requisition should be clocked in to document specimen receipt.

PNEUMATIC TUBE SYSTEMS

Many hospitals use **pneumatic tube systems** to transport patient records, messages, letters, bills, medications, x-rays, and laboratory test results. Reports from health care institutions differ, however, as to the effectiveness of using tube systems for transporting blood specimens. Considerations in the use of pneumatic tubes for transporting specimens are mechanical reliability, distance of transport, speed of carrier, control mechanisms, landing mechanism, radius of loops and bends, shock absorbency, sizes of carriers, and laboratory assessment of chemical and cellular components in transported specimens versus hand-carried specimens. It is generally recommended that blood collection tubes be placed in the pneumatic tube with shock-absorbent inserts padding the sides and with the tubes separated from one another to prevent spillage or breakage. Plastic clear liners are also commercially available so that if leaks do occur, they are visible and are contained to prevent contamination of the tube system, the carrier, and the personnel handling the specimens.

TRANSPORTATION BY VEHICLE

Some manufacturers provide transport systems that are automated, motorized, or computerized. Delivery of specimens can be by means of a small container car attached to a network of track that is routed to appropriate sites in the laboratory, nursing stations, or other specimen collection areas. Again, a thorough evaluation of such automated delivery systems needs to include mechanical reliability, transportation distances, speed of the carriers, control mechanisms, soft-landing provisions, radius of loops and bends, shock absorbency, size of carriers, method of cleaning containers, and overall time- and cost-effectiveness. When plans are made to renovate a laboratory area so that it includes this type of transport system, extra space above the ceiling tiles should be considered because the transport vehicles require a sizable right-of-way.

OTHER TRANSPORT EQUIPMENT

Health care workers involved in specimen collection may also be required to order and use special transport containers. All should be evaluated for cost, protective ability, temperature control, sterilizing potential, appearance, labeling system, breakage, leakage, and tamper resistance.

Some hospitals send specimens to reference laboratories for special analysis. When packaging or receiving one of the specimens in a special transport container, care must be taken to pay attention to the following details:

1. Specimens, such as human or animal feces, blood, body fluids, or tissue, should be properly labeled and be placed in containers that protect individuals from contamination.
2. Specimens containing viable microorganisms must be specially packaged so that they can withstand leakage of contents, pressure and temperature changes, and rough handling. It is recommended that the specimen be placed in a primary con-

tainer surrounded by absorbent packing material. This container should be labeled with pertinent information and instructions about the specimen contents. It can then be placed in a secondary container. Thus, if the specimen contents are released, they are maintained in the primary container. Biohazard and mailing labels should be affixed to the outside container.[5]

3. Specimen requisition forms or special instructions should accompany the specimen.

4. Containers holding dry ice should be labeled—for example, "DRY ICE, FROZEN BIOHAZARDOUS MEDICAL SPECIMEN." Biohazard labels should be affixed so that they are easily visible to anyone handling the container.

5. It is recommended that, when shipping biohazardous material, the address and telephone number of the Centers for Disease Control and Prevention (CDC), Atlanta, GA, be affixed to the container. In the event of damage or leakage, individuals outside the health care professions may need advice on how to dispose of or clean up a biohazardous spill.

6. After receiving an intact specimen from an outside source, the container must be identified by name, number, and source. This information should match that on the accompanying requisition, and the specimen can then be processed accordingly.

7. If a leaky or broken specimen is received, it should be handled cautiously and according to safety procedures.

■ REPORTING MECHANISMS

WRITTEN REPORTS

The laboratory report is a feedback mechanism for transmitting vital data from the laboratory to the physician requesting the information. Both the JCAHO and the CAP state that the results should be confirmed, dated, and accompanied by permanent report copies that are kept in the laboratory, as well as added to the patient's medical record. The CAP also states that each report should contain adequate patient identification, be stamped to record the date and hour when the procedures were completed, and be signed and initialed by the laboratory personnel performing the procedure. When computer-generated report forms are used, laboratory documentation on worksheets by personnel performing the procedures is sufficient. The CAP has suggested that health care personnel consider the following when designing a report form:[3]

1. Identification of patient, patient location, and physician.
2. Date and time of specimen collection.
3. Description, source of specimen, and labeled precautions.
4. Compactness and ease of preparing the package for shipment.
5. Consistency in format.
6. Clear understandability of instructions or orders.
7. Logical location in patient's chart for reference laboratory reports.
8. Sequential order of multiple results on single specimens.
9. Listing of reference ranges or normal and abnormal values.
10. Assurance of accuracy of request transcription.
11. Administrative and record-keeping value.

Any unique institutional requirements for an acceptable report should be stated in the laboratory procedure manual and may include such criteria as QC limits, absolute limits, and delta checks. If these criteria cannot be met on the report form, a written policy including these requirements should be available when needed.

Results can be documented in one of the following three ways: manual recording of test results, laboratory instrument–printed reports, and computer-generated reports. As previously mentioned, in most manual systems, combination test requisition–report forms are used. These forms may include multiple copies. Most laboratory instruments in use today contain microprocessors that can generate digital outputs and printed reports. In addition, hospital computer systems can provide patient laboratory trends over a designated period of time.

VERBAL REPORTS

The use of verbal and telephone reports has declined in recent years because computer access to laboratory data is prevalent in most health care environments. If laboratory personnel take an active role in educating clerical, nursing, and physician staff on the acquisition of computerized data, the number of phone requests will decrease.

Verbal reports, although useful for reporting stat results and "panic" values, may become a problem in laboratories. The possibility of error is so great that at a minimum, a laboratory should always require proper identification of the patient and the name of the person receiving the report. Written documentation of verbally issued reports is recommended and should include the following information: patient name and hospital number, name of person receiving the report, date, information given, and name of person issuing the report (Box 6–7).

BOX 6–7.   SAMPLE FORM USED BY A MICROBIOLOGY LABORATORY TO ISSUE VERBAL CULTURE RESULTS

CULTURE RESULTS—TELEPHONE REQUEST

PATIENT NAME: _____

PATIENT ID NUMBER: _____

PHYSICIAN: _____

PERSON REQUESTING INFORMATION: _____

DATE	SOURCE	CULTURE #	INFO GIVEN

TIME OF INQUIRY: _____

DATE OF INQUIRY: _____

TECHNOLOGIST: _____

COMPUTERIZED REPORTS

Various computer-transmission devices can provide a rapid on-line report system and are, in general, more reliable than verbal reports and faster than waiting for the written report. A hospital with an on-line laboratory computer system can have terminals located in each patient unit. After the tests have been completed and verified in the laboratory, the results can be immediately displayed in each patient unit. A printer can be attached to each terminal to generate a temporary hard-copy report. Another transmission method electronically transmits a handwritten report, which is generated in a similar form at the receiving end. A third transmission device transmits fax results. All these methods can provide a written report that is accurate, dependable, and consistent.

INTERIM REPORTS AND CUMULATIVE SUMMARIES

Interim laboratory reports are typically used on hospital units at specified times during the day (e.g., 10:00 AM and 2:00 PM). These reports may include test results completed or in progress. This type of reporting system is often used in facilities that are only partially computerized or as a backup process if the hospital computer system is malfunctioning or down.

Cumulative summaries are a compilation of laboratory reports on one patient over a designated period or after a certain number of tests have been performed on the patient. They are printed at designated times during the week and facilitate the medical record-charting process. They are helpful to nurses and physicians because groups of similar tests are reported together. Trends that reveal laboratory and physiologic changes can be detected more easily than if each laboratory value were reported separately and charted in the medical record at random.

■ DISTRIBUTION OF RESULTS

The final communication involved in the laboratory communication network is the distribution of test results. Those who receive the laboratory data include nurses, phlebotomists, clerical and medical record personnel (chart attachment); the hospital business officers (patient billing); and laboratory personnel (department record).

CHARTING REPORTS

Manual Methods

So that a chronological type of reporting system is used on the patient's chart, the laboratory reports have traditionally been shingled one upon another. Color coding by the laboratory originating the results aids in coordinating them on a carrier page. The laboratory may also key chronological reports by having a master card prepared in the laboratory for each patient, beginning with the admitting laboratory test results. The results of each day are added to the card, which can be photocopied and sent to the physician.

Computerized Medical Records

A health care facility's computer system can easily provide daily laboratory reports and cumulative reports for the patient's computerized medical record. All reports should be available at times convenient for making clinical decisions by the medical staff.

The business office of the health care facility also receives data on-line regarding laboratory procedures. This office must be notified of all laboratory charges, according to data requested and procedural code for patient billing. It is financially advantageous to send reports promptly. Also laboratory copies of test results from previous days, months, or years should be accessible because they are often requested to confirm charges for the hospital stay.

SELF STUDY

KEY TERMS

Bar Codes

Clinical (or Medical) Record

E-Mail

Fax Machine

Pneumatic Tube Systems

Reference Ranges

Requisition Form

STUDY QUESTIONS

The following may have *one* or *more* answers:

1. The key elements common to most medical records are which of the following:
   - a. face sheet
   - b. medical history and physical evaluation
   - c. physician's order sheet
   - d. discharge plan

2. Medical records serve what purpose?
   - a. allow coordination of care
   - b. meet accrediting and licensing requirements
   - c. provide legal protection
   - d. provide research data

3. Guidelines for documentation in health care include which of the following:
   - a. accuracy
   - b. personal opinions of the situation
   - c. completion about each event or procedure
   - d. objectivity

4. Which of the following data should be considered confidential?
   - a. laboratory test results
   - b. radiology reports
   - c. patient's diagnosis
   - d. universal precautions

5. Bar codes can be used for which type(s) of information?
   - a. identification of patient names
   - b. identification of patient numbers
   - c. designation of test to be performed
   - d. inventory of supplies

6. What is the most error-free method for requesting a laboratory test?
   - a. handwritten requisition
   - b. computerized method
   - c. verbal method
   - d. verbal stat method

7. Sources of preanalytic error can be categorized as follows:
   a. processing variables
   b. specimen variables
   c. physician's attitude
   d. patient variables

8. Telephone responsibilities for health care workers usually include:
   a. using effective customer service manners
   b. using an intercom system
   c. transferring calls
   d. placing people on hold

9. A specimen should be protected from light for which of the following determinations?
   a. bilirubin concentration
   b. hemoglobin level
   c. glucose level
   d. blood cultures

10. A specimen should be chilled for which of the following analyses?
   a. complete blood count (CBC)
   b. bilirubin level
   c. blood gas
   d. glucose level

References

1. Clinical Skillbuilders: *Better Documentation*. Spring House, PA: Spring House Corporation; 1992.

2. Hamann LJ: Pre-analytical Variability: A Phlebotomy Perspective. Presented at Current Issues in Phlebotomy. Baltimore, MD; March 6, 1997.

3. College of American Pathologists (CAP): *Standards for Accreditation of Medical Laboratories*. Skokie, IL: CAP; 1990.

4. National Committee for Clinical Laboratory Standards (NCCLS): *Procedures for Handling and Transport of Diagnostic Specimens and Etiologic Agents*. NCCLS Document H5-A3, Villanova, PA: NCCLS; 1994.

5. National Committee for Clinical Laboratory Standards (NCCLS): *Procedures for the Collection of Diagnostic Blood Specimens by Venipuncture*. NCCLS Document H3-A4, Villanova, PA: NCCLS; June, 1998.

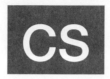

PHLEBOTOMY CASE STUDY

■

Accidental Injury

Sally Landers had been on the job for only 8 months. She was a phlebotomist at a rural hospital in the Southwest where she had been hired to do early morning blood collections and deliver specimens to the centralized laboratory. She was tired when she went to work one Friday morning. She drew blood from a frail middle-aged man, Mr. Johnson. She had trouble with the collection procedure in that she had to stick him twice before she acquired the blood specimen. She was relieved when she finally finished the procedure. As she began to clean up and discard the used equipment, she noticed that the biohazard container was full. She decided, however, that it could probably hold the needles she had used on Mr. Johnson. She used her fingers to push the used needles and needle holders into the container and she felt a sharp puncture. She realized that she had stuck herself with a contaminated sharp object. She gathered the specimens she had drawn and quickly left. She immediately reported the injury to her supervisor.

QUESTIONS:

1. Describe what Sally did correctly and incorrectly?
2. What procedures would need to be reviewed with Sally?
3. What additional education would you recommend for Sally?

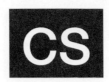

PHLEBOTOMY CASE STUDY

■

Transporting Specimens From Homebound Patients to the Laboratory

The medical assistant, Larry Smith, works for Mackin Home Health Agency. His job is multifaceted because he performs history and physical assessments, and when required to, he draws blood for laboratory testing. One day he went to collect blood and urine samples on Mr. Gonzales, an 80-year-old man who spoke very little English. He greeted Mr. Gonzales and found the bathroom and a suitable spot to draw blood from him. He felt confident that Mr. Gonzales had understood his communication. He was successful on the first attempt to collect the blood sample, and he helped Mr. Gonzales to the bathroom to collect the urine. Mr. Gonzales followed directions except he did not close the urine bottle tightly because he lacked the strength. Larry did not notice that the lid was not on tightly. He placed all the specimens in the container he had brought. He decided to leave the lid open because he knew his next stop was just 1 block away. On the way to the next house, a car ran a stop sign so Larry had to jam on his brakes, and the container with specimens fell off the seat of the car. The urine specimen spilled all over the floor of his vehicle.

QUESTIONS:

1. What could Larry have done to avoid the situation?
2. What should Larry do now?

EQUIPMENT AND PROCEDURES

HLEBOTOMY PRACTICE IS BEST DESCRIBED by what phlebotomists do. Part III answers the following technical questions:

- What tools (supplies and equipment) do I need?
- How do I prepare myself and the patient?
- How do I perform a venipuncture?
- How do I perform a finger stick?
- What can go wrong, and how can I prevent it from happening?

Building on the knowledge from the first six chapters, Part III highlights technical skills, supplies, and equipment. It is divided into four chapters that describe the supplies, equipment, techniques, and complications associated with phlebotomy practice.

Chapter 7, Blood Collection Equipment, describes and illustrates the latest supplies and equipment necessary for the collection of blood. Emphasis is on anticoagulated and nonadditive blood collection tubes, the importance of color coding, and the use of gloves, syringes, needles, microcollection equipment, specimen collection chairs and trays, and other supplies needed for a safe and effective collection procedure. Safe handling of blood specimens is highlighted.

Chapter 8, Venipuncture Procedures, provides a comprehensive description and illustrations of each step of the blood collection process. It includes a discussion of patient identification, as well as the venipuncture procedure itself. Emphasis is on safe and proper preparation, technique, and collection.

Chapter 9, Skin Puncture Procedures, provides a detailed description and illustrations of each step of the skin puncture procedure. Emphasis is on site selection, finger sticks, and blood smear preparation.

Chapter 10, Complications in Blood Collection, describes the complications that occur during the blood collection process and the reasons for their occurrence. Emphasis is on recognition and prevention of these complications, the effects of the patient's physical disposition on the integrity of the specimen, and the interfering effects of drugs and other substances in the blood. Guidelines for specimen rejection are also presented.

Blood Collection Equipment

CHAPTER OUTLINE

CHAPTER OBJECTIVES

Upon completion of Chapter 7, the learner is responsible for the following:

1. List the various types of anticoagulants used in blood collection, their mechanisms for preventing blood from clotting, and the vacuum collection tube color codes for these anticoagulants.

2. Describe the latest phlebotomy safety supplies and equipment, and evaluate their effectiveness in blood collection.

3. Identify the various supplies that should be carried on a specimen collection tray when a skin puncture specimen must be collected.

4. Identify the types of equipment needed to collect blood by venipuncture.

5. Describe the special precautions that should be taken and the techniques that should be used when various types of specimens must be transported to the clinical laboratory.

■ VACUUM (EVACUATED) TUBE SYSTEMS

Venipuncture with a **vacuum (evacuated) tube** (VACUTAINER [Becton-Dickinson VACUTAINER Systems, Franklin Lakes, NJ]), as shown in Figure 7–1 is the most direct and efficient method for obtaining a blood specimen. The evacuated tube system requires three components: the evacuated sample tube, the double-pointed needle, and a special plastic **holder (adapter).** One end of the double-pointed needle enters the vein, the other end pierces the top of the tube, and the vacuum aspirates the blood (Fig. 7–2). Vacuum tubes may contain silicon to decrease the possibility of hemolysis and prevent the clot from adhering to the wall of the tube. This convenient system eliminates the need for syringes and

Figure 7–1.   Vacuum tube (VACUTAINER).

(Courtesy of Becton-Dickinson VACUTAINER Systems, Franklin Lakes, NJ.)

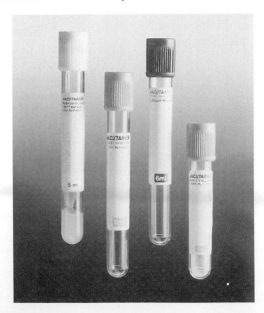

Figure 7–2. Holder-needle combination with inserted VACUTAINER.

(Courtesy of Becton-Dickinson VACUTAINER Systems, Franklin Lakes, NJ.)

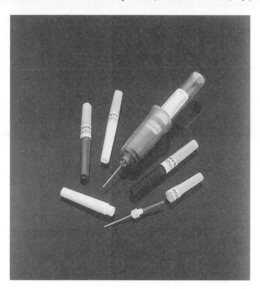

consists of disposable needles and tubes. The tubes are available in different sizes and can be purchased in glass or unbreakable plastic. The external tube diameter and length plus the maximum amount of specimen to be drawn into the vacuum tube are the two criteria used to describe vacuum tube size (Table 7–1). The smaller sizes (e.g., 2 mL) are useful for pediatric and geriatric collections and can be purchased with different types of anticoagu-

Table 7–1. Typical Sizes of Blood Collection Vacuum Tubes

EXTRA DIAMETER × LENGTH (mm)	DRAW VOLUMES (mL)
10.25 × 50	2.0
10.25 × 64	3.0
10.25 × 82	4.0
13 × 75	2.0
13 × 75	4.0
13 × 75	5.0
13 × 100	4.2
13 × 100	6.0
13 × 100	7.0
13 × 100	15.0
16 × 75	7.0
16 × 100	10.0
16 × 125	15.0

lants, as well as chemically clean or sterile glassware. Each vacuum tube is color coded according to the anticoagulant contained within the tube (Table 7–2).

Many tubes are specifically designed to be used directly with chemistry, hematology, or microbiology instrumentation. In these cases, the tube of blood is identified by its bar code and is pierced by the instrument probe, and some sample is aspirated into the instrument for analyses. Use of these *closed systems* minimizes laboratory personnel's risk of exposure to blood. In addition, some tubes have plastic tops or screw-on enclosures around the rubber stopper to minimize exposure to blood left on the top of the cap or blood splatters that can occur during cap removal.

Evacuated tubes are also used for transferring blood from a syringe into the tubes. The syringe needle is simply pushed through the top of the tube, and blood is automatically pulled into the tube because of the vacuum. The plunger must not be pushed down if the tubes are being filled from the syringe because it is extremely hazardous. Also, pushing the plunger may damage cellular components because of the forceful expulsion of blood. Specialized tubes and bottles that may fit the adapter are also available for blood culture collection.

The expiration dates of tubes should be monitored continuously. Such monitoring is most easily accomplished with a computerized inventory system; however, routine rotation of

Table 7–2.   Specimen Type and Collection Vacuum Tubes

SPECIMEN TYPE	COLLECTION TUBES (STOPPER COLOR/TYPE)	ADDITIVE
Clotted blood/serum	Gray and red	Polymer barrier
	Yellow and red	Polymer barrier
	Gold	Polymer barrier
	Red	None
Whole blood/plasma	Green and gray	Polymer barrier and lithium heparin
	Green and red	Polymer barrier and lithium heparin
	Light green	Polymer barrier and lithium heparin
	Light blue	Trisodium citrate
	Lavender (purple)	EDTA (K_3) or EDTA (K_2) or EDTA (Na_2)
	Gray	Sodium fluoride and potassium oxalate
	Green	Lithium heparin
	Green	Sodium heparin
	Royal blue	Sodium heparin or EDTA (Na_2)-sterile tube for toxicology and nutritional studies
Clotted blood/serum	Royal blue	No additive; but sterile tube for trace elements, toxicology, and nutritional studies
	Brown	No additive or sodium heparin, but lead-free glass and sterile for lead determinations
Whole blood	Lavender (purple)	EDTA (K_3) or EDTA (K_2) or EDTA (Na_2)
	Green	Lithium heparin, sodium heparin, or ammonium heparin
	Black	Sodium citrate
	Yellow	Sodium polyanetholesulfonate (SPS)

stocked supplies and careful checking of phlebotomy trays and carts should also be the responsibility of each phlebotomist.

Clinical Alert

The holder of the evacuated tube system has a large opening for the blood vacuum tube and a small opening at the other end for needle insertion. Various manufacturers have modified the adapter to reduce the risk of accidental needle sticks. For instance, Becton-Dickinson VACUTAINER Systems (Franklin Lakes, NJ) developed the Safety-Lok Needle Holder (Fig. 7–3), which has a protective shield so that the blood collector can slide the protective shield over the needle and lock it in place after the needle is withdrawn from the puncture site. This single-use adapter is fairly large and requires a large biohazardous sharps container for disposal. However, it provides effective, immediate containment of a used needle.

Another protective holder that provides effective, immediate containment of a used needle is the Saf-T Clik holder (Winfield Medical, San Diego, CA) (Fig. 7–4). It reduces the risk of cross-contamination and fits any standard blood collection needle.

Figure 7–3.   Safety-Lok Needle Holder.

(Courtesy of Becton-Dickinson VACUTAINER Systems, Franklin Lakes, NJ.)

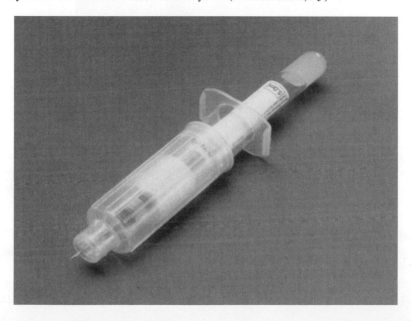

Figure 7–4.   Saf-T Clik shielded blood needle adapter.

(Courtesy of Winfield Medical, San Diego, CA.)

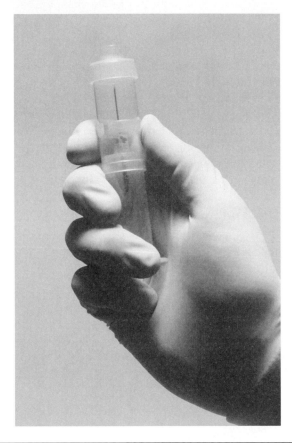

The Safety-Gard Phlebotomy System (Becton-Dickinson VACUTAINER Systems, Franklin Lakes, NJ) has been developed as a safety device for blood collection (Fig. 7–5). The blood collector can single-handedly retract a used blood collection needle and then safely recover the needle while it is enclosed and locked inside the holder. This holder system provides safe disposal of the needle because it remains locked within the Safety-Gard Needle Holder. A companion biohazardous container (Fig. 7–6), for use with the Safety-Gard Needle Holder, is also available. This system provides protection from needle sticks by removing used needles from the holder without user contact with the needles.

Another vacuum tube assembly developed to prevent needle stick injuries is the Proguard II (Care Medical Products, Ontario, CA). It is a single-use vacuum tube/needle holder. The used needle is manually retracted into the holder.

Sarstedt, Inc. has the S-Monovette (Sarstedt, Inc., Newton, NC) Blood Collection System (Fig. 7–7) that is a safety device for vacuum collection or the syringe collection technique.

Figure 7–5. Safety-Gard Phlebotomy System.

(Courtesy of Becton-Dickinson VACUTAINER Systems, Franklin Lakes, NJ.)

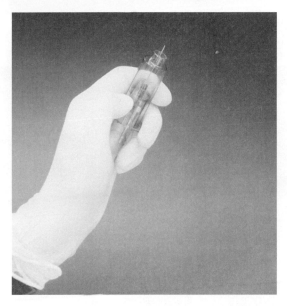

Figure 7–6. Safety-Gard Needle Disposal Container that permits one-handed disposal of enclosed needle.

(Courtesy of Becton-Dickinson VACUTAINER Systems, Franklin Lakes, NJ.)

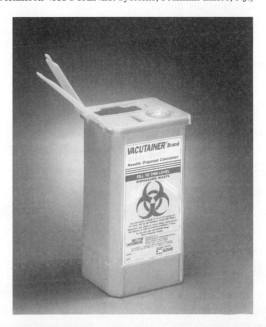

Figure 7–7. S-Monovette.

(Courtesy of Sarstedt, Inc., Newton, NC.)

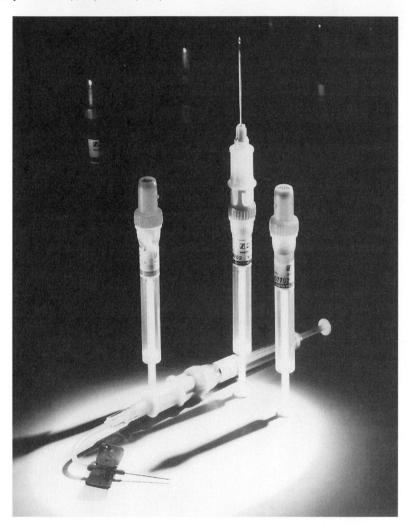

It is unique in that the sample collection, transportation, and centrifugation tube is a combined unit.

■ ANTICOAGULANTS AND BLOOD COLLECTION TUBES

Traditionally, in most clinical laboratories, serum, plasma, or whole blood has been used to perform various assays. More recently, though, heparinized whole blood has become the specimen of choice for the latest clinical laboratory instruments used in stat (immediate) situations. Using whole blood as a specimen decreases the time involved in acquiring the test result because centrifugation is not required prior to laboratory testing.

Many coagulation factors are involved in blood clotting, and coagulation can be prevented by the addition of different types of anticoagulants. These **anticoagulants** often contain preservatives that can extend the metabolism and life span of the red blood cells (RBCs) after blood collection. Anticoagulants and preservatives are used extensively in blood donations to ensure the biochemical balance of certain components of RBCs, such as hemoglobin, pH, adenosine triphosphate (ATP), and glucose. Once transferred, anticoagulants, such as **citrate–phosphate–dextrose (CPD)** and **acid–citrate–dextrose (ACD),** ensure that the RBCs provide the recipient with the means of delivering oxygen (O_2) to the tissues.

Another major use of anticoagulants and preservatives is in the collection of plasma for laboratory analysis. Specific anticoagulants or preservatives must be used depending on the test procedure ordered. Anticoagulants cannot be substituted for one another. Table 7–3 lists the various laboratory assays along with the types of anticoagulants required and the approximate milliliters of blood that must be collected for each assay.

Coagulation of blood can be prevented by the addition of **oxalates, citrates, ethylene-diamine tetra-acetic acid (EDTA),** or **heparin.** Oxalates, citrates, and EDTA prevent the coagulation of blood by removing calcium and forming insoluble calcium salts. These three anticoagulants cannot be used in calcium determinations; however, citrates are frequently used in coagulation blood studies. EDTA prevents platelet aggregation and is, therefore, used for platelet counts and platelet function tests. Fresh EDTA-anticoagulated blood allows preparation of blood films with minimal distortion of white blood cells (WBCs). Heparin, a mucopolysaccharide used in assays, such as ammonia and plasma hemoglobin, prevents blood clotting by inactivating the blood-clotting chemicals—thrombin and thromboplastin.

Clinical Alert

In addition to using the correct anticoagulant for a specific laboratory assay, using the correct amount or dilution of anticoagulant in the blood specimen is important. The blood collection vacuum tubes have been designed for a certain amount of blood to be drawn into the tube by vacuum according to the amount of prefilled anticoagulant in the tube. If an insufficient amount of blood is collected in a tube with anticoagulant, the laboratory test results may be erroneous because of an incorrect blood-to-anticoagulant ratio.

"Partial collection" tubes are available through manufacturers for patient blood collections in which it is anticipated that a "short draw" will be collected. These partial collection tubes will provide accurate laboratory results even though a short draw is collected.

GRAY-TOPPED TUBES

Gray-topped vacuum tubes usually contain (1) potassium oxalate and **sodium fluoride** or (2) **lithium iodoacetate** and heparin. This type of collection tube is used primarily for glycolytic inhibition tests. Thus, sometimes *antiglycolytic agent* is the term for this tube's addi-

(*text continues on p. 198*)

Table 7–3.   Laboratory Assays and the Required Types of Anticoagulants

TEST NAME	SPECIMEN TUBE (TYPE/COLOR)	WHOLE BLOOD, MINIMUM VOLUME FOR ADULTS (mL)
A_{1c} hemoglobin (see glycosylated hemoglobin)		
ABG (see Blood gases)		
ABO group and type	Whole blood (purple) or serum (red)	5
Acetaminophen (Tylenol)	Serum (speckled)	1
Acetone	Serum (speckled)	2
Acetylcholine receptor–binding antibodies	Serum (speckled)	3
Acid hemolysis (PNH)	Plasma (light blue)	3
Acidified serum test (see Hamm's test)		
Acid phosphatase, prostatic isoenzyme	Serum (speckled)	2
ACTH (adrenocorticotropic) hormone	Whole blood (purple)	10
Activated partial thromboplastin time (see Partial thromboplastin time)		
Adenovirus antibody	Serum (speckled)	3
Adrenal cortical antibody	Serum (red)	3
Albumin	Serum (speckled)	2
Alcohol (ethanol)	Whole blood (gray)	2
Aldolase	Serum (speckled)	2
Aldosterone	Serum (speckled) or plasma (purple or green) *Ice needed for transportation *Patient should be recumbent for at least 30 minutes prior to blood collection	7
Alkaline phosphatase (Alk p'tase)	Serum (speckled)	2
Alkaline phosphatase isoenzymes	Serum (speckled)	2
Alpha$_1$-antitrypsin	Serum (speckled)	1
Alpha-fetoprotein (AFP)	Serum (speckled)	3
Alpha$_2$-macroglobulin	Serum (red)	1
Aluminum	Whole blood (royal blue)	7
Amebiasis	Serum (speckled)	3
Amikacin	Serum (speckled)	1
Amino acid	Serum (speckled)	3
Amiodarone	Serum (speckled)	10
Amitriptyline	Serum (red)	3
Ammonia	Plasma (green)	3
Ampicillin	Serum (red)	5
Amylase	Serum (speckled)	2
Androstenedione	Serum (speckled) *Deliver immediately	5

(continued)

Table 7–3. *(continued)*

TEST NAME	SPECIMEN TUBE (TYPE/COLOR)	WHOLE BLOOD, MINIMUM VOLUME FOR ADULTS (mL)
Angiotensin–converting enzyme (ACE)	Serum (speckled) *Ice needed for transportation	5
Antibody to hepatitis A virus (anti-HAV)	Serum (speckled)	5
Antibody to hepatitis B core antigen	Serum (red)	3
Antibody to hepatitis BE antigen	Serum (red)	3
Antibody to hepatitis B surface antigen	Serum (red)	3
Antibody identification	Whole blood (red)	7
Antibody screen and blood grouping	Whole blood (red)	5
Antibody titer	Whole blood (red)	5
Anticonvulsants (Dilantin, Mysoline, phenobarbital, carbamazepine, valproic acid)	Serum (speckled)	7
Antidiuretic hormone (ADH, vasopressin)	Whole blood (purple)	3
Anti–DNase B	Serum (speckled)	3
Antinuclear antibodies, fluorescent (ANA)	Whole blood (red)	5
Anti–smooth muscle antibody (ASMA)	Serum (speckled)	3
Antithrombin III	Plasma (light blue)	1
APTT	Plasma (light blue)	1.8
Arboviruses (St. Louis encephalitis)	Serum (speckled)	3
Arsenic (As)	Whole blood (royal blue)	7
Ascorbic acid (see Vitamin C)		
ASO (anti–streptolysin O) titer	Serum (speckled)	3
Aspirin (see Salicylate)		
Autologous blood	Whole blood (red)	5
Bactrim (see Sulfonamides)		
Barbiturates	Serum (speckled)	2
B-cell antigen	Whole blood (red)	3
Benzodiazepines	Serum (speckled)	2
Beta$_2$-microglobulin	Serum (speckled)	3
Bilirubin, total and direct	Serum (speckled) *Protect blood from light	1
Blastomycosis, complement fixation (fungal serology)	Serum (speckled)	4
Bleeding time	Patient	Test performed on patient's arm
Blood packed red blood cells	Whole blood (red)	5
Blood cell count, CBC survey (WBC, RBC, Hgb, Hct, MCV, MCH, MCHC)	Whole blood (purple)	3

(continued)

Table 7–3. *(continued)*

TEST NAME	SPECIMEN TUBE (TYPE/COLOR)	WHOLE BLOOD, MINIMUM VOLUME FOR ADULTS (mL)
Blood cell count, differential	Blood smear	Blood smear
Blood cell count, eosinophil	Whole blood (purple)	3
Blood cell count, erythrocyte (RBC)	Whole blood (purple)	3
Blood cell count, leukocyte (WBC)	Whole blood (purple)	3
Blood cell count, platelets	Whole blood (purple)	3
Blood cell count, reticulocyte	Whole blood (purple)	3
Blood gases, arterial (ABG) (pH, pCO_2, pO_2, HCO_3^-, base excess [BE])	Arterial blood (heparinized syringe)	0.6
Bordetella pertussis antibody (whooping cough)	Serum (red)	3
Borrelia burgdorferi antibody (Lyme disease)	Serum (red)	3
Bromide	Serum (red)	2
Brucella	Serum (speckled)	2
BUN (blood urea nitrogen)	Serum (speckled)	1
Cadmium (Cd)	Whole blood (green, purple) *Use acid-washed syringes	2
Calcitonin	Plasma (green)	3
Calcium	Serum (speckled)	1
Calcium, ionized	Plasma (green)	3
Candida serology, qualitative	Serum (speckled)	3
Carbamazepine (see Tegretol)		
Carbon dioxide (CO_2)	Serum (speckled)	1
Carcinoembryonic antigen (CEA)	Serum (speckled)	3
Cardiac troponins (cTnI, cTnT)	Serum (speckled)	3
Cardiolipin antibodies (anti–cardiolipin antibody IgG and IgM)	Serum (speckled)	3
Carotene	Serum (speckled)	3
Catecholamines	Whole blood (purple) *Ice needed for transportation	20
Ceruloplasmin	Serum (speckled)	3
Chemistry screen (T. protein, Alb, Ca, I phos, Glu, BUN, uric acid, Creat, T. bil, Alk p'tase, LDH, ALT)	Serum (speckled)	3
Chickenpox titer	Serum (speckled)	3
Chloramphenicol	Serum (speckled)	4
Chloride	Serum (speckled)	1
Cholesterol	Serum (speckled)	1
Cholinesterase	Serum (speckled)	3
Chromium (Cr)	Serum (royal blue) *Avoid chromium-plated needles; use platinum needles and acid-washed syringes	2

(continued)

Table 7–3. *(continued)*

TEST NAME	SPECIMEN TUBE (TYPE/COLOR)	WHOLE BLOOD, MINIMUM VOLUME FOR ADULTS (mL)
Chromosome analysis	Sterile whole blood (green) (Na heparin)	7
Circulating anticoagulants	Plasma (light blue)	3
Clonazepam	Serum (red) or plasma (purple)	2
CMV, IFA serology	Serum (speckled)	3
Coccidioides immitis (San Joaquin fever)	Serum (speckled)	3
Cold agglutinins	Whole blood (speckled) *Place in warm water and deliver immediately	3
Complement, total	Serum (speckled)	5
Complement—C3	Serum (speckled)	5
Complement—C4	Serum (speckled)	5
Coombs' test, direct (direct antiglobulin test)	Whole blood (red)	3
Coombs' test, indirect (indirect antiglobulin test)	Whole blood (red)	5
Copper (Cu)	Serum (speckled) or whole blood (royal blue)	3
Cortisol	Plasma (green)	1
Coxiella burnetii (Q fever)	Serum (speckled)	3
Coxsackievirus (Bornholm disease)	Serum (speckled)	3
C-peptide	Serum (speckled)	3
CPK (CK)	Serum (speckled)	1
CPK isoenzymes (CK isoenzymes) (CK-MB)	Serum (speckled)	3
C-reactive protein	Serum (speckled)	2
Creatinine	Serum (speckled)	1
Cross-match	Whole blood (red)	3
Cryofibrinogen	Plasma (green)	1
Cryoglobulin	Serum (speckled) *Immediately place in warm water and transport to lab	4
Cryptococcal antigen	Serum (red)	3
Cyclosporine	Serum (speckled)	3
Cysticercus cellulosae (pork tapeworm)	Serum (red)	3
Cytomegalovirus (CMV), IFA serology	Serum (speckled)	3
D-dimer (D-D$_1$)	Whole blood (blue)	3.5
Dengue virus antibody (breakbone fever)	Serum (speckled)	3
Deoxycorticosteroids	Serum (speckled) or plasma (green)	3
Depakene (see Valproic Acid)		
Desipramine	Serum (speckled) or plasma (green)	5

(continued)

Table 7–3. *(continued)*

TEST NAME	SPECIMEN TUBE (TYPE/COLOR)	WHOLE BLOOD, MINIMUM VOLUME FOR ADULTS (mL)
DHEA	Serum (red) *Immediately place in ice slurry and transport to lab	10
Diazepam (see Valium)		
Digitoxin	Serum (speckled)	2
Digoxin (Lanoxin)	Serum (speckled)	2
Dilantin (phenytoin)	Serum (speckled)	1
Directogen for *Haemophilus influenzae, Streptococcus pneumoniae, Neisseria meningitidis*	Serum (speckled)	3
DNA antibody (anti-DNA)	Serum (speckled)	3
Drug screen	Serum (speckled)	10
EBV–early antigen	Serum (speckled)	3
EBV-IgM	Serum (speckled)	3
EBV-NA	Serum (speckled)	3
EBV-VCA	Serum (speckled)	3
Echinococcus (hydatid disease)	Serum (red)	3
Electrolytes (Na, K, Cl, HCO_3)	Plasma (green) or whole blood (green)	2
Electrophoresis (hemoglobin)	Whole blood (purple)	1
Electrophoresis (immuno)	Serum (speckled)	3
Electrophoresis (SPE)	Serum (speckled)	3
Elution studies	Whole blood (purple)	2
Entamoeba histolytica	Serum (speckled)	3
Eosinophil count	Whole blood (purple)	1
E-rosette	Whole blood (purple)	3
E-rosette receptor	Whole blood (purple)	3
Erythrocyte fragility	Whole blood (purple)	1
Erythrocyte osmotic fragility	Whole blood (green)	2
Erythromycin	Serum (speckled)	5
Erythropoietin	Serum (speckled)	5
ESR (sedimentation rate, sed rate)	Whole blood (purple)	3
Estradiol (E_2)	Serum (speckled) or plasma (green)	3
Estriol	Serum (speckled) or plasma (green)	3
Estrogens, total	Serum (speckled)	7
Ethanol (alcohol)	Whole blood (gray)	2
Ethosuximide (Zarontin)	Plasma (green)	3
Euglobulin lysis	Plasma (blue)	4.5
Factor assays	Plasma (blue)	4.5
Fasting blood glucose (FBG)	Plasma (gray)	1
Fatty acids, free	Serum (speckled) *Transport in ice water	10
Febrile agglutinins	Serum (speckled)	7

(continued)

Table 7-3. (*continued*)

TEST NAME	SPECIMEN TUBE (TYPE/COLOR)	WHOLE BLOOD, MINIMUM VOLUME FOR ADULTS (mL)
Ferritin	Serum (speckled)	2
Fetal hemoglobin	Whole blood (purple)	2
Fibrin degradation products (FDP) (FSP)	Plasma (blue)	2
Fibrinogen	Plasma (blue)	1.8
Fibrinogen antigen	Plasma (blue)	4.5
Fibrinopeptide A	Whole blood with special tube from hematology	5
Fitzgerald factor	Plasma (blue)	4.5
Flecainide	Serum (red)	3
Fletcher factor (prekallinkrein)	Plasma (blue)	4.5
Fluorescent antinuclear antibody	Serum (speckled)	3
Fluorescent treponemal antibody test (MHA-TP)	Serum (red or speckled)	3
Fluoride	Serum (red)	6
Folate, serum	Serum (speckled)	3
Folate, whole blood (RBC and serum)	Whole blood (purple)	3
Follicle-stimulating hormone (FSH)	Serum (speckled) or plasma (green)	3
Fragility, erythrocyte (RBC)	Whole blood (purple)	2
Francisella tularensis antibody (tularemia)	Serum (speckled)	3
Free, T_4 (see Thyroxine, free)		
Free thyroxine index (see Thyroid studies)		
Fungal serology	Serum (speckled)	3
Gamma-glutamyl transpeptidase (GGT) (GT)	Serum (speckled)	3
Gastrin	Serum (speckled)	7
Gentamicin	Serum (speckled)	1
Glucagon	Whole blood (purple)	3
Glucose (FBS and tolerance)	Plasma (gray) or serum (speckled)	1
Glucose-6-phosphate dehydrogenase (G6PD), quantitative	Whole blood (green)	1
Glucose, 2-hour postprandial	Plasma (gray) or serum (speckled)	1
Glycosylated hemoglobin	Whole blood (purple)	1
Gonadotropin HCG-beta (immuno test)	Serum (speckled)	7
Growth hormone (HGH)	Serum (speckled)	1.5
Hamm's test (PNH) confirmation	Plasma (green)	5
Haptoglobin	Serum (speckled)	1
HDL (high-density lipoprotein) cholesterol	Serum (speckled)	5

(*continued*)

Table 7–3.   (continued)

TEST NAME	SPECIMEN TUBE (TYPE/COLOR)	WHOLE BLOOD, MINIMUM VOLUME FOR ADULTS (mL)
Heinz body preparation	Whole blood (purple) or (green)	3
Helper T	Whole blood (purple)	2
Hematocrit	Whole blood (purple)	1
Hematology profile (Hct, Hgb, WBC, RBC, MCV, MCH, MCHC)	Whole blood (purple)	1
Hemoglobin	Whole blood (purple)	1
Hemoglobin, plasma	Plasma (purple)	1
Heparin	Plasma (blue)	3
Hepatitis A Ab IgM (Anti–HAV-IgM)	Serum (speckled)	5
Hepatitis B core antibody (HB$_c$Ab) (Anti-HB$_c$)	Serum (speckled)	3
Hepatitis B surface Ab (Anti-HB$_s$)	Serum (speckled)	4
Hepatitis B surface antigen (HB$_s$Ag)	Serum (speckled)	3
Hepatitis C Ab (HCV)	Serum (speckled)	5
HCV RNA	Serum (red)	1
Hepatitis delta antibody and antigen	Serum (speckled)	3
Hepatitis G test	Serum (red)	10
Herpes simplex, virus serology	Serum (speckled)	3
Heterophile antibody (see Monospot)		
Histamine	Serum (speckled)	5
Histoplasmosis	Serum (speckled)	5
HI titer (St. Louis encephalitis)	Serum (speckled)	3
HIV antibody screen	Serum (speckled)	5
HIV antigen	Serum (speckled)	3
HLA typing (microcytotoxicity)	Whole blood (green)	5
Human chorionic gonadotrophin (HCG)	Serum (speckled)	6
Human growth hormone (HGH) (see Growth hormone)		
Human T-cell lymphotropic virus type I (HTLV-1) antibody	Serum (speckled)	2
Hydroxybutyric dehydrogenase (HBD)	Serum (speckled)	5
IgA	Serum (speckled)	1
IgD	Serum (speckled)	1
IgG	Serum (speckled)	1
IgM	Serum (speckled)	1
Imipramine (Tofranil)	Serum (red)	10
Infectious mononucleosis (see Monospot)		
Inhibitor assay	Plasma (blue)	4.5
Insulin (on ice)	Plasma (purple)	4.5

(continued)

Table 7–3. (*continued*)

TEST NAME	SPECIMEN TUBE (TYPE/COLOR)	WHOLE BLOOD, MINIMUM VOLUME FOR ADULTS (mL)
Intrinsic factor antibody	Serum (speckled)	3
Iron profile (iron, TIBC, and saturation)	Serum (speckled)	3
Kanamycin	Serum (speckled)	5
Lactate dehydrogenase (LD) and LD isoenzymes (LD-1)	Serum (speckled)	3
Lactic acid (on ice)	Plasma (gray)	1
Lanoxin (see Digoxin)		
LDL (low-density lipoprotein) cholesterol	Serum (speckled)	10
Lead, blood	Blood (royal blue) or special tube from chem	2
LE cell test	Whole blood (green)	3
Legionnaires' serology	Serum (speckled)	3
Leishmania antibody	Serum (speckled)	3
Leptospira agglutination	Serum (speckled)	3
Leucine aminopeptidase (LAP)	Plasma (green)	2
Leukocyte alkaline phosphatase (LAP) stain		Six fresh blood smears
LGV-psittacosis titer	Serum (speckled)	5
LH (see Luteinizing hormone)		
Lidocaine	Serum (speckled)	5
Lipase	Serum (speckled)	2
Lipid profile	Serum (speckled)	10
Lithium	Serum (speckled)	1
Low-density lipoprotein (LDL) cholesterol	Serum (speckled)	5
Lupus anticoagulant (tissue thromboplastin inhibition test)	Plasma (blue) *Deliver immediately	5
Luteinizing hormone (LH)	Serum (speckled)	2
Lyme disease serology	Serum (speckled)	4
Lymphocyte blastogenesis (LBR)	Whole blood (green)	7
Lymphogranuloma venereum	Serum (speckled)	3
Lysozyme, serum	Serum (speckled)	2
Magnesium, serum	Serum (speckled)	1
Malaria antibody	Serum (speckled)	2
Malaria smear		Blood smear
Manganese (Mn)	Whole blood (royal blue) or serum *Use acid-washed syringes	5
Mercury (Hg)	Whole blood (royal blue)	5
Methemalbumin	Serum (speckled)	2
Methemoglobin	Serum (speckled)	3
Methicillin	Serum (speckled)	5
Methotrexate	Serum (red)	2
MHA-TP	Serum (speckled or red)	3

(*continued*)

Table 7–3. (continued)

TEST NAME	SPECIMEN TUBE (TYPE/COLOR)	WHOLE BLOOD, MINIMUM VOLUME FOR ADULTS (mL)
Molecular diagnostic lab tests	Whole blood (purple) *Immediately transport in ice slurry	3 × 10 mL
Monocyte antigens	Whole blood (purple)	2
Monospot (Ortho Diagnostics, Raritan, NJ) (infectious mononucleosis	Serum (speckled)	4
Mumps serology	Serum (speckled)	3
Mycoplasma pneumoniae	Serum (speckled)	2
Myelin antibodies	Serum (speckled)	3
NAPA (see Procainamide)		
Nickel (Ni)	Plasma, serum, whole blood *Must prepare collection vials by acid-washing syringes	5
5′-Nucleotidase	Serum (speckled)	2
Nutritional panel	Serum (speckled)	2
Opiates (methadone, codeine, morphine)	Serum (speckled)	3
Osmolality, serum	Serum (speckled)	2
Parathyroid hormone (PTH)	Serum (speckled)	2
Partial thromboplastin time (PTT) (APTT)	Plasma (blue)	1
Penicillin	Serum (red)	5
Pentobarbital	Serum (speckled)	5
pH, blood (see Blood gases)		
Phenobarbital	Serum (speckled)	2
Phenylalanine	Whole blood *Filter paper with low background fluorescence	Droplets used to saturate filter paper (< 0.5)
Phenytoin (Dilantin)	Serum (speckled)	1
Phenytoin (free)	Serum (speckled)	5
Phosphorus	Serum (speckled)	1
Plasminogen antigen	Whole blood (blue)	5
Platelet function profile	Whole blood (purple) Whole blood (blue)	1 / 7
Pneumocystic serology	Serum (red)	3
Potassium	Plasma (green)	2
Prealbumin	Serum (speckled)	3
Precursor T	Whole blood (purple)	2
Primidone (Mysoline)	Serum (speckled)	2
Procainamide, N-acetylprocainamide (NAPA)	Serum (speckled)	2
Progesterone	Clotted whole blood (red) *Avoid serum separator tube in speckled tube top	3
Prolactin	Serum (speckled)	2
Pronestyl (procainamide)	Serum (speckled)	2

(continued)

Table 7–3.   *(continued)*

TEST NAME	SPECIMEN TUBE (TYPE/COLOR)	WHOLE BLOOD, MINIMUM VOLUME FOR ADULTS (mL)
Propranolol	Serum (speckled) or plasma (purple)	3
Protein, total	Serum (speckled)	1
Protein, total A/G ratio	Serum (speckled)	1
Proteus OX 19	Serum (speckled)	2
Prothrombin consumption time	Serum (speckled)	3
Protime (International Technidyne Corporation, Edison, NJ) (prothrombin time, PT)	Plasma (blue)	2
Prostatic acid phosphatase (PAP) (see Acid phosphatase)		
PSA (prostatic specific antigen)	Serum (speckled)	1
PTH (see Parathyroid hormone)		
Pyruvate	Whole blood (gray) *Transport immediately in ice water	5
Q fever antibodies	Serum (speckled)	3
Quinidine	Serum (speckled)	1
Rabies virus antibody	Serum (speckled)	3
Renin activity	Plasma (purple) *Transport immediately in ice water	2
Reptilase time	Whole blood (blue)	3.5
Reticulocyte	Whole blood (purple)	5
Rheumatoid factor assay	Serum (speckled)	2
Rickettsial *Proteus* antibodies (*Proteus* OX 19)	Serum (speckled)	3
RPR	Serum (speckled)	2
Rubella	Serum (speckled)	4
Rubeola serology	Serum (speckled)	1
Russell viper venom (RVV) time (Stypven time)	Plasma (blue)	3
Salicylate (aspirin)	Serum (speckled)	2
Salmonella antibody	Serum (speckled)	5
Sedimentation rate (ESR) (erythrocyte sedimentation rate)	Whole blood (purple)	3
Selenium (Se)	Plasma, whole blood, serum (royal blue with heparin or EDTA or no anticoagulant)	3
Serotonin blood (5-hydroxytryptamine)	Whole blood or special tube from chem	10
SGOT (AST)	Serum (speckled)	1
SGPT (ALT)	Serum (speckled)	1
Sickling screen	Whole blood (purple)	2
Sjögren's antibody	Serum (red)	7
Sodium, serum	Serum (speckled)	1

(continued)

Table 7–3.   *(continued)*

TEST NAME	SPECIMEN TUBE (TYPE/COLOR)	WHOLE BLOOD, MINIMUM VOLUME FOR ADULTS (mL)
SPE (serum protein electrophoresis)	Serum (speckled)	3
Special stains		
Acid phosphatase	Blood smear	
Alkaline phosphatase	Blood smear	
Esterases	Blood smear	
Heinz bodies	Blood smear	
Iron	Blood smear	
Lipid	Blood smear	
PAS for glycogen	Blood smear	
Peroxidase	Blood smear	
Sudan black	Blood smear	
Toluidine blue	Blood smear	
Streptozyme (Carter-Wallace, Inc., New York, NY) (multiple strep Ab screen)	Serum (speckled)	3
Stypven time (RVV time)	Plasma (blue)	3
Sucrose presumptive (PNH)	Whole blood (blue)	3
Sulfonamides	Serum (speckled)	5
Suppressor	Whole blood (purple)	3
Syphilis (RPR)	Serum (speckled)	2
T_3 uptake	Serum (speckled)	2
Tegretol (carbamazepine)	Serum (speckled)	2
Teichoic acid antibody	Serum (speckled)	5
Testosterone	Serum (speckled)	7
Theophylline (aminophylline)	Serum (speckled)	2
Thiamine	Whole blood (green)	10
Thiocyanate	Serum (speckled) or plasma (green) or plasma (purple)	8
Thrombin time (Fibrindex [Ortho Pharmaceutical Corporation, Raritan, NJ])	Plasma (blue)	3
Thyroglobulin	Serum (speckled)	5
Thyroid antibodies	Serum (speckled)	3
Thyroiditis, antithyroglobulin, and antimicrosomal fraction	Serum (speckled)	5
Thyroid studies (T_3, T_4, TSH)	Serum (speckled)	4
Thyroxine (T_4)	Serum (speckled)	2
Thyroxine (T_4), free	Serum (speckled)	3
Tobramycin	Serum (speckled)	1
Tofranil (see Imipramine)		
TORCH titers	Serum (speckled)	5
Total T_3 (triiodothyronine)	Serum (speckled)	2
Toxoplasmosis serological test, IFA	Serum (speckled)	3
Transaminase (ALT, SGPT)	Serum (speckled)	1
Transaminase (AST, SGOT)	Serum (speckled)	1

(continued)

Table 7–3. *(continued)*

TEST NAME	SPECIMEN TUBE (TYPE/COLOR)	WHOLE BLOOD, MINIMUM VOLUME FOR ADULTS (mL)
Transferrin	Serum (speckled)	2
Trichinella agglutination	Serum (speckled)	3
Tricyclic antidepressants (amitriptyline, nortriptyline)	Serum or plasma (red, green, or purple) [a]Avoid gel separator	3
Triglycerides (fasting)	Serum (speckled)	1
Troponin I (cTnI) troponin T (cTnT)	Serum (speckled)	3
TSH (thyroid-stimulating hormone, or thyrotropin)	Serum (speckled)	2
Tylenol (see Acetominophen)		
Urea nitrogen (BUN)	Serum (speckled)	1
Uric acid	Serum (speckled)	1
Valium (diazepam)	Serum (red)	2
Valproic acid (Depakene)	Serum (speckled)	5
Vancomycin	Serum (speckled)	1
Varicella-zoster immune status	Serum (speckled)	2
Varicella-zoster serology	Serum (speckled)	2
VDRL (RPR) syphilis	Serum (speckled)	2
Vitamin A	Serum (speckled) *Protect blood from light	3
Vitamin B_6	Whole blood (purple)	10
Vitamin B_{12}	Serum (speckled)	2
Vitamin B_{12} binding capacity	Serum (speckled)	3
Vitamin C (ascorbic acid)	Whole blood (green) *Immediately transport in ice slurry	5
Vitamin D (25-OH)	Whole blood (purple)	7
Vitamin E level	Serum (speckled)	5
von Willebrand's factor assay (Rristocetin cofactor)	Whole blood (blue) *Deliver immediately	5
D-Xylose	Serum (red)	3
Zinc	Draw blood with syringe; transfer to special plastic tube from chemistry	5

[a]*Note:* For toxicology and therapeutic drugs, the speckled-topped gel serum separator tube should be evaluated to determine whether the gel serum separator interferes in test results before these tubes are used in drug analysis collections. (See Chapter 9.)

Abbreviations: A/G, albumin/globulin (ratio); Alb, albumin; Alk p'tase, alkaline phosphatase; ALT, alanine aminotransferase; APTT, activated partial thromboplastin time; AST, aspartate aminotransferase; Ca, calcium; CBC, complete blood (count); CMV, cytomegalovirus; CPK, creatine phosphokinase; Creat, creatinine; EBV, Epstein-Barr virus; ESR, erythrocyte sedimentation rate; FBS, fasting blood sugar; Glu, glucose; HB$_s$Ag, hepatitis B surface antigen; HCG, human chorionic gonadotropin; Hct, hematocrit; Hgb, hemoglobin; IFA, indirect fluorescent antibody (test); IgA, immunoglobulin A; IgD, immunoglobulin D; IgG, immunoglobulin G; IgM, immunoglobulin M; I phos, inorganic phosphorus; LD, lactate dehydrogenase; MCH, mean corpuscular hemoglobin; MCHC, mean corpuscular hemoglobin concentration; MCV, mean corpuscular volume; PAS, periodic acid–Schiff; PNH, paroxysmal nocturnal hemoglobinuria; RBC, red blood cell; RPR, rapid plasma reagin; RVV, Russell viper venom (time); SGOT, serum glutamic oxaloacetic transaminase; SGPT, serum glutamic pyruvic transaminase; SPE, serum protein electrophoresis; T. bil, total bilirubin; TIBC, total iron-binding capacity; T. protein, total protein; VDRL, Venereal Disease Research Laboratory; WBC, white blood cell.

tive. Because fluoride destroys many enzymes, this additive should not be used in blood collections for enzyme determinations (e.g., creatine kinase [CK], alanine aminotransferase [ALT], aspartate aminotransferase [AST], and alkaline phosphatase [ALP] determinations). Likewise, oxalate distorts cellular morphologic features. Thus, gray-topped tubes should not be used for hematology studies.

GREEN-TOPPED TUBES

The anticoagulants sodium heparin, ammonium heparin, and lithium heparin are found in green-topped vacuum tubes. These tubes are used in various laboratory assays requiring plasma or whole blood, which are mainly chemistry tests. For potassium measurement, heparinized plasma or whole blood, rather than serum, is preferred because sporadic increased potassium levels can occur in serum as a result of potassium released from platelets during blood clotting.[1] Lithium heparin tubes may be used for glucose, blood urea nitrogen (BUN), ionized calcium, creatinine, and electrolyte studies; however, this anticoagulant is not suitable for tests involving the measurement of lithium levels.[2] Similarly, sodium heparin tubes should not be used for assays that measure the sodium concentration. In other cases, a particular procedure will require sodium heparin without lithium or vice versa.

Green-topped vacuum tubes should not be used for collections for blood smears that are to be stained with Wright's stain because the heparin causes the Wright's stain to have a blue background. When used for cytogenetic studies, these tubes must be sterile.

PURPLE-TOPPED AND LIGHT BLUE–TOPPED TUBES

The purple-topped vacuum tubes (containing EDTA) are used for most hematology procedures. If a purple-topped tube is underfilled, the patient will have erroneously low blood cell counts and hematocrits, staining alterations, and erroneous morphologic changes to RBCs. Many coagulation procedures are done on blood collected in light blue–topped vacuum tubes, which contain sodium citrate at a concentration of 3.8 percent. If a light blue–topped tube is underfilled, coagulation results will be erroneously prolonged.

RED-TOPPED, ROYAL BLUE–TOPPED, AND BROWN-TOPPED TUBES

The red-topped tubes indicate a tube without anticoagulant for the collection of serum. Thus, the collected blood will clot in this tube. The royal blue–topped tubes are used to collect samples for nutritional studies, therapeutic drug monitoring, and toxicology. The royal blue–topped tube is the trace element tube. The brown-topped tube contains heparin or no additive and is used for blood lead values.

BLACK-TOPPED TUBES

From certain manufacturers, a black-topped tube with buffered sodium citrate is available for blood collections used to determine the erythrocyte sedimentation rate (ESR).

BLOOD CULTURE COLLECTION TUBES

Sterile blood specimens are also ordered for blood cultures when the patient is suspected of having septicemia (symptoms of sepsis). A major problem with collecting blood for culture is that the patient's sample can become contaminated with microorganisms from the skin. Thus, the blood must be collected in a sterile container (vacuum vial or syringe) under aseptic conditions. (See Chapter 12 for blood culture collections.)

As shown in Figure 7–8, blood can be collected directly into vacuum vials that contain culture media. This type of collection minimizes the risk of specimen contamination. The vacuum vials can be purchased with different types of culture media, an unplugged venting unit for aerobic incubation, or a plugged venting unit for anaerobic incubation.

SEPARATION TUBES (MOTTLED-TOPPED AND SPECKLED-TOPPED TUBES)

Another collection method is to draw blood into a serum separation tube, such as the Monoject Corvac (Sherwood, Davis & Geck, St. Louis, MO). Blood is collected in the vacuum Monoject Corvac Serum Separator tube by conventional blood-collecting means. As illustrated in Figure 7–9, this tube contains a gel with a specific gravity intermediate to serum and coagulation. During centrifugation, the gel forms a stable barrier between serum and coagulum.

■ SYRINGES

Some patients' veins are too fragile for blood collection with vacuum tubes. Thus, syringes must be used for the collection process. Syringes are also used for drawing blood from central venous catheter (CVC) lines. This procedure is discussed in detail in Chapter 12. A syringe, without the needle, consists of the barrel, the plunger, and the tip. The barrel and the plunger are made to fit together tightly so that when the plunger is in the barrel and drawn back, a vacuum is created. This vacuum allows blood or other fluids to be aspirated, or sucked, into the barrel as the plunger is pulled back. The barrel of the syringe has gradu-

Figure 7–8. BACTEC culture vials.

(Courtesy of Becton-Dickinson Diagnostic Instrument Systems, Sparks, MD.)

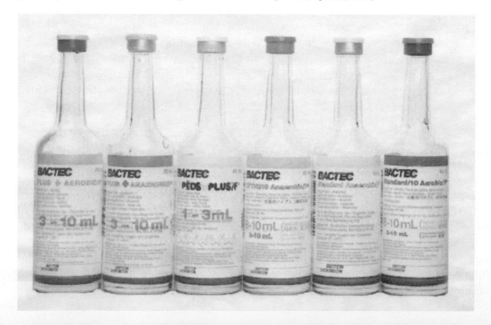

Figure 7–9. Monoject Corvac Serum Separator tube.

(Courtesy of Sherwood, Davis & Geck, St. Louis, MO.)

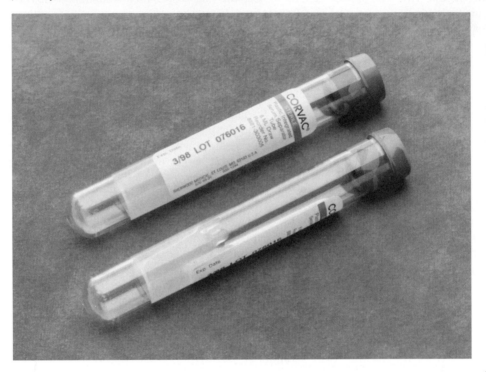

ated measurements in milliliter increments. Sizes range from approximately 0.2 to 50.0 mL; however, for specimen collection purposes, 5- to 20-mL syringes are used most often. A needle is usually attached directly on the smooth tip of the syringe. Some syringes have Luer-Lok tips (Becton-Dickinson VACUTAINER Systems, Franklin Lakes, NJ), which lock the needle onto the tip for a firm hold. In addition, the health care worker should ensure that the syringe is the correct size for the amount of blood to be collected.

 Clinical Alert

To avoid possible needlestick injuries, it is highly advisable to use safety syringes, such as the S-Monovette Blood Collection (Sarstedt, Inc., Newton, NC), B-D Safety Lok (Becton-Dickinson VACUTAINER Systems, Franklin Lakes, NJ), Monoject with needle guard (Sherwood, Davis & Geck, St. Louis, MO), and Bio-Plexus (Tolland, CT) Punctur-Guard needle products. These products are designed to reduce needlesticks by either sliding a cover over the needle after venipuncture or by making the needle "blunt," thereby reducing exposure to a sharp contaminated object.

Although disposable plastic syringes are used most frequently, on occasion a glass syringe may be needed for blood collection for a special procedure. In such cases, the glass plunger and barrel should be inspected carefully before use to check for possible cracks or chips.

■ NEEDLES

The gauge and length of a needle used on a syringe or a vacuum tube is selected according to the specific task. For example, larger (18-gauge) needles are used for collecting donor units of blood (450 mL or less), whereas smaller (21- and 22-gauge) needles are used for collecting specimens for laboratory assays. When blood is collected from children, a 21- to 23-gauge needle is usually used with a tuberculin, or 3-mL, syringe or with a winged infusion set. The **gauge number** indicates the diameter of the needle; the smaller the gauge number, the larger the needle. The length of the needle depends on the depth of the vein to be punctured. Needles are usually available as either 1 or 1.5 inch.

Needles are sterilized and packaged by vendors in sealed shields that maintain sterility. These shields are packaged in individual containers that are color coded according to the gauge size of the needles and must be twisted apart before the needles are used in blood collection.[2]

The tip of each needle should be checked for damage. A blunt or bent tip can be harmful to the patient's vein and may result in failure to collect blood.

Different types of needles are used for single- and multiple-sample collections. **Multiple-sample needles** are used with vacuum collection tubes and the holder to allow for multiple tube changes without blood leakage within the plastic holder. The multiple-sample needle has a plastic cover over the tube-top puncturing portion of the needle; this cover creates a leakage barrier. The **single-sample needle** is usually used for collecting blood with a syringe.

THE BUTTERFLY NEEDLE (BLOOD COLLECTION SET)

The butterfly needle, also referred to as a blood collection set or winged infusion set, is the most commonly used intravenous device. It is a stainless steel beveled needle and tube with attached plastic wings. The most common butterfly needle sizes are 21, 23, and 25 gauge. The butterfly needle is sometimes used in the collection of blood from patients who are difficult to stick by conventional methods (e.g., geriatric patients, cancer patients, pediatric patients).

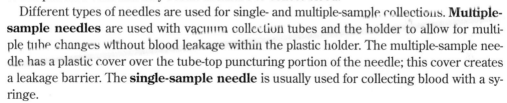

Clinical Alert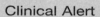

Winged infusion sets, however, account for the *highest* percentage of needlestick injuries.

Numerous types of safety butterfly needles are now available. These safety needles each have a shield that automatically covers the contaminated needle point upon withdrawal from the patient's vein. One example is the Angel Wing blood collection set (Fig. 7–10) from

Figure 7–10. Angel Wing blood collection set.

(Courtesy of Sherwood, Davis & Geck, St. Louis, MO.)

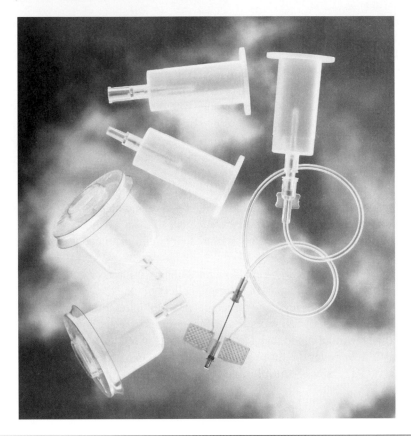

Sherwood, Davis & Geck (St. Louis, MO). It has a stainless steel safety shield that automatically resheaths the needle during withdrawal from the patient. The system includes multisample needle-shielded tube holders and sets for use in drawing blood specimens directly into blood collection tubes and blood culture bottles, as well as multisample needle-shielded transfer tube holders and sets for transferring blood from syringes into collection tubes and blood culture bottles.

The Shamrock safety winged set (Winfield Medical, San Diego, CA) has a luer hub that can be connected to a syringe or a multiple-sample luer adapter with a preattached Saf-T Holder (Winfield Medical, San Diego, CA) (Fig. 7–11). Another example of a winged infusion set is the Luer-Lok blood collection device (Fig. 7–12) manufactured by Becton-Dickinson VACUTAINER Systems. Bio-Plexus (Tolland, CT) also produces the Punctur-Guard winged-infusion set. The safety device uses an internal hollow blunt built within the sharp

Figure 7–11. Shamrock safety winged set. **A.** The luer hub can be connected to a syringe or a multiple-sample luer adapter with a preattached Saf-T Holder. **B.** After withdrawal from the patient's vein, the needle is simply and securely pulled back into its protective shield. **C.** The audible click and the visual indicator ensure that the needle has been locked into its protective shield for safe disposal.

(Courtesy of Winfield Medical, San Diego, CA.)

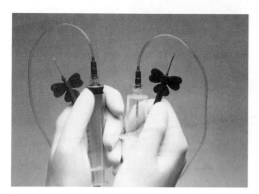

A

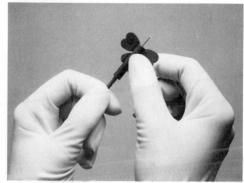

B

C

Figure 7–12. Luer-Lok blood collection device.

(Courtesy of Becton-Dickinson VACUTAINER Systems, Franklin Lakes, NJ.)

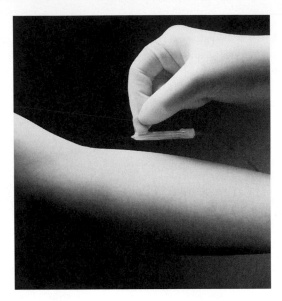

outer needle. When the blood samples have been withdrawn, the "internal blunt" is activated *prior* to removing the needle from the vein, thus reducing exposure to a sharp contaminated needle. No matter what type of blood collection set is used, it is imperative to use a luer adapter from the same manufacturer to avoid possible blood leakage and exposure.

NEEDLE DISPOSAL

As shown in Figure 7–13, Datar, Inc. (Long Lake, MN) produces a phlebotomy resheather and tube holder. This system allows needles to be resheathed safely, and it acts as a holder for vacuum tubes. Because the unit can be autoclaved, it can be reused. In addition, Datar, Inc. offers a pocket resheather (Fig. 7–14) that allows the phlebotomist to resheath needles safely with the "one-handed technique." The IV Pole Resheather (IV-R), also by Datar, Inc., provides a safe one-handed method (Fig. 7–15) for recapping needles from intermediate intravenous (IV) tubing and syringes. It can connect directly to an IV pole or be used as a portable stand-alone resheather.

Datar, Inc. also produces several sizes of needle-disposal containers (Fig. 7–16) for use at the bedside, on the cart, in isolation, during surgery, on home health care trays, and so on. Needles and syringes must be discarded in rigid plastic containers, which reduces the possibility of needle sticks for the phlebotomist. Each unit is disposable as biohazardous waste.

Figure 7–13. Phlebotomy resheather and tube holder.   **Figure 7–14.** Pocket resheather.

(Courtesy of Datar, Inc., Long Lake, MN.)   (Courtesy of Datar, Inc., Long Lake, MN.)

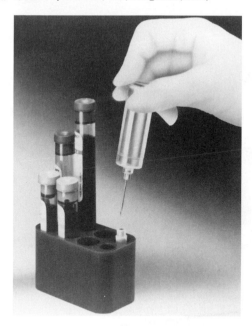 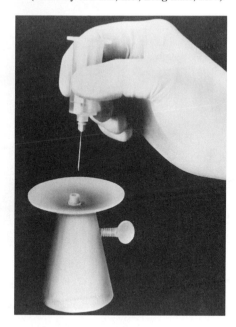

Figure 7–15. IV Pole Resheather.

(Courtesy of Datar, Inc., Long Lake, MN.)

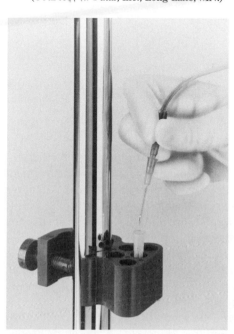

Figure 7–16. Needle disposal systems.

(Courtesy of Datar, Inc., Long Lake, MN.)

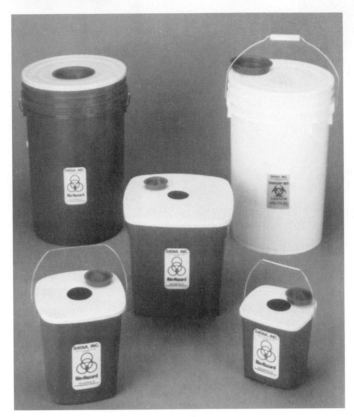

■ SAFE ACCESS TO BLOOD SAMPLES

After blood collection, the health care worker must gain access to the blood in the vacuum tube for testing purposes. To protect laboratory personnel against blood exposure during this hazardous step, manufacturers developed several different types of items.

An example is the Becton-Dickinson VACUTAINER tube with Hemogard. This device is a vacuum blood collection tube with a plastic shield over the stopper. The shield protects the health care worker from splattering blood when the stopper is removed from the tube.

The Pumpette (Helena Laboratories, Beaumont, TX) is a device that can provide access to the needed blood sample without uncapping the blood collection tube. The sample is aspirated by pressing the accordion-style pump on top of the stopper. Safety and efficiency are increased by using this device.

Another device that was developed to reduce the possibility of infection, contamination, and aerosol spray is the Aerotrap (Innovative Laboratory Products, Ltd., Citrus Heights, CA, distributed by Fisher Scientific, Citrus Heights, CA). It is used in laboratories to remove the stopper from vacuum tubes. The Aerotrap allows laboratory personnel to handle the vacuum tubes without touching the stoppers, and it reduces the amount of contamination that is hand carried throughout the laboratory.

After blood is drawn by syringe, it should immediately be transferred to a dry, chemically clean tube. The blood should be allowed to clot for a minimum of 15 minutes at room temperature, or longer if it is refrigerated. If the clot is allowed to retract for a longer period, the chances for hemolysis are decreased and the yield of serum is enhanced. The longer the blood cells remain in contact with the serum, the greater the shift of substances from blood cells to serum through the metabolic process of glycolysis.

■ TOURNIQUETS

The tourniquet is a key to successful venipuncture: it provides a barrier to slow down venous flow. Tourniquets are used in specimen collection to apply enough pressure to the arm to slow the return of venous blood to the heart. This slowing of venous return causes pooling of blood in the veins, which makes the veins more visible and easier to feel and find. A tourniquet should *not* restrict arterial blood flowing into the arm. Blood should enter the arm at a normal rate and, with the use of a tourniquet, return to the heart at a slower rate.

Tourniquets that are usually used include the pliable strap, the Velcro type, and the blood pressure cuff. The blood pressure cuff can be used successfully when veins are difficult to find. The most efficient blood barrier provides a resistance that is less than systolic blood pressure but greater than diastolic; or, stated another way, blood flows in but not out. The blood pressure cuff can determine these pressures; consequently, it is a perfect tourniquet.[4]

Another type of tourniquet is the Seraket (Propper Manufacturing Co., Inc., Long Island City, NY), which uses a seat-belt design. It allows the phlebotomist to release the venous pressure partially by using a lever that releases some pressure, but not all. Thus, if the phlebotomist needs to tighten the tourniquet again, the lever can be used to adjust the tourniquet. Because errors in laboratory test results can occur from prolonged tourniquet pressure, the Seraket provides a solution to this problem. One drawback of this type of tourniquet, however, is the difficulty in cleaning and decontaminating it if it is soiled with blood.

Velcro-type tourniquets are popular because they are easy to apply and comfortable for the patient. Alternatively, because of major concern for infection control in health care institutions, many facilities now use a disposable natural latex tourniquet strap (The Hygenic Corp., Akron, OH) to help prevent cross-contamination. If the tourniquets used in the health care facility are not disposable, they must be wiped frequently with 70 percent isopropyl alcohol.

■ BLEEDING-TIME EQUIPMENT

Bleeding time is an assay used to assess the contributions of platelet function and blood vessel integrity to primary blood-clotting abilities.[5] The test is performed by making a minor standardized incision in the forearm or earlobe and recording the length of time required for bleeding to stop. Many procedures have been used to measure bleeding time. Recent advances have led to the development of mechanical devices that are used to create uniform skin incisions for bleeding-time determination. One such device is the Hemalet (Medprobe

Laboratories, New York, NY), which has an automatic blade-retraction mechanism. Another such device is the Surgicutt (International Technidyne Corporation, Edison, NJ), which provides a uniform surgical incision. The procedure for determining bleeding time is provided in Chapter 12.

■ GLOVES FOR BLOOD COLLECTION

Safety guidelines have been established for health care workers to help them prevent the possibility of acquiring infections, such as hepatitis or those associated with AIDS. These guidelines include the use of gloves during collection of blood from patients. Examples of gloves being used by health care workers include Ultraderm sterile surgeon's gloves (Baxter Travenol Laboratories, Inc., Deerfield, IL), talc-free Eudermic surgical gloves (Becton-Dickinson and Company, Franklin Lakes, NJ), Medi-Pak latex gloves (General Medical Corp., Richmond, VA), and Lab Safety Supply nonirritating surgical gloves (Lab Safety Supply, Janesville, WI), which are made without talc. It is recommended that phlebotomists not use gloves with talc powder containing calcium because tubes of patients' blood may become contaminated with this powder, and such contamination can result in falsely elevated calcium values. Researchers have found that latex gloves provide better protection than vinyl gloves.[6] The Safeskin hypoallergenic latex glove (Safeskin Corporation, Coral Gables, FL) outperformed all other brands in the referenced study. Phlebotomists should not, however, use petroleum products or other skin protectants when wearing latex gloves because these substances break down the latex and decrease the active barrier.[7] If a health care worker develops allergenic dermatitis to gloves, she or he should try other brands of gloves or wear cotton gloves under the latex gloves. Stahmer Weston Scientific (Portsmouth, NH) developed UltraFIT glove liners (Fig. 7–17) for individuals who are extrasensitive to latex. These liners are made with 100 percent durable nylon material and can be washed several times for reuse. Another approach suggested by the US Food and Drug Administration (FDA) is to wear latex gloves between two vinyl gloves.[8]

 Clinical Alert

If the patient is allergic to latex, the phlebotomist should wear nonlatex gloves or latex gloves between two vinyl gloves. Also, in such cases, latex bandages or tourniquets should not be used on the patient. Instead, a cloth tourniquet and latex-free tape should be used.

Glove liners have also been developed that provide hand protection from cuts, nicks, and abrasions (Vigard Medical Products, Lovell-Schenck, Inc., Charlotte, NC). These glove liners are available in three styles—reusable, disposable, and clinical.

Uarco, Inc. (Barrington, IL) developed adhesive labels that do not stick to gloves. These

Figure 7–17.   UltraFIT glove liner.

(Courtesy of Stahmer Weston Scientific, Portsmouth, NH.)

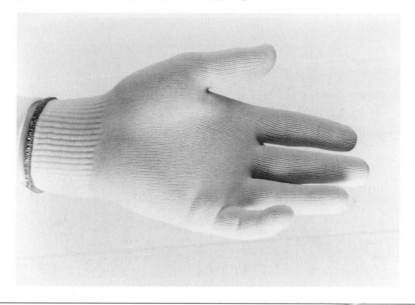

Glove-Free labels adhere firmly to glass, plastic, and paper, but they do not stick to vinyl or latex gloves. The labels, coated with a special adhesive, aid laboratory safety by eliminating the problem of torn gloves caused by trying to remove an adhering label.

■ ANTISEPTICS, STERILE GAUZE PADS, AND BANDAGES

The health care worker needs **antiseptics, sterile gauze pads,** and bandages for blood collection by either venipuncture or microcollection. Therefore, 70 percent isopropyl alcohol preparation and povidone–iodine (Betadine) swab sticks or pads (for blood cultures) are essential items for blood collection.

Clinical Alert

In home health care and other ambulatory health care environments where soap and water may not be readily available for the blood collector to wash his or her hands, an antimicrobial safety scrub (Fig. 7–18) should be carried with other blood collection items and used before and after blood collection.

Figure 7–18.   Safety-Soft antibacterial foam hand scrub.

(Courtesy of Bio-Medical Products Corp., Mendham, NJ.)

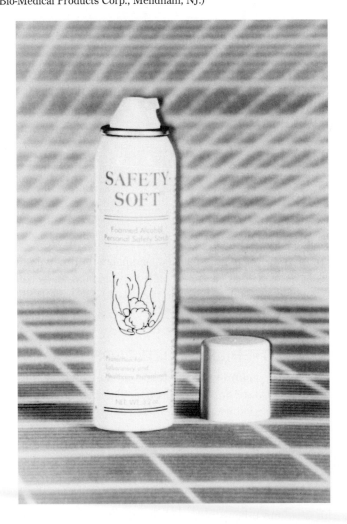

■ MICROCOLLECTION EQUIPMENT

Usually, skin puncture blood-collecting techniques are used on infants because venipuncture is excessively hazardous. Skin puncture collection is also indicated for adults and older children when they are severely burned, have veins that are difficult to stick because of their small size or location, must undergo bedside clinical testing, are extremely obese, or must perform home glucose testing.

The volume of plasma or serum that generally can be collected from a premature infant is approximately 100 to 150 μL, and about two times that amount can be taken from a full-term newborn. Larger volumes are obtained from older children and adults.[9]

Clinical Alert

A **disposable sterile lancet** should be used to puncture the skin for skin puncture collection. To avoid possible blood-borne pathogen exposure, it is highly recommended to use a "retracting lancet." Surgical blades should not be used for skin puncture due to hazards to the patient and phlebotomist.

For newborns, lancets with tips 2.4 mm or less in length, such as the Microtainer safety flow lancet (Becton-Dickinson VACUTAINER Systems, Franklin Lakes, NJ) (Fig. 7–19), are required to avoid penetrating bone.[10] Research indicates that for some infants (including premature infants) a puncture depth of 2.4 mm may be excessive and that the appropriate puncture depth for infants requires more study.[11] The Monolet OPD lancet (Sherwood, Davis & Geck, St. Louis, MO), as shown in Figure 7–20, is a lancet available for safe skin

---

Figure 7–19. Microtainer safety flow lancet.

(Courtesy of Becton-Dickinson VACUTAINER Systems, Franklin Lakes, NJ.)

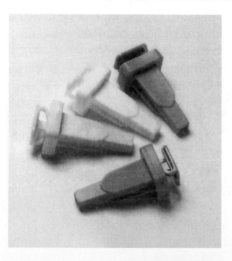

Figure 7–20. Monolet and Monojector lancet device.

(Courtesy of Sherwood, Davis & Geck, St. Louis, MO.)

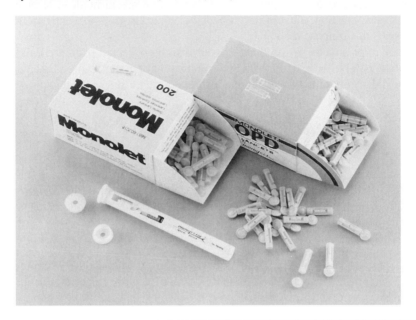

puncture of neonates. In addition, Sherwood, Davis & Geck manufactures the Monoject Monolettor safety lancet that automatically retracts and locks after puncture.

International Technidyne Corporation (Edison, NJ) has produced fully automated, single-use, automatically retracting, disposable devices that provide safety both for the neonate and for the health care worker (Fig. 7–21). Tenderlett jr. for children, Tenderlett for adults, and Tenderlett toddler for infants and toddlers are engineered to incise to the least invasive but most effective depth for optimal blood flow. The Tenderlett incises 1.75-mm deep, Tenderlett jr. incises 1.25-mm deep, and Tenderlett toddler incises only 0.85-mm deep. The retracting blade of each of these devices eliminates potential injury from an exposed blade contaminated with blood.

The Unistik 2 microcollection lancet is available in three penetration ranges (1.8, 2.4, and 3.0 mm) and automatically retracts after incision. The devices are color coded for easy identification of penetration depth. The Unistik 2 line of single-use capillary sampling devices now has four versions: Neonatal, Normal, Extra, and Super.

Other devices for microcollection are the Autolet II Clinisafe (Fig. 7–22) and the Autolet Lite Clinisafe (Fig. 7–23), both by Owen Mumford Inc., Marietta, GA. The Autolet II Clinisafe is a spring-activated puncture device that allows easy ejection of the lancet and platform, providing safety for both patient and phlebotomist. The Autolet platform can be chosen for the patient's level of comfort and the needed blood volume. These platforms are available in three color-coded depths: white (1.8 mm) for shallow penetration, yellow (2.4 mm) for normal penetration, and orange (3.0 mm) for deeper incisions.

Figure 7–21.   Tenderlett Automated Skin Incision Device.

(Courtesy of International Technidyne Corp., Edison, NJ.)

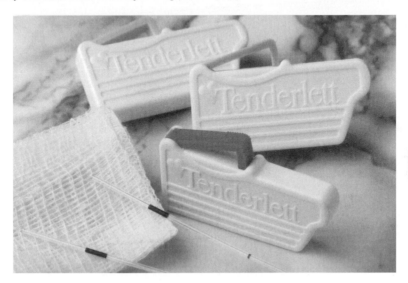

Figure 7–22.   Autolet II Clinisafe blood-drawing device.

(Courtesy of Owen Mumford, Inc., Marietta, GA.)

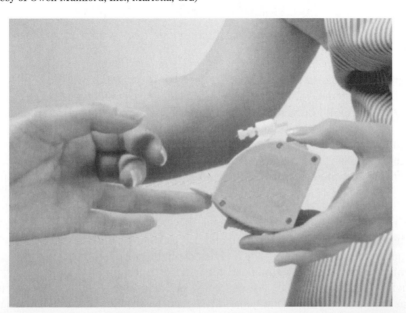

Figure 7–23.   Autolet Lite Clinisafe.

(Courtesy of Owen Mumford, Inc., Marietta, GA.)

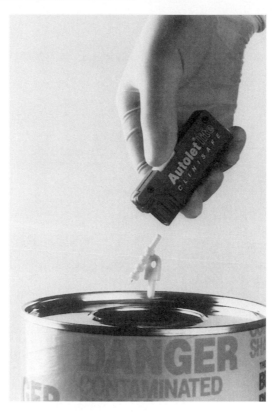

The Autolet Lite Clinisafe features a safety mechanism that inhibits the use of the device unless it is first reloaded with a new lancet and platform. Complying with FDA and Centers for Disease Control and Prevention (CDC) guidelines, both the lancet and the platform can be used only *once* and are simultaneously ejected at the touch of a button.

Superlite lancets have been developed with a slimmer needle and a new bevel to allow for smooth and easy skin penetration, which provides more comfort for the patient. Blades that do not provide appropriate control of the cutting edge and depth of puncture should not be used.

Two laser-based devices have been undergoing clinical evaluations. They are the Lasette (Cell Robotics, Albuquerque, NM) and Laser Lancet (Transmedica, Little Rock, AR). The laser penetrates to a depth of 1 to 2 mm and 250 μm wide. This is a smaller puncture hole than other devices make. Up to 100 μL of blood can be collected.[12]

The **microcontainers** recommended for use for collections for blood gas, electrolyte, and general chemistry analyses are described in Table 7–4. Usually, microspecimens for blood gas analysis are collected in heparinized glass Natelson tubes. These tubes may have

Table 7–4.   Containers for Blood Collection

CONTAINER[a]	REMARKS
Blood gases (pH, pCO$_2$, pO$_2$):	
Natelson glass collecting pipettes, 250-μL volume, lithium heparin; heparinized glass capillary tubes, 100 to 250 μL.	To mix, insert metal "fleas," or mixing bars, after filling.[b] Seal with plastic caps or sealing wax. Mix by use of a magnet. Source: many laboratory suppliers.
Blood-collecting pipette kits and component parts, supplied by manufacturers of blood gas apparatus.	Kits containing glass capillaries, sealing wax, metal mixing bars, and magnets. Source: laboratory suppliers of Corning, IL, and radiometer equipment.
Caraway glass tubes, 370-mL volume, sodium or lithium heparin.	Mix and seal as above, or by inversion. Source: many laboratory suppliers.
Electrolytes (CO$_2$, Cl, K, Na) and general chemistry:	
Microhematocrit glass capillary tubes 1.1–1.2 mm inner diameter, 75-mm long, ammonium heparin; other sizes.	Plasma obtained. Mix and seal as above.
Microsample tubes, polyethylene, 300 μL, lithium heparin; larger sizes (400 to 550 μL) for general chemistry, with and without heparin.	Plasma obtained. Seal with attached cap. Mix by inversion.[c] Source: Kew Scientific and Beckman Instruments, Inc., Fullerton, CA.
Microtainer, polypropylene, 600 and 700 mL, silicone separator, with and without lithium heparin.	Serum obtained. Seal with accompanying cap. Centrifuge at 6000 $\times$ g. Source: Becton-Dickinson VACUTAINER Systems, Franklin Lakes, NJ.

[a]Containers listed here are all commercially available.
[b]Mixing without a flea is also possible by gently inverting the capillary before sealing.
[c]Shake the first drop entering the tube to its bottom. All further drops should then flow along the path of the first drop if the tube is held in a nearly vertical position.
From Meites S (ed): *Pediatric Clinical Chemistry,* 3rd ed. Washington, DC; American Association for Clinical Chemistry; 1989, p 10, with permission.

a color band indicating the presence and type of anticoagulant. The band also identifies the top part of the pipette in reference to sample handling. A red band indicates an ammonium heparin coating in the tube, and a green band indicates a sodium or lithium heparin coating. Because ammonium ions can falsely change the blood pH of the collected blood, sodium or lithium heparin should be used in collections for blood gas analysis. The blood collected in these tubes must be mixed with the heparin by a small metal "flea," or bar, with a magnet. After mixing, the ends are sealed with sealing wax or plastic caps.

AVL Scientific Corporation (Graz, Austria) has developed the AVL microsampler for collection of two 120-μL **arterial blood gas** samples from children or adults. It has a 26-gauge microneedle, which reduces the chances of puncture pain and hematoma formation. The tubes are coated with heparin to prevent clotting, and they automatically fill without bubble formation. This microsampler is used on the radial, brachial, or femoral artery.

Microhematocrit **capillary tubes** are disposable narrow-bore pipettes that are used for packed red cell volume in microcentrifugation. These tubes also have colored bands; a red band indicates a heparin-coated tube, and a blue band indicates no anticoagulant. The Safe-Crit™ (Statspin/IRIS, Norwood, MA) is a microhematocrit tube made of plastic to avoid the hazard of glass breakage.

Plastic microcollection devices for general laboratory collections (e.g., chemistry, immunology) are usually color coded according to the established protocol for blood collection vacuum tube tops. Thus, purple-topped (lavender-topped) tubes contain EDTA, green-topped tubes contain heparin, red- or pink-topped tubes have no additive, and gray-topped tubes have sodium fluoride to inhibit blood enzymes that destroy glucose.

Sherwood, Davis & Geck (St. Louis, MO) manufactures the Samplette capillary blood collector (Fig. 7–24), which is offered with a full range of anticoagulants and serum and plasma separation gels. One of their collectors is an amber capillary blood separator that provides protection for light-sensitive analytes (e.g., bilirubin).

Electrolytes and general chemistry microspecimens can be collected in the Microtainer tube (Becton-Dickinson VACUTAINER Systems, Franklin Lakes, NJ), which has its own capillary blood collector, self-contained serum separator, and plastic top (Fig. 7–25). This system can collect as much as 600 μL of blood. Alternatively, two or more capillary tubes can be used for electrolyte and general chemistry collection. One advantage of these tubes is that if blood hemolyzes in one capillary tube, another capillary tube containing the patient's sample can be used for the chemical analyses.

The Multivette capillary blood collection system (Sarstedt, Inc., Newton, NC) is another microcollection system that is offered with a full range of anticoagulants and serum separation gel. This system can be used to collect, store, and separate samples in the same unbreakable, disposable container.

RAM Scientific Co. (Needham, MA) has developed an unbreakable plastic capillary-receptacle system called the SAFE-T-FILL capillary blood collection system. The device consists of a plastic capillary inserted into a microtube receptacle (Fig. 7–26). With the attached receptacle, blood flows directly to the bottom of the tube. This system makes the

Figure 7–24.   Samplette capillary blood collector.

(Courtesy of Sherwood, Davis & Geck, St. Louis, MO.)

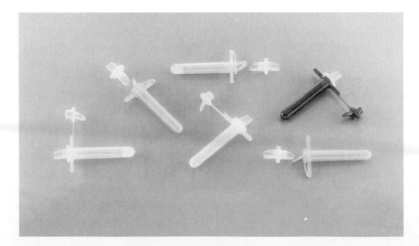

Figure 7–25.   Microtainer tube.

(Courtesy of Becton-Dickinson VACUTAINER Systems, Franklin Lakes, NJ.)

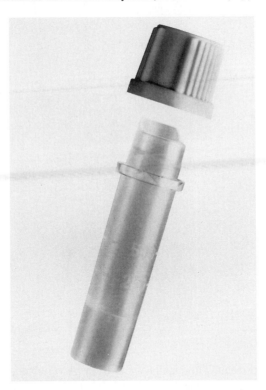

Figure 7–26.   Safe-T-Fill Capillary Blood Collection Device.

(Courtesy of Ram Scientific, Inc., Needham, MA.)

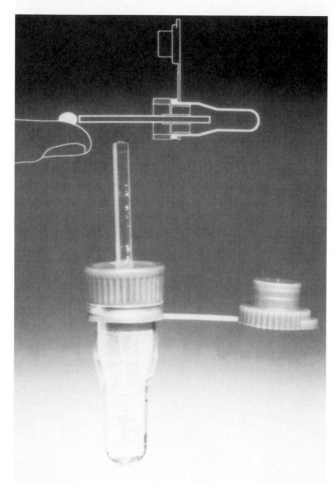

blood drawing safe and clean. The capillary can then be removed, and the tube is closed with the appropriate color-coded cap.

For most chemical assays, lithium and ammonium salts of heparin are the anticoagulants of choice for microcollections. They have rarely been reported to interfere with the determination of electrolytes and most other chemical assays.[10]

Another type of microcollection device is the Unopette (Becton-Dickinson VACUTAINER Systems, Franklin Lakes, NJ), shown in Figure 7–27. This device serves as a collection and dilution unit for blood samples and, thus, increases the speed and simplicity of laboratory procedures. These devices are prefilled with specific amounts of diluents or reagents, or

Figure 7–27.   Unopette, a collection and dilution unit for blood samples.

(Courtesy of Becton-Dickinson VACUTAINER Systems, Franklin Lakes, NJ.)

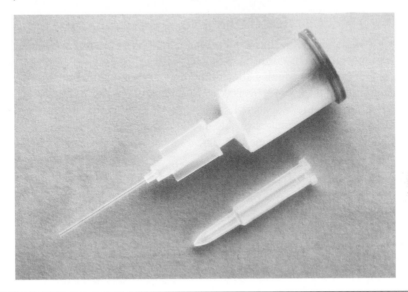

both, for different types of laboratory assays. Some of the more prevalent procedures in which Unopette devices are used include the WBC count, RBC count, platelet count, hemoglobin, RBC fragility, sodium and potassium, and lead determinations.

The standard Unopette test comprises (1) a disposable, self-filling diluting pipette consisting of a straight, thin-walled, uniform-bore, glass capillary tube fitted into a plastic holder and (2) a plastic reservoir containing a premeasured volume of reagent for diluting. For quick and easy visual identification, each capillary pipette is color coded according to its capacity. Color coding for all disposable self-filling Unopette capillary pipettes is as follows: 3 μL—green, 3.3 μL—gray, 10 μL—pink, 20 μL—yellow, 25 μL—blue, and 44.7 μL—black.

SEALING ITEMS FOR MICROCOLLECTION TUBES

For capillary pipettes and tubes, sealing wax or caps are necessary when the blood is drawn into the tube. Putty-like sealants and plastic closures are available from various manufacturers. The phlebotomist must be sure to follow the instructions with the sealant in order to provide safe sealing during microcentrifugation. A capillary tube device that was developed to reduce the opportunity for blowout of the sealant during microcentrifugation is the Safecap capillary and Safeplug (Safe-Tec, Inc.). Safecap capillary has a self-sealing plug called

Safeplug that was manufactured to permit a more accurate measurement of the packed cell volume and to decrease biohazardous risk to blood splatters and aerosol spray during microcentrifugation.

TRANSPORTING MICROSPECIMENS

Glycolysis in RBCs and WBCs causes a decrease in blood pH that can be detected after a blood gas sample has been stored at room temperature for approximately 20 minutes. Therefore, blood gas microsamples should be immersed in a slurry of ice water from the time of collection until they are delivered to the clinical laboratory. Plastic containers that are small enough to hold these specimens with ice and water should be carried on the specimen collection tray. Ice is usually available on the patient ward. Other items to be carried on a microcollection tray include the following:

1. Seventy percent isopropyl alcohol and Betadine pads.
2. Marking pens for labels.
3. Microtainer blood serum separator tubes (600 μL).
4. Microtainer capillary whole blood cell collectors with 0.23 mg of EDTA (200 μL).
5. Lancets for skin puncture.
6. Sterile gauze pads or bandages.
7. Unheparinized plastic microcentrifuge tubes.
8. Heparinized plastic microcentrifuge tubes (250, 400, and 500 μL).
9. Heparinized Natelson tubes (75 μL).
10. Unopette devices for collection and dilution procedures.
11. Disposable gloves.
12. Cloth towel or washcloth.
13. Thermometer.
14. Biohazardous waste containers for sharps.
15. Glass microscope slides.
16. Capillary tube sealer.
17. Antimicrobial hand gel or foam to wash hands without water and soap.

■ BLOOD-DRAWING CHAIR

 Clinical Alert

 In an outpatient clinic that requires blood collections, a **blood-drawing chair** must be available for patients. The chair is designed for maximum safety and comfort of the patient plus easy accessibility to either arm of the patient. The chair should have an armrest for the patient's use during blood drawing. The armrest should lock in place so that the patient cannot fall from the chair if he or she becomes faint. Also, the armrest should adjust in an up-and-down position so that the best venipuncture position for each patient can be achieved.

Figure 7–28. Infant phlebotomy station.

(Courtesy of Custom Comfort, Inc., Orlando, FL.)

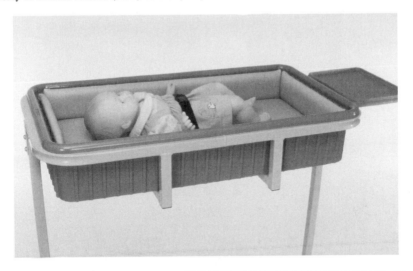

There are many chair styles and options available for making phlebotomy procedures easier and safer. Options include adjustable arm rests, leg extensions, neck pillows or supports, scale mounts, storage cabinets, hydraulic lifts, and foot covers (Custom Comfort, Orlando, FL).

■ INFANT PHLEBOTOMY STATION

As health care services are increasingly being provided at ambulatory sites, including home visits, a safe site is frequently needed for infant blood collections. An infant phlebotomy station (Custom Comfort, Inc., Orlando, FL) provides safety for infant blood collections at off-site locations (Fig. 7–28).

■ SPECIMEN COLLECTION TRAYS

The health care worker needs a specimen tray (Fig. 7–29) to take on blood-collecting rounds. The tray is usually made of plastic and must be amenable to sterilization. The tray should include all necessary collection equipment, and its contents usually differ from one hospital or clinic to another, depending on the patient population. For example, if the phlebotomist works in a children's hospital, he or she needs trays containing microcollection equipment, such as that described earlier. For home health care providers and reference laboratory couriers, the necessary collection supplies, equipment, and collected blood must be carried in an enclosed container with the biohazard symbol shown on the outside. For example, the Loc-Top Lab Tray (Healthmark Industries Co., Detroit, MI), shown in Figure 7–30, is lockable to protect the contents from tampering or accidental contamination. It also

Figure 7–29.   Specimen collection tray.

(Courtesy of Becton-Dickinson VACUTAINER Systems, Franklin Lakes, NJ.)

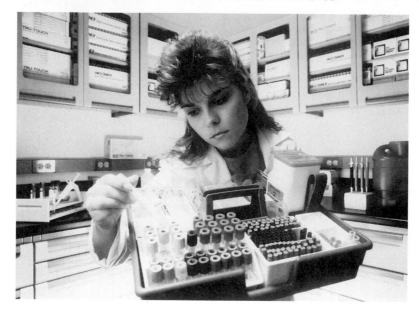

Figure 7–30.   Loc-Top Lab Tray.

(Courtesy of Healthmark Industries, Co., Detroit, MI.)

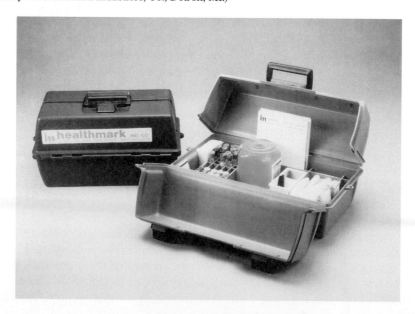

has a tight seal to reduce the risk of infection from blood-borne pathogens due to spills or accidents.

Health care workers who collect blood from adults usually have the following equipment on their trays or in their safety container:

1. Marking pens or pencils.
2. Vacuum tubes containing the anticoagulants designated in the clinical laboratory blood collection manual.
3. Holders for vacuum tubes.
4. Needles for vacuum tubes and syringes.
5. Syringes.
6. Tourniquet.
7. Blood collection sets (Butterfly needle assembly).
8. Seventy percent isopropyl alcohol, iodine, and Betadine pads or swab sticks.
9. Sterile gauze pads.
10. Bandages.
11. Biohazardous waste containers for used needles and lancets.
12. Lancets for skin puncture.
13. Unopette devices for fingerstick blood collection.
14. Microtainer blood serum separator tubes (600 µL).
15. Microtainer capillary whole blood collectors with 0.23 mg of EDTA (200 µL).
16. Disposable gloves.
17. Cloth towel or washcloth.
18. Thermometer.
19. Antimicrobial hand gel or foam to wash hands without water and soap.

SELF STUDY

KEY TERMS

Acid–Citrate–Dextrose (ACD)
Anticoagulants
Antiseptics
Arterial Blood Gas
Blood-Drawing Chair
Capillary Tubes
Citrates
Citrate–Phosphate–Dextrose (CPD)
Disposable Sterile Lancet
Ethylenediamine Tetra-acetic Acid
   (EDTA)

Gauge Number
Heparin
Holder (Adapter)
Lithium Iodoacetate
Microcontainers
Multiple-Sample Needles
Oxalates
Single-Sample Needle
Sodium Fluoride
Sterile Gauze Pads
Vacuum (Evacuated) Tube

STUDY QUESTIONS

The following may have *one* or *more* answers:

1. Which of the following anticoagulants prevent coagulation of blood by removing calcium through the formation of insoluble calcium salts?

  a. EDTA
  b. ammonium oxalate
  c. sodium citrate
  ~~d.~~ sodium heparin

2. Which of the following anticoagulants is found in a green-topped blood-collection vacuum tube?

  a. EDTA
  b. ammonium oxalate
  c. sodium citrate
  d. sodium heparin

3. For capillary collection from newborns, a lancet of which of the following lengths should be used to avoid penetrating bone?

  a. 2.40 mm
  b. 2.75 mm
  c. 3.00 mm
  d. 3.25 mm

4. Which of the following blood chemical constituents is light sensitive?

  a. glucose
  b. bilirubin
  c. phosphorus
  d. blood gases

5. When blood is collected from a patient, the serum should be separated from the blood cells as quickly as possible to avoid

  a. hemoconcentration
  b. hemolysis
  ~~c.~~ glycolysis
  d. hemostasis

6. The color coding for needles indicates the

   a. length   c. manufacturer
   b. gauge   d. anticoagulant

7. From the listed needle gauges, which one has the largest diameter?

   a. 19   c. 21
   b. 20   d. 23

8. Which of the following is/are skin puncture equipment?

   a. Tenderlett   c. Samplette
   b. Autolet Lite   d. AVL microsampler

9. Which of the following laboratory tests requires that the blood be transported in a slurry of ice water to the laboratory?

   a. bilirubin   c. blood gas analysis
   b. CK   d. complete blood cell (CBC) count

References

1. Hyman D, Kaplan N: The difference between serum and plasma potassium (letter). *N Engl J Med.* 1985;313:642.

2. National Committee for Clinical Laboratory Standards (NCCLS). *Evacuated Tubes and Additives for Blood Specimen Collection.* 4th ed. Approved Standard. NCCLS Document H1-A4, Villanova, PA: NCCLS; 1996.

3. National Committee for Clinical Laboratory Standards (NCCLS). *Procedures for the Collection of Diagnostic Blood Specimens by Venipuncture.* 4th ed. Approved Standard. NCCLS Document H3-A4, Villanova, PA: NCCLS; June, 1998.

4. Scranton PE. *Practical Techniques in Venipuncture.* Baltimore: Williams & Wilkins; 1977, p 66.

5. Harker LA, Slichter SI. The bleeding time as a screening test for evaluation of platelet function. *N Engl J Med.* 1972;287:155.

6. Brown JW, Backwell H. Putting on gloves in the fight against AIDS. *Med Lab Observ.* 1990;November:47.

7. Personius CD. Patients, health care workers and latex allergy. *Med Lab Observ.* 1995;March:30–32.

8. Strickland DA. Latex sensitivity prompts alert. *Med World News.* 1991;April:13.

9. National Committee for Clinical Laboratory Standards (NCCLS). *Procedures for the Collection of Diagnostic Blood Specimens by Skin Puncture.* NCCLS Document H4-A3, Villanova, PA: NCCLS; 1991.

10. Meites S (ed). *Pediatric Clinical Chemistry.* 3rd ed. Washington, DC: American Association for Clinical Chemistry; 1989.

11. Reiner CB, Meites S, Hayes J. Optimal sites and depths for specimens by skin puncture of infants and children as assessed from anatomical measurements. *Clin Chem.* 1990;36:574.

12. News & Views: Lasers to replace lancets? *Lab Med.* 1997;28:11,689.

8

EIGHT

■

Venipuncture Procedures

CHAPTER OUTLINE

CHAPTER OBJECTIVES

Upon completion of Chapter 8, the learner is responsible for the following:

1. Describe the patient identification process for inpatients, emergency room patients, and ambulatory patients.
2. List essential information for test requisitions.
3. List supplies that would be used in a typical venipuncture procedure.
4. Identify the most common sites for venipuncture, and describe situations when these sites might not be acceptable sites for venipuncture. Identify alternative sites for the venipuncture procedure.
5. Describe the process and the time limits for applying a tourniquet to a patient's arm.
6. Describe the decontamination process and the agents used to decontaminate skin for routine blood tests and blood cultures.
7. Describe the actual venipuncture procedure and the steps that are different using the evacuated tube method, the syringe method, and the butterfly or winged infusion system.
8. Describe the order of draw for collection tubes when using the evacuated tube method, the syringe method, and the butterfly or winged infusion system.
9. List examples and explain reasons for the importance of collecting "timed specimens" at the requested times.
10. Describe the proper method for hand washing.
11. Describe what the terms *fasting* and *STAT* mean when referring to blood tests.

■ BLOOD COLLECTION

In preparing for blood collection, each health care worker generally establishes a routine that is comfortable for him or her. Several essential steps, however, are part of every successful collection procedure. This chapter discusses the following steps in which a health care worker would progress through the blood collection process. These steps were developed from several sources and represent typical scenarios in the blood collection process. Individual facilities may vary the sequence of steps based on the characteristics of their patient populations.[1,2] In some cases, steps may occur simultaneously (e.g., assessing the patient's physical disposition while confirming his or her identity).

1. Preparation of the health care worker.
2. Assessing the patient's physical disposition.
3. Identifying the patient.
4. Approaching the patient.
5. Selecting and preparing equipment and supplies.
6. Finding a puncture site.
7. Preparing the puncture site.
8. Choosing a venipuncture method.
9. Collecting the samples in the appropriate tubes and in the correct order.
10. Labeling the samples.

11. Assessing the patient after withdrawal of the blood specimen.
12. Considering any special circumstances that occurred during the phlebotomy procedure.
13. Assessing criteria for sample recollection or rejection.
14. Prioritizing patients and sample tubes.

■ HEALTH CARE WORKER PREPARATION

Prior to performing any type of specimen collection, the health care worker should have all protective equipment, supplies, forms, and so forth ready for the procedure. If patient information is incomplete on test requisitions, the health care worker may not be able to identify the patient correctly or he or she may not know in which tubes to collect the blood. In such cases, assistance from a laboratory supervisor or a nurse is required.

■ EXERCISING UNIVERSAL STANDARD PRECAUTIONS

Clinical Alert

All health care workers must be familiar with current recommendations and hospital policies on precautions for handling blood and body fluids. *All specimens should be treated as if they are hazardous and infectious,* according to the universal standard precautions described in detail in Chapters 4 and 5 (Fig. 8–1). Hands should be washed before and after specimen collection procedures (Fig. 8–2). A clean pair of gloves should be put on in the presence of the patient[1]; as a safety-conscious, reassuring gesture for the patient and the health care worker. A clean, pressed uniform with a laboratory coat also instills a sense of commitment to safety and cleanliness, which is gratifying to patients and promotes a safer work environment for health care workers.

■ ASSESSING, IDENTIFYING, AND APPROACHING THE PATIENT

PHYSICAL DISPOSITION OF THE PATIENT

Factors related to the physical or emotional disposition of the patient often have an impact on the blood collection process or the integrity of the specimen. If the phlebotomist is aware of them, she or he may be able to prepare more adequately for the venipuncture. Sometimes the phlebotomist can get clues about the patient's disposition upon entering a hospital room. For example, if there is an empty food tray by the patient's bedside, it is likely that the patient has eaten recently. At other times, the cues come after talking to the patient or after the identification process has taken place. It is important that phlebotomists use pro-

Figure 8–1. Universal standard precautions.

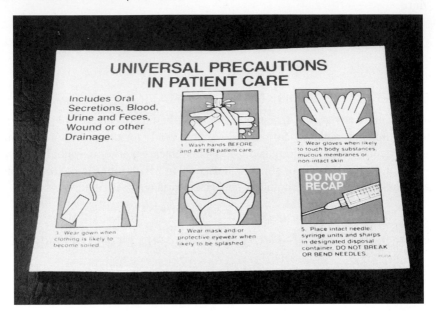

Figure 8–2. Hand-washing technique. **A.** Hand-washing techniques should involve soap lather, friction between hands, and thorough washing between fingers. Foot pedals are preferable for controlling the flow of water. (*continued*)

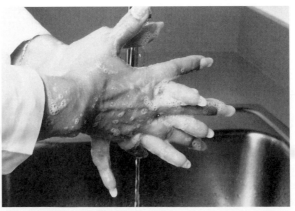

A

Figure 8–2. (*continued*)   **B.** Washing should include the wrist areas. **C.** Lather should be rinsed. Rinsing should continue until all soap is removed. If the water must be turned off by hand, a clean paper towel should be used to grab the faucet.

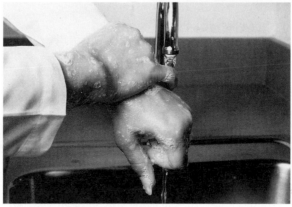

B

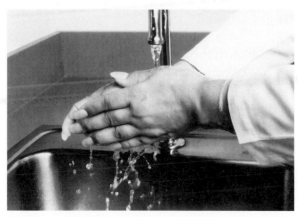

C

fessional judgment in asking or confirming issues related to disposition. These factors include:

- Diet   Many body substances are affected by the ingestion of foods and beverages. Therefore, it is important to note whether the patient has been fasting or not.
- Stress   Excessively anxious or emotional patients may need extra time to calm down prior to, during, or after the procedure. The phlebotomist should be keenly aware of these emotional needs and know how to deal with them. (Refer to Chapter 1.)
- Age   Elderly patients may have more "difficult" or frail veins from which to choose the venipuncture site.

- Weight   Obese patients may require special equipment, such as a large blood pressure cuff for the tourniquet or a longer needle to penetrate the vein.

Effects of these and other factors on blood collection are discussed in more detail in Chapter 10.

PATIENT IDENTIFICATION PROCESS

Clinical Alert

Prior to any specimen collection procedure, the patient must be correctly identified by using a two-step process:

1. The patient should be asked to state his or her first and last names.
2. More important, a confirmatory match should be made among the patient's response, the test requisition form, and some type of identification, such as a hospital identification bracelet, a driver's license, or another identification card.

INPATIENT IDENTIFICATION

A hospitalized patient should always wear an identification bracelet indicating his or her first and last names and a designated hospital number (often called a *unit number*). Hospital identification numbers help hospital personnel to distinguish between patients with the same first or last names.

Clinical Alert

To practice the two-step identification process, the health care worker should, upon entering the room, ask the patient what his or her name is. The health care worker should *not* ask, "Are you Ms. Doe?" because an ill patient on medication may mistakenly utter something, nod, or answer yes. Consequently, the best tactic is to ask, "What is your name?" and let the patient reply. *The patient must be correctly identified by his or her identification bracelet.*

Information on the bracelet may also include the patient's room number, bed assignment, and physician's name (Fig. 8–3). A three-way match should be made with the identification bracelet, the test requisition form, and the patient's statement of his or her name. The name card on the bed or door should never be used for confirming identity because it is often the last to be changed when patients are discharged and new patients are admitted.

Figure 8–3. Identification bracelet, requisition form, specimen label.

(Adapted from College of American Pathologists: *So You're Going to Collect a Blood Specimen: An Introduction to Phlebotomy,* 6th ed. Northfield, IL, Author, 1994, with permission.)

TEST REQUEST SLIP	HAPPY HOSPITAL Department of Laboratory Medicine			DATE REQUESTED 5/22/98 TIME REQUESTED 7 15/AM
	TEST	RESULT	PERFORMED BY	DATE COLLECTED 5/22/98 TIME COLLECTED 7 30/AM
				NAME Peter McLaughlin
				ADDRESS 4129 University Blvd.
				Houston, Texas
				PATIENT ROOM NO. 1708 BED NO. 2
				AGE 35 SEX M HOSPITAL I.D. NO. 601537
				PHYSICIAN Dr. McGarry
				TODAY ☐ ROUTINE ☐
				EMERGENCY ☐ SIGNED DG

Sample Requisition Form

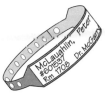

Sample Identification Bracelet

Printed information should include the following: patient's name, hospital number, room number, and patient's physician.

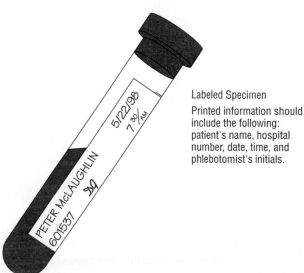

Labeled Specimen

Printed information should include the following: patient's name, hospital number, date, time, and phlebotomist's initials.

Clinical Alert

If the patient does not have an identification bracelet, the nurse responsible for the patient must be asked to make the identification. In such cases, the situation and the nurse's name should be documented on the requisition form. Specimens should *not* be collected until a positive identification can be made and documented. Drawing blood from the wrong patient can lead to serious consequences, such as incorrect treatment or therapy, and it is a violation for which the health care worker may be counseled or dismissed.

There are rare cases that usually involve severe burns or patients in isolation, where the identification may be attached to the patient's bed. These are the *only* circumstances in which a phlebotomist may use a bed-labeled identification tag to confirm identity. This step should be followed up by a nurse's confirmation as well. It should also be documented.

IDENTIFICATION OF INFANTS AND YOUNG CHILDREN

See Chapter 11, Pediatric Phlebotomy.

EMERGENCY ROOM PATIENT IDENTIFICATION

Health care workers must also be careful when identifying emergency room patients. Often, when patients come to the emergency room, they are unconscious and/or unidentified. Each hospital has policies and procedures for dealing with these cases. Usually, standard procedure involves assigning the patient an identification tag with a hospital or medical record number. This tag may be a multipart form that can be used by health care workers who need some type of temporary identification.

Clinical Alert

The "emergency identification" tag should be attached to the patient's body by wrist band or other similar device. The temporary identification number will be cross-referenced with the permanent identification number when the patient's identity is confirmed.[1]

AMBULATORY PATIENT IDENTIFICATION

Patient identification for ambulatory patients is usually more difficult to monitor. Most outpatient clinics, however, distribute identification cards to patients before any specimens are collected. If this is the case and the patient has the card available, positive identification can occur in the same manner as with hospitalized patients. These cards can also be used to make an imprinted label for the specimen if an Addressograph machine (Addressograph Company, Chicago, IL) is used. Alternatively, some ambulatory clinics issue identification bracelets to patients. If the patient does not have a patient identification bracelet or card, it is *strongly recommended* that another form of identification (e.g., driver's license) be checked and documented prior to specimen collection.

Clinical Alert

Some home-bound patients, infants, or children, may not have any form of identification available. In this situation, someone else, for example, the nurse or a relative, or the home-bound patient should be asked to confirm the identification by verifying the name, address, and birth date. The phlebotomist should compare this information with the test requests and document the identification process prior to specimen collection. Misidentification of patient's specimens can result in serious medical consequences, including patient death.

TEST REQUISITIONS

Laboratory tests must be ordered by physicians. The documented requests are usually transmitted in the form of a requisition form or by computer. Computer-generated requests contain the same required information as paper requisition forms. In either case, the requisition should contain the following information:

1. Patient's full name.
2. Patient's identification (or medical record) number.
3. Patient's date of birth.
4. Types of tests to be performed.
5. Date of test.
6. Room number and bed.
7. Physician's name and/or code.
8. Test status (timed, **stat,** fasting, etc.).
9. Billing information (optional).
10. Special precautions (potential bleeder, faints easily, etc.).

When requisitions are received in a centralized laboratory department, computer-generated labels that, in some laboratories, also serve as the requisition are often printed (Fig. 8–4). The numerous types, colors, and styles of labels (e.g., bar-coded labels) and requisitions are discussed further in Chapter 6.

Regardless of whether the requisitions are computer-generated or multipart forms, the health care worker should be familiar with the forms and with the procedures for generating, printing, and using the forms properly. Collection requests should be checked prior to

Figure 8–4. Labels and requisition forms.

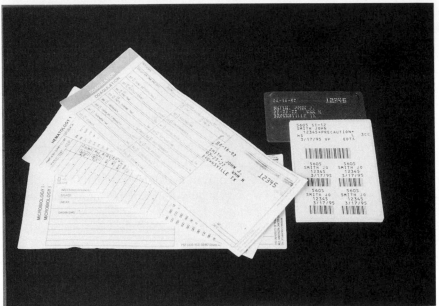

> ### Clinical Alert
>
> If the health care worker does not understand the test ordered, a supervisor, a laboratory technologist, or a nurse should be consulted prior to the phlebotomy procedure. Knowing which tests are requested helps the health care worker to prepare the patient appropriately and to collect the specimen in the appropriate tubes and in the correct order. Failure to do so results in preanalytical errors and misleading test results.

the venipuncture procedure to ensure that there are no discrepancies or duplicates in the test orders.

APPROACHING THE PATIENT

In addition to being prepared with the proper equipment and supplies, and safety precautions, the health care worker must be emotionally prepared. Such preparation involves adopting a professional appearance and behavior, as well as exercising good communication skills, both as a listener and as a speaker. (Refer to Chapter 1 for more information about professional behavior and communication skills.)

Several professional and courteous behaviors and phrases can help make the patient–health care worker encounter a smooth interaction. The first of these is a polite knock on the patient's door prior to entering the patient's room. The health care worker should introduce him- or herself and state that he or she is from the laboratory and has come to collect a blood sample. As stated previously, making a correct identification is crucial. Once this has occurred, the process may continue. Sometimes, the health care worker may need to explain to the patient that the physician ordered the laboratory test or tests. The health care worker may also need to explain the procedure as supplies are being set up. During setup, the specimen collection tray should *not* be placed on the patient's bed or eating table. As supplies are being readied and the vein is being palpated, the health care worker may try to alleviate some of the patient's fears. Chapter 1 covers verbal and nonverbal cues for detecting apprehension in patients. Box 8–1 presents a typical scenario of a health care worker–patient interaction.

BOX 8–1. TYPICAL HEALTH CARE WORKER–PATIENT INTERACTION

Knock on the patient's door.

Health care worker: Good morning. I am Ms. Smith from the laboratory. I have come to collect a blood sample.

Pause to give the patient an opportunity to speak. If the lights are off or dimmed, explain that you need to turn the lights on. Doing so gives the patient a moment to adjust to the idea of bright lights if he or she has been asleep.

Health care worker: What is your name, please? (*In general, it is not wise to ask a patient. "How are you?" because most patients in the hospital do not feel well.*)

Patient: I am John Jones.

Health care worker: May I please see your identification (ID) armband?

Check armband against laboratory requisitions and patient's verbal identification. If all three match, proceed.

Health care worker: This will take only a few minutes.

Patient: Will it hurt?

Health care worker: It will hurt a little, but it will be over soon. Please allow me to look at your arm veins.

Proceed with the remainder of the procedure, maintaining a highly professional atmosphere and a respectful attitude.

For certain tests, you may need to ascertain whether the patient has been fasting.

Health care worker: Mr. Jones, when was the last time you ate or drank anything? (*Do not use the term* fast *because some patients may not understand it completely.*)

At the end of the procedure, say the following:

Health care worker: Thank you, Mr. Jones.

■ EQUIPMENT SELECTION AND PREPARATION

SUPPLIES FOR VENIPUNCTURE

Supplies for venipuncture differ according to the method used (i.e., **syringe method, evacuated tube system,** or **winged infusion/butterfly system**). All methods of venipuncture involve the use of gloves, a **tourniquet,** alcohol pads or disinfectants, cotton balls, bandages or gauze pads, glass microscope slides, needles, syringes or evacuated tube holders, winged infusion sets, capillary tubes, tube sealer, blood collection tubes, laboratory request slips or labels, marking pens, and discard buckets (Fig. 8–5). Supplies should be readily available and selected just prior to the procedure. These supplies are discussed in more detail in Chapter 7.

POSITIONING OF THE PATIENT AND VENIPUNCTURE SITE SELECTION

It is important to choose the least hazardous site for blood collection by skin puncture or venipuncture. Several techniques can facilitate the selection of a suitable site.

 Clinical Alert

Proper positioning is important to both the health care worker and the patient for a successful venipuncture or skin puncture, and efforts to make sure that the patient is comfortable are worthwhile. Patients should *not* stand or sit on high stools during the procedure because of the possibility of fainting. A reclining (supine) position is preferred; however, sitting in a sturdy, comfortable chair with arm supports is also acceptable. Refer to Chapter 7 for more information about blood collection chairs and recliners. The health care worker can position him- or herself in front of the chair to protect the patient from falling forward in the event of fainting. A slight rotation of the patient's arm or hand may help expose a vein and prevent it from rolling as the needle is inserted. The visibility of veins varies with each individual's skin color, weight, physiologic conditions, gender, and physical features (Fig. 8–6). Therefore, the health care worker must rely on the sense of touch (palpation) to locate the vein. A pillow may be used for arm support of a bedridden patient if the patient is too weak to hold the arm in one position. Equipment should be placed in an accessible spot where it is unlikely to be disturbed by the patient. The phlebotomist can then palpate and trace the path of veins with the index finger.

The most common sites for venipuncture are in the antecubital area of the arm, where the median cubital, cephalic, and basilic veins lie close to the surface of the skin and are most prominent. Palpating this area usually helps the health care worker get an idea of the size, angle, and depth of the vein. The patient can assist in the process by opening and closing the fist tightly.[2] It is important to remember that veins may also be used for transfusion, infusion, and therapeutic agents. Thus, sometimes veins have restricted use for those purposes.

Figure 8–5. Supplies for venipunctures.

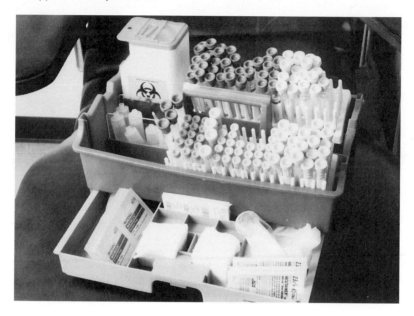

Figure 8–6. Differences in the visibility of veins. **A.** Veins are easily visible on a 45-year-old healthy male. (*continued*)

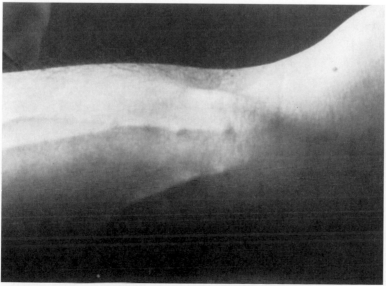

A

Figure 8–6. (*continued*)   **B.** On a 50-year-old healthy female, the veins are often more difficult to visualize.

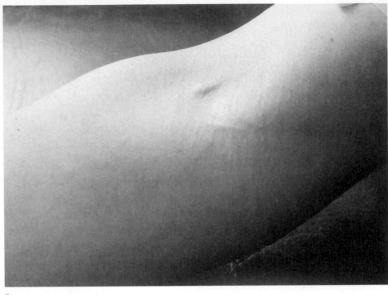

B

The dorsal side of the hand or wrist, ankle, and foot veins should be used only if arm veins have been determined unsuitable (Figs. 8–7 and 8–8).

 Clinical Alert

Reasons for *not* using the patient's arm veins include the following:

- Intravenous (IV) lines in both arms.
- Burned or scarred areas.
- Cast(s) on arm(s).
- Thrombosed veins.
- Edematous arms.
- Partial or radical mastectomy on one side.

Hand veins or the veins on the dorsal surface of the wrist are preferred over foot or ankle veins because coagulation and vascular complications tend to be more troublesome in the lower extremities, especially for diabetic patients.

Figure 8–7. Hand and foot veins.

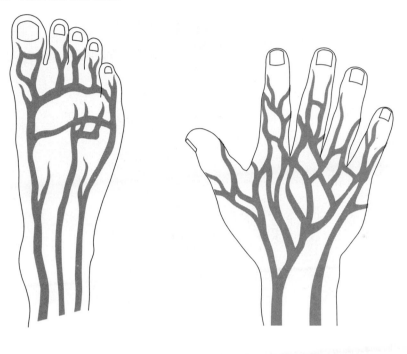

Figure 8–8. Differences in the patterns of hand veins. **A.** Male. (*continued*)

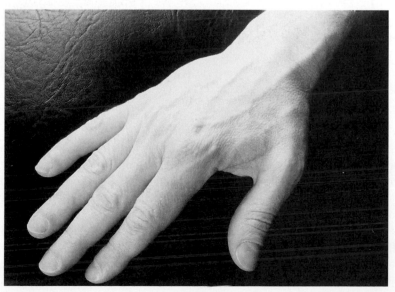

A

Figure 8–8. (*continued*)   **B.** Female.

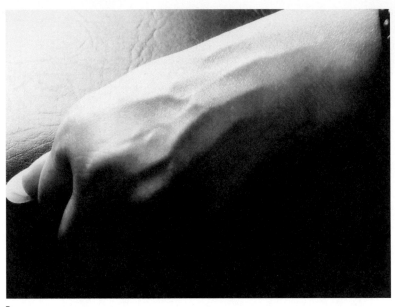

B

⬡! Clinical Alert

For hand vein punctures, the posterior surface of the wrist is preferred. *Do not use the anterior side or the palmar venous network* in the wrist, because nerves lie very close to the palmar venous network and can easily be injured by needle probing.

Veins in the wrist or ankle tend to move, or "roll," aside as the needle is inserted; therefore, it may be helpful to have the patient extend the foot or hand into a position that helps hold the vein taut (see Fig. 8–8). Veins of the extremities, however, should be avoided if they are edematous. Some hospitals do not allow health care workers to use the lower extremities for blood-sampling sites. Other hospitals allow sampling from these sites only after permission is granted from the patient's physician. Venipuncture in small veins is facilitated by the use of a 21- to 25-gauge butterfly needle (or winged infusion set) (Fig. 8–9).

It is also important to know that arteries do not feel like veins. Arteries pulsate, are more elastic, and have a thick wall. Thrombosed veins lack resilience, feel like a cord, and roll easily.

Figure 8–9.   Winged infusion set, or butterfly needle.

(Courtesy of Becton-Dickinson VACUTAINER Systems, Franklin Lakes, NJ.)

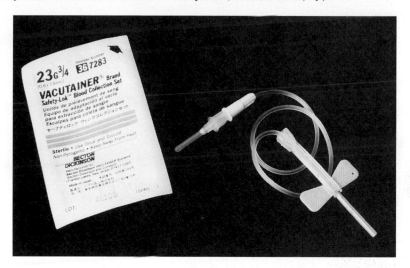

WARMING THE PUNCTURE SITE

Warming the puncture site helps facilitate phlebotomy by increasing arterial blood flow to the area and, in some cases, by making the veins more prominent. Although several methods of warming are available commercially, a surgical towel or a washcloth heated with warm water to 42°C will not burn the skin. When the towel or cloth is wrapped around the site for 3 to 5 minutes, the skin temperature can increase several degrees. The wrap can be encased in a plastic bag to help retain heat and keep the patient's bed dry. The health care worker may leave the warm wrap on the patient while he or she collects specimens from other patients, and then return to the original patient after several minutes.

TOURNIQUET APPLICATION

A tourniquet or blood pressure cuff may be used to help find a site for venipuncture. The use of a tourniquet makes the veins more prominent and easier to puncture due to venous filling.[2] A soft rubber tourniquet about 1-in. (2.5-cm) wide and about 15- to 18-in. (45-cm) long is most comfortable. To apply it, the health care worker should stretch the ends around the patient's arm about 3 in. (7.6 cm) above the venipuncture area; both ends of the tourniquet can be held in one hand while the other hand tucks in a section next to the skin and makes a partial loop with the tourniquet. The tourniquet should be tight but not painful to the patient (Fig. 8–10). It should not be placed over sores or burned skin, but, depending on the policies of each health care facility, it may be placed over a hospital gown sleeve or a piece of gauze. The partially looped tourniquet should allow for easy release by the health care worker during the venipuncture procedure. During the venipuncture, the health care worker should be able to release the tourniquet with one hand because the other hand will be holding the needle and tubes.

Figure 8–10. Performing a venipuncture procedure. **A.** Greeting the patient and confirming identification. **B.** Equipment preparation. **C.** Site selection. **D.** Tourniquet application. **E.** Palpating the site. **F.** Decontamination with alcohol. (*continued*)

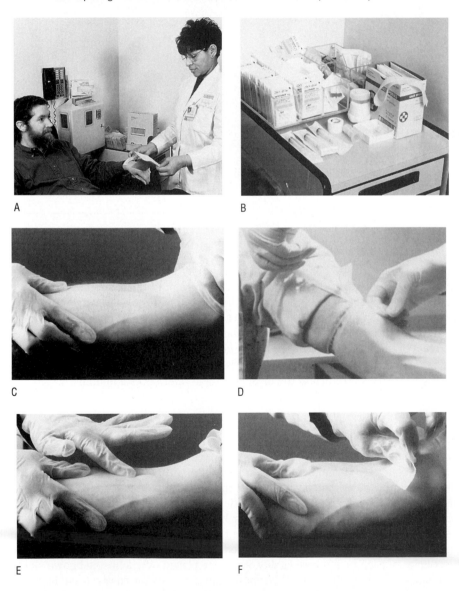

Figure 8–10. (*continued*)   **G.** The venipuncture procedure. **H.** Removal of tourniquet. **I.** Tube and needle removal. **J.** Application of pressure. **K.** Waste disposal. **L.** Application of bandage.

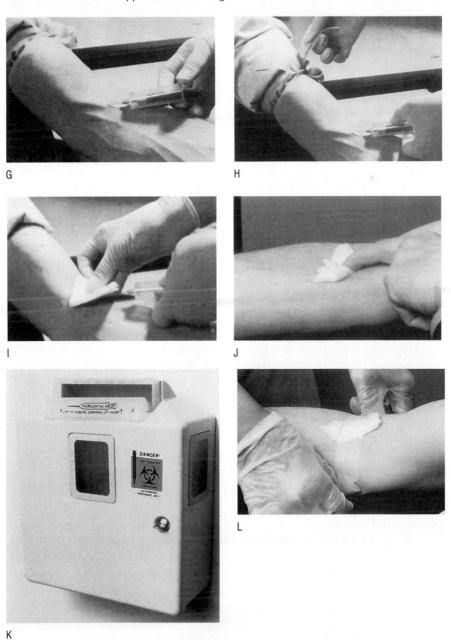

Figure 8–10. (*continued*)   **M.** Immediate labeling of tube. **N.** Adding initials, time, and date.

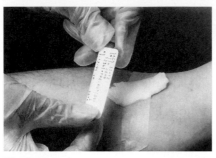 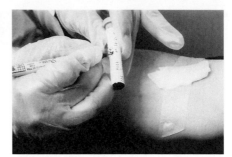

M   N

! Clinical Alert

The tourniquet should *not* be left on for more than 1 minute because it becomes uncomfortable and causes **hemoconcentration**—that is, increased blood concentration of large molecules, such as proteins, cells, and coagulation factors (see Chapter 10). The patient may be asked to clench and unclench the fist only a *few* times because excessive clenching also results in hemoconcentration. If no vein becomes apparent or "pops up," the patient may be asked to dangle the arm for 1 to 2 minutes to allow blood to fill the veins to capacity, then the tourniquet may be reapplied and the area palpated again. The health care worker should *never* stick a vein unless it can be felt. It is better to defer the patient to someone else who can search for the vein than to take a blind chance.

DECONTAMINATION OF THE PUNCTURE SITE

Once the site is selected, it should be **decontaminated** with a sterile swab or sponge soaked in 70 percent isopropanol (isopropyl alcohol), or with a commercially packaged alcohol pad (see Fig. 8–10 F). This prevents microbiological contamination of either the patient or the specimen. The health care worker should rub the site, working in concentric circles from the inside out. If the skin is particularly dirty, the process should be repeated. The health care worker should also decontaminate his or her own gloved finger if he or she intends to palpate the site again.

Clinical Alert

The decontaminated area should *never* be touched with any nonsterile object. The alcohol should be allowed to dry (approximately 30 to 60 seconds) or should be wiped off with sterile gauze or cotton after the site is prepared; otherwise, the puncture site will sting, and the alcohol can interfere with test results, such as blood alcohol levels. Blowing on the site to hasten the drying process is not advised because doing so may recontaminate the site.[2]

Povidone–iodine (Betadine) preparations are primarily used for drawing blood for blood gas analysis and blood cultures (see Chapter 12, Arterial and Special Collection Procedures). For some patients, iodine causes skin irritation. Efforts should be made to remove iodine from the skin with sterile gauze after decontamination because excess iodine can interfere with some laboratory tests.

■ VENIPUNCTURE METHODS

VENIPUNCTURE

Once the puncture site is cleansed, the health care worker may hold the patient's arm below the site, pulling the skin tightly with the thumb. A syringe, butterfly, or VACUTAINER (Becton-Dickinson VACUTAINER Systems, Franklin Lakes, NJ) assembly can be used for venipuncture. (If a syringe is used, before the needle is inserted the plunger should be moved back and forth to allow for free movement and to expel all air.) The whole assembly can be held between the thumb and the third or fourth finger. (The index finger may rest on the hub of the needle to guide the needle entry.) The needle should run in the same direction as the vein and should be inserted quickly and smoothly at approximately a 15-degree angle with the skin.[1] To avoid startling the patient, just before inserting the needle, the health care worker should mention to the patient that he or she will "feel a stick." This warning cautions patients and usually alerts them to be still. The health care worker may also need to tell the patient, "Please be very still." Also, there should be no foreign objects (food, chewing gum, a thermometer) in the patient's mouth at the time of the puncture. The needle should be inserted with the *bevel side upward* and directly above a prominent vein or slightly below the palpable vein. The health care worker may need to palpate with one hand after needle insertion if the vein has not been hit. Often, the health care worker can feel a slight "pop" as the needle enters the vein. As the blood begins to flow, the patient may open the fist. The tourniquet can be released immediately or after the blood has been collected, but before needle withdrawal. (Refer to Figure 8–10G–I.)

Box 8–2 describes the specific laboratory procedure used to perform a routine venipuncture.

EVACUATED TUBE SYSTEM

If the evacuated tube (e.g., VACUTAINER) system is used, first the needle should be threaded onto the holder; second, the test tube should be pushed *carefully* into the holder

BOX 8–2. SAMPLE PROCEDURE FOR PERFORMANCE OF A ROUTINE VENIPUNCTURE

Performance of a Venipuncture

1. Greet the patient in a friendly, professional manner.

   In an outpatient setting:

   Ask the patient a direct question, "What is your name, sir/madam?" "What is your date of birth?" Compare the name and date of birth stated by the patient with information on the identification card, computer labels, and laboratory request slips. When a blood specimen is required for blood components, an identification bracelet must be worn by the patient.

   In a hospital setting (inpatients):

   Knock on the patient's door and enter the room. Compare your request slip or computer labels with the patient's name and hospital number found on the door of the patient's room to make sure you are in the right room. Identify yourself to the patient, stating that you have come to draw blood for some laboratory tests ordered by his or her physician. Compare information on the patient's identification bracelet with that on your computer labels and laboratory request slips. **This information must be identical.** Request a nurse to identify a patient who does not have an identification bracelet. The nurse should also place a bracelet on the patient's wrist except in cases when this is not feasible. Sometimes a patient cannot wear an ID bracelet because his or her wrist is irritated or too edematous for an ID bracelet to fit.

   If this is the case, on the requisition make a note of the nurse who identified the patient.

2. Try to gain the patient's confidence and remind the patient that the venipuncture may be slightly painful. Patient's should never be told, "This will not hurt." Exercise Universal Standard Precautions, including use of gloves.

3. Position the patient:

   Procedure for seating the patient (usually outpatients):

   The patient should be seated comfortably in a chair and should position his or her arm on an armrest, extending the arm so as to form a relatively straight line from the shoulder to the wrist. The arm should be supported firmly by the armrest and should be only slightly bent at the elbow.

   Procedure for having the patient lie down (usually inpatients):

   The patient lies comfortably on his or her back. If additional support is needed, a pillow may be placed under the arm from which the specimen is to be drawn. The patient extends the arm so as to form a relatively straight line from the shoulder to the wrist.

4. Assemble the following supplies for collecting a blood specimen: gloves, blood-collecting tubes, needles, syringe or VACUTAINER holder, tourniquet, 70 percent isopropyl alcohol, and gauze pads or alcohol preparation, pads, povidone–iodine and acetone alcohol swab sticks (if blood cultures are to be drawn), and gauze bandage rolls, or paper tape and cotton balls.

5. Select a vein site. Place a tourniquet on the patient's arm. Choose the vein that feels fullest. Look at both arms. Ask the patient to make a fist that makes the veins more prominent and easier to enter. Vigorous hand exercise "pumping" should be avoided because it may affect some test values. Use your index finger to palpate and trace the path of the vein. Thrombosed veins lack resilience, feel cordlike, and roll easily. Feel firmly, but do not tap or rub your finger lightly over the skin because you may feel only small surface veins. Always feel for the median cubital vein first; it is usually bigger and anchored better, and it bruises less. The cephalic vein (depending on size) is the second choice over the basilic vein because it does not roll and bruise as easily. The bend of the elbow is the best place to make a puncture. When this is not possible, other sites include the surface of the forearm, dorsal wrist area above the thumb, volar area of the wrist, knuckle of the thumb or index finger, back of the hand, and back of the lower arm. If a "good" vein cannot be found, try the following:

   • Try the other arm unless otherwise instructed.

   • Ask the patient to make a fist again.

   • Apply the tourniquet, remembering that the tourniquet should never be left on the arm for more than 2 minutes.

(continued)

BOX 8–2. *(continued)*

- Massage the arm from wrist to elbow.
- Tap a few times at the vein site with your index finger.
- Apply heat to the vein site.
- Lower the arm over the bedside or venipuncture chair.

6. Cleanse the venipuncture site. Using an alcohol preparation pad or cotton ball saturated with alcohol, cleanse the area by moving the pad in a circular motion from the center of the vein site outward. The area must be allowed to dry. *Never* touch the skin after the site is cleansed unless you have prepared your gloved finger.

7. Inspect the needle, syringe, or evacuated tube before performing the venipuncture. The appropriate needle is attached to the syringe or the evacuated tube holder and threaded into the holder until it is secure; the needle sheath will lock onto the holder. The cover of the needle must not be removed until you are ready to draw blood so that the needle does not become contaminated. If the needle touches anything but the sterile site, it should be changed.

8. Perform the venipuncture:

Evacuated tube method:

Grasp the patient's arm firmly, using your thumb to draw the skin taut. The vein is entered with the bevel of the needle upward. One hand should hold the evacuated tube while the other depresses the tube to the end of the holder.

The tube should be filled until the vacuum is exhausted and the blood flow ceases to ensure a correct ratio of anticoagulant to blood. After each tube is drawn, an additive should be mixed immediately by inverting the tube at least five times. Gentle inversion will prevent hemolysis. *Never* shake a tube of blood after collecting a blood specimen.

Occasionally, a faulty tube will have no vacuum. If a tube is not filling and the needle is inside the vein, another tube should be used. If a tube starts to fill but then stops, the needle should be moved slightly forward or backward. Usually, this adjustment will increase the blood flow. The needle can then be rotated half a turn, and the tourniquet, which may have been applied too tightly, is loosened. Probing is not recommended because it is painful to the patient. If none of these procedures is helpful, the needle should be removed, and an alternate site used.

Syringe method:

A syringe and needle should be used to collect blood from patients with more difficult veins. If the puncture has been made and the blood is not flowing, determine whether you are pulling too hard on the plunger and collapsing the vein. The needle should be drawn back while the plunger is being pulled slightly. Make sure that the bevel is covered by the skin. With the syringe in the right hand, you can use the index finger of the left hand to feel for the vein. After the vein is relocated, keep your finger gently on the vein, and guide the needle to that point. Then, pull gently on the plunger. As soon as the blood starts to flow into the syringe, the needle should not be moved.

Other methods:

A winged infusion set with leur adapters can be used instead of a syringe and needle for very difficult veins. The winged collection set is a closed system. Blood flows from the vein, through the set directly into a Vacutainer tube.

If all possibilities have been exhausted, and you have not successfully performed a venipuncture on a patient after two attempts, enlist the aid of a co-worker or a supervisor. Inform the nurse caring for the patient that you have made two unsuccessful attempts to draw blood from the patient. Make a notation of the circumstances on a worksheet.

9. The tourniquet is released after the blood is drawn and the patient has opened his or her hand. Releasing the tourniquet allows for normal blood circulation and a reduction in the amount of bleeding at the venipuncture site. Fold a gauze pad or place a cotton ball over the needle, then gently remove the needle. The gauze pad or cotton ball should be held firmly over the venipuncture site.

10. All tubes should be appropriately mixed and labeled at the patient's bedside. Labels must include the patient's first and last names and ID number, the date, the time of collection, and the phlebotomist's initials.

11. Dispose of contaminated materials and supplies in designated containers.

12. Wash hands.

13. Thank the patient.

14. Deliver specimens to the appropriate laboratory.

so that the test tube cap is punctured by the inside needle and blood can enter the evacuated tube. If multiple sample tubes are to be collected, each tube should be *gently removed* from the VACUTAINER holder and replaced with another tube. Experienced health care workers are able to mix a full tube in one hand while holding the needle apparatus and waiting for another tube to fill. Some health care workers use the dominant hand to change tubes while the other hand keeps the needle apparatus steady. This approach may require the health care worker to switch hands after needle insertion. The position that is the most comfortable for the patient and the health care worker should be used while the needle is simultaneously kept as stable and motionless as possible during tube fillings. (As mentioned previously, remember to release the tourniquet once blood begins to flow into the tubes.) Multiple tubes can be filled in less than 1 minute if the needle remains stable in the vein and the vein does not collapse. So that the proper dilution of blood and additive in the tube is ensured, each tube should be allowed to fill until the blood flow stops. Tubes do not fill completely, so the health care worker must be attentive to when the blood flow ceases. To change tubes, the health care worker should remove the full one from the needle apparatus with a gentle twist-and-pull motion, then replace it with an empty tube, using a gentle push onto the needle apparatus. During the tube exchange, the needle apparatus should be held firmly so that the needle remains in the vein and is not pushed through or pulled out of the vein.

 Clinical Alert

When all tubes have been filled, the needle should be carefully but quickly withdrawn. *Depending on the needle manufacturer,* the safety device should be activated either prior to or immediately upon withdrawal of the needle (Refer to Chapter 7 for details on equipment safety devices that prevent accidental needlesticks.)

SYRINGE METHOD

If a syringe is used, the same approach to needle insertion should take place as is used for the evacuated tube method. Once the needle is in the vein, the syringe plunger can be drawn back slowly until the required amount of blood is drawn. (It may be helpful to turn the syringe slightly so that the graduated markings are visible.) Care must be taken not to accidentally withdraw the needle while pulling back on the plunger and not to pull hard enough to cause **hemolysis** (e.g., rupture of the cells) or collapse of the vein.

After tourniquet release and collection of the appropriate amount of blood, the entire needle assembly should be withdrawn quickly. Again, the safety device should be activated immediately, depending on the manufacturer's specifications.

WINGED INFUSION SYSTEM OR BUTTERFLY METHOD

A **winged infusion set,** butterfly needle assembly, or scalp needle set can be used for particularly difficult venipunctures. (Refer to Figure 8–11.) This type of method is useful for the
following circumstances:

- Patients with small veins (hand or wrist).
- Pediatric patients.
- Geriatric patients.
- Patients having numerous needlesticks (i.e., cancer patients).
- Patients in restrictive positions (i.e., traction, severe arthritis).
- Patients who are severely burned.
- Patients with fragile skin and veins.

The use of this type of system has been reported to be less painful to patients. Also, these
devices are useful for short-term infusion therapy.

The needles range from ½ to ¾ inch in length and from 21 to 25 gauge in diameter. Attached to the needle is a thin tubing with a luer adapter at the end so that it can be used on
a syringe or an evacuated tube system from the same manufacturer. Since the tubing con-

Figure 8–11. Performing a venipuncture procedure with the combination butterfly (double-pointed)
needle and evacuated tube system.

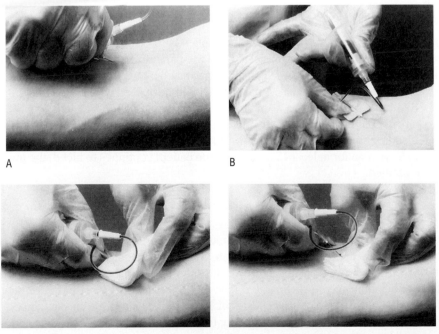

A

B

C

D

tains air, it will underfill the first evacuated tube by 0.5 mL. Therefore, a red-topped tube should be filled prior to any tube with additives. After the first tube, the order of the tube draw should correspond with the adapter type (evacuated tube or syringe used with the butterfly needle). When using the winged infusion system, each tube should be held horizontally or slightly down to avoid transfer of additives from one tube to the next. It is also suggested that small evacuated collection tubes (i.e., 13×75 mm or 4 mL) be used with winged infusion sets to avoid collapsing fragile veins. Or if using a syringe attached to the luer adapter, a small syringe, such as 5 or 10 mL, should be used for the same reason. Usually a 21- or 23-gauge needle is better than a 25-gauge needle because the small diameter may lead to hemolysis as the specimen is withdrawn. For an infant, however, the 25-gauge needle is the best choice for small veins.

Health care workers should be extra cautious as the needle is removed from the patient because it tends to hang loose on the end of the tubing. Therefore, the safety device that is built into the system should be activated according to the manufacturer's instructions. This may involve a retractable safety enclosure that allows for resheathing or covering the needle once it has been withdrawn (Becton-Dickinson VACUTAINER Systems, Franklin Lakes, NJ) or rotating a device on the needle set that advances a safety blunt prior to withdrawal of the needle from the vein (Puncture Guard Technology, Bio-Plexus, Tolland, CT). (Refer to Chapter 7, Blood Collection Equipment.)

Use of winged infusion or butterfly systems requires training and practice, but they are very popular because they are less painful. Use of this system is, however, more hazardous for health care workers than use of conventional needles. Failure to activate the safety devices correctly as described by the manufacturers may result in a higher incidence of needlestick injuries.

BANDAGE FOR THE PUNCTURE SITE

A dry, sterile gauze or cotton ball should be applied with pressure to the puncture site for several minutes or until bleeding has ceased. If the patient has a free hand, he or she may be asked to apply the pressure. The patient's arm may be kept straight, slightly bent at the elbow, or elevated above the heart. A bandage should be applied, and the patient should be instructed to leave it on for at least 15 minutes.

If the patient continues to bleed, the phlebotomist should apply pressure her- or himself until the bleeding stops. A gauze bandage can then be applied, and the patient should be instructed to leave it on for at least 15 minutes. If the patient continues to bleed, the unit nurse should be notified.

PROPER DISPOSAL

All disposable or contaminated equipment should be discarded into appropriate containers. Paper and plastic wrappers can be thrown into a wastebasket. Needles and lancets should *not* be thrown into a wastebasket, however, but into a sturdy, puncture-proof, disposable container to be autoclaved or incinerated (see Fig. 8–10K). Any items that have been contaminated with blood should be disposed of in biohazardous disposal containers as explained in the universal precautions (see Chapter 4, Infection Control. Also refer to Chapter 7, Blood Collection Equipment.)

ORDER OF TUBE COLLECTION

Very often, multiple blood assays are ordered on patients. Whether the health care worker chooses to use a multiple-draw evacuated tube collection system or a plastic syringe, there are certain guidelines for delivery of blood into the proper collection tubes.

Evacuated Tube Collection System

The **National Committee for Clinical Laboratory Standards (NCCLS)** and Becton-Dickinson (B-D), the tube manufacturer, recommends the following specific order for collection of tubes. Although steps 1–3 are the same, their recommendations for step 4 specifically state the order of collection for tubes with additives.[2,3] (It may be helpful to check with each manufacturer about their recommendations for the order of tube draw.)

Order of draw:
1. Blood culture tubes (yellow stopper), or culture bottles.
2. Nonadditive or serum tube (red stopper).
3. Citrate (light blue stopper), or coagulation tubes.

4. Recommendations for additive tubes:
   NCCLS[2]
   - Gel separator tube
   - Heparin (green stopper)
   - Ethylenediamine tetracetic acid (EDTA) (lavender stopper)
   - Oxalate/fluoride (gray stopper)

   Recommendations for additive tubes:
   B-D[3]
   - Heparin (green stopper or light green Hemogard)
   - EDTA (lavender Hemogard)
   - Gel separator tubes and PLUS serum tubes containing silica clot activators (mottled gold Hemogard or PLUS red-top tube).
   - Other additives.

The blood cultures are always drawn first to decrease the possibility of bacterial contamination. The procedure for collection of blood cultures is discussed in Chapter 12 in greater detail. Whenever coagulation studies are ordered for diagnostic purposes (prothrombin time [PT], partial thromboplastin time [PTT]), it is preferable that at least one other tube of blood should be drawn before the coagulation test specimen. This diminishes contamination with tissue fluids, which *may* initiate the clotting sequence. Recent studies, however, suggest that accurate results may be obtained using the *first* tube.[4,5] This is particularly important when coagulation studies are the *only* tests ordered. The findings suggest that collecting and discarding the first of two tubes may no longer be necessary in all cases. According to NCCLS recommendations, if *only* a coagulation tube is to be drawn for routine coagulation tests (APTT and PT tests) the first tube drawn may be used for testing. For special coagulation tests (e.g., Factor VIII) the second or third tube should be used.[2] Each health care worker should clearly understand the procedure adopted by his or her own facility. If numerous tubes are to be collected, the tube that has an anticoagulant in it should be drawn last so that it can be mixed as soon after collection as possible. Care should be taken so that the anticoagulant present in the tube does not come into contact with the multisample needle when changing tubes, as some may be carried into the next tube and cause erroneous test results. For example, it is recommended that blood for serum iron be drawn before other specimens with chelating anticoagulants (e.g., EDTA) are collected in tubes. This will avoid interference in testing the serum iron level. Also, electrolyte determinations include measurement of potassium (K) and sodium (Na). Since the chelating anticoagulant EDTA is usually bound to potassium as $EDTA(K_3)$ or to sodium (Na) as $EDTA(Na_2)$, it is important to collect specimens that require EDTA after a specimen is collected in heparin for electrolytes. The K_3 and Na_2 from the EDTA may falsely elevate the patient's K or Na values. To minimize transfer of anticoagulants from tube to tube, holding the tube horizontally or slightly downward during blood collection is recommended.

Plastic Syringe Collection

When a health care worker chooses to use a syringe, the order of delivery of blood into the tubes changes. It should be as follows:

1. To minimize contamination, blood culture tubes are filled first.
2. Before proceeding, tubes for coagulation studies are filled and mixed.
3. Other anticoagulated tubes then are filled and mixed as quickly and safely as possible.
4. Lastly, tubes without anticoagulants are filled (Fig. 8–12).

Again, care should be taken not to transfer anticoagulants from one tube to another. Blood should always be delivered gently to the tubes to avoid hemolyzing the cells. This is done by directing the flow from the needle or the syringe hub along the side of the tube without allowing the blood to foam or without putting extra pressure on the plunger. Remember that evacuated tubes fill themselves; therefore, the blood does *not* need to be forcefully ejected from the syringe.

Sometimes, when a large volume (more than 20 mL) of blood has been drawn, there is a possibility that some of the blood may be clotted. If this occurs, the needle can be *carefully* removed from the hub of the syringe, the top can be removed from the tube, and then the blood can be *carefully* expelled into the tube. Again, it is suggested that the tube be filled by letting the blood run *gently,* not forcefully, down the inside of the tube to avoid hemolysis. If two syringes of blood have been withdrawn, NCCLS recommends taking blood from the second syringe for coagulation studies.[2]

SPECIMEN IDENTIFICATION AND LABELING

Specimens should be labeled immediately at the patient's bedside or ambulatory setting, and the labels should consistently include the following information[1,2] (see Figure 8–3):

1. Patient's full name.
2. Patient's identification number.
3. Date of collection.
4. Time of collection.
5. Health care worker's initials.
6. Patient's room number, bed assignment, or outpatient status are optional information.

For hospitalized patients, the tubes should be labeled immediately after the specimen is

Figure 8–12. Collection priority. Depending on the method used, the order of tube collection changes. When the evacuation tube method is used, the plain red-topped tube is used first, followed by the light blue–topped tube, the purple-topped tube, and any others that are needed. When the syringe deposit method is used, the blood should be expelled into the light blue–topped tube first, followed by other anticoagulated tubes, and finally the plain red-topped tube. If two syringes of blood have been withdrawn, the anticoagulated tubes should be filled as soon as possible with the second syringe of blood.

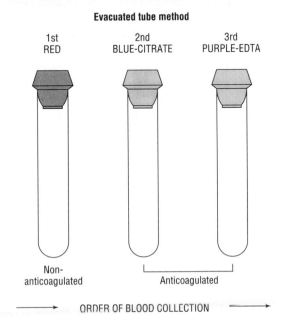

Evacuated tube method

| 1st
RED | 2nd
BLUE-CITRATE | 3rd
PURPLE-EDTA |

Non-anticoagulated · Anticoagulated

⟶ ORDER OF BLOOD COLLECTION ⟶

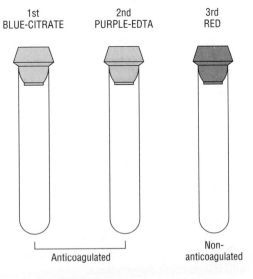

Syringe deposit method

| 1st
BLUE-CITRATE | 2nd
PURPLE-EDTA | 3rd
RED |

Anticoagulated · Non-anticoagulated

⟶ ORDER OF BLOOD DEPOSITED FROM SYRINGE ⟶

collected. Tubes should *not* be prelabeled because they may not be used, then they might be erroneously picked up and used for another patient. Also, a different health care worker may complete the venipuncture if the initial health care worker is unsuccessful. In that case, the prelabeled tubes may contain the initials of the first health care worker and, therefore, be inaccurate. In addition, if the prelabeled tubes are not used, tearing off the old or unused label may be difficult because of the adhesive; thus, either a new label (from a different patient) would have to be placed on the tube with a partially torn label, *or* the unused tube would have to be discarded. Either option is unsatisfactory, messy, and wasteful.

For the ambulatory care setting, there are mixed opinions about when to label the blood collection tube. The NCCLS suggests that the health care worker "must apply a label to each of the necessary tubes" prior to the actual collection process. Many health care workers (the authors included), however, believe that the same risks exist with prelabeled tubes in the outpatient setting as in the inpatient setting. Therefore, each laboratory procedure manual should contain explicit instructions on labeling requirements, and supervisors should spend ample time not only training new employees in correct identification and labeling practices, but also observing these trainees as they execute such practices.

For unidentified or unconscious patients who come to a hospital through the emergency room or other unusual circumstances, a temporary identification number can be assigned. The identification tag should be a multiple-part form with the same identification number on each part. One part can be attached to the patient's arm, and the other can be used for the specimens. When the hospital's permanent identification number is assigned to the patient, it can be cross-referenced to the temporary number.

The health care worker should confirm all the information before leaving the patient's hospital room or before drawing blood from another clinic outpatient. The date and time are necessary because requisition forms may indicate the date and time when a laboratory test was *ordered,* rather than the date and time when it was *collected.* For timed specimens (e.g., specimens for glucose tolerance testing), the actual collection time is critical to the test. The health care worker's initials are necessary to help clarify questions about the specimen if any arise during laboratory processing or testing.

No foolproof method exists for labeling specimens. The health care worker may write directly on the container. Alternatively, commercial collection tubes may have blank affixed labels for this purpose. Similarly, hospitals often use computer-generated labels for collection tubes; however, capillary tubes, microcollection tubes and vials, or other containers without labels must be identified, either by labeling them directly with a permanent felt-tipped pen, wrapping an adhesive label around them, or placing them into a larger labeled test tube for transport. In some cases, small computerized adhesive labels with printed information are available with and detachable from the requisition form.

OTHER CONSIDERATIONS

Because the health care team members (including doctors, medical technologists, clerks, secretaries, and nurses) are all working for the welfare of the patient, they should strive to reduce the total number of daily phlebotomies. To do this, all health care workers involved in patient care duties could follow these suggestions:

- Doctors could write orders on the same line on the chart.
- Orders could be coordinated among all staff physicians working with the patient.

- The laboratory could be notified when multiple timed tests are ordered. For example, if a patient needs a hemoglobin test at 2:00 PM and a glucose test at 3:00 PM., coordinating the times and drawing both specimens during one venipuncture may be possible.
- Therapeutic drug monitoring should be coordinated among laboratory, nursing, and pharmacy personnel.
- Nurses and ward secretaries could organize laboratory orders as much as possible to avoid sending frequent requests minutes apart for multiple venipunctures.
- When orders are transcribed, all of them should be requested at the same time.
- The laboratory should be notified of patient transfers.
- An up-to-date log of room numbers and patients' names should be available on the ward as a resource for laboratory personnel.

Health care workers collecting blood specimens should organize requisition forms by patient and floor. Any identification discrepancies should be communicated to a nurse.

One hospital has suggested several slogans for their health care personnel regarding phlebotomy:

- A stick in time saves nine.
- We care—several pokes are no joke.
- For their sake, let's stick together.

Other items that should be considered for inclusion in policies and procedures are

1. The number of times that a patient can be punctured by the same health care worker. Generally, a health care worker should not puncture a patient more than twice before calling for a second opinion.
2. The number of times that a patient can be punctured in 1 day. Staff physicians, nurses, and health care workers should coordinate their efforts to minimize the number of patient venipunctures.
3. The total volume of blood that can be drawn daily from a patient, especially a patient in pediatrics or in the nursery (see Table 8–1).
4. The type of information that a health care worker may provide to the patient about the laboratory tests ordered. In general, the use of good judgment is required. Providing basic information about the tests that have been ordered is acceptable *if* the health care worker is knowledgeable. The health care worker should always emphasize, however, that the patient's physician ordered the tests.
5. The steps to take if a patient refuses to have blood collected. All patients have a right to refuse treatment. In these cases, the health care worker should use good, sound judgment in explaining to the patient that laboratory results are used to help the physician make an accurate diagnosis, establish proper treatment, and monitor the patient's health status. The health care worker should explain that the patient's cooperation would be greatly appreciated. If the patient continues to refuse, the health care worker must remain professional and acknowledge the right to refuse. The health care worker should indicate to the patient that he or she will make a note of the refusal and notify the patient's physician.

ASSESSING THE PATIENT BEFORE LEAVING

Before leaving the patient's side, the health care worker must check the puncture site to make sure that the bleeding stopped. All tubes must be appropriately labeled, and the in-

Table 8–1.   Maximum Amounts of Blood to Be Drawn From Patients Younger Than 14 Years

PATIENT'S WEIGHT		MAXIMUM AMOUNT TO BE DRAWN AT ANY ONE TIME (mL)	MAXIMUM AMOUNT OF BLOOD (CUMULATIVE) TO BE DRAWN DURING A GIVEN HOSPITAL STAY (1 MONTH OR LESS) (mL)
lb	kg (approx)		
6–8	2.7–3.6	2.5	23
8–10	3.6–4.5	3.5	30
10–15	4.5–6.8	5	40
16–20	7.3–9.1	10	60
21–25	9.5–11.4	10	70
26–30	11.8–13.6	10	80
31–35	14.1–15.9	10	100
36–40	16.4–18.2	10	130
41–45	18.6–20.5	20	140
46–50	20.9–22.7	20	160
51–55	23.2–25.0	20	180
56–60	25.5–27.3	20	200
61–65	27.7–29.5	25	220
66–70	30.0–31.8	30	240
71–75	32.3–34.1	30	250
76–80	34.5–36.4	30	270
81–85	36.8–38.6	30	290
86–90	39.1–40.9	30	310
91–95	41.4–43.2	30	330
96–100	43.6–45.5	30	350

Adapted from Becan-McBride K. *Textbook of Clinical Laboratory Supervision.* New York: Appleton-Century-Crofts; 1982.

formation on the labels confirmed. All supplies and equipment that were brought in should be removed or discarded appropriately, and the health care worker should thank the patient. An adhesive bandage may be applied. Such bandages, however, are not recommended for infants or young children because of possible irritation and the potential of swallowing or aspirating a bandage.

■ SPECIMEN REJECTION

Each clinical laboratory should establish its own guidelines for specimen rejection. In general, the following factors should be considered:[6,7]

- Discrepancies between requisition forms and labeled tubes (names, dates, times).
- Unlabeled tubes.
- Inadequate volume of blood.
- Hemolyzed specimens (except for tests in which hemolysis does not interfere).
- Specimens in the wrong collection tubes.
- Specimens that were improperly transported (chilled or unchilled).

- Anticoagulated specimens that contain blood clots.
- Use of outdated equipment, supplies, or reagents.
- Contaminated specimens.

When a problem arises, the appropriate investigational channels should be followed. The health care worker who drew the specimen and his or her supervisor should try to solve the problem initially. Errors should be acknowledged and documented with corrective actions. Other personnel may be involved as needed. Communication, honesty, and ethical professional behavior are the keys to an efficient and reliable health care environment. Chapter 10 addresses complications in blood collection.

■ PRIORITIZING PATIENTS

In the course of a day's work at a busy hospital or clinic, a health care worker may have to make decisions about the order in which blood work is obtained. Priorities must be set and adhered to, whether they concern the order in which certain blood tests are drawn on a particular patient or which patients are to be drawn from first among a group. If these distinctions are not made properly, test results can be affected and interpretation of the results may be difficult.

PATIENT PRIORITIES

Timed Specimens

Whenever a test is ordered to be drawn at a particular time, the health care worker is responsible for drawing the blood as near to the requested time as possible. The most common requests for timed specimens are for glucose level determination for which blood should be drawn 2 hours after a meal. The glucose value in the blood is constantly changing, so the blood must not be drawn too early, which yields a falsely elevated result, or too late, which yields a falsely normal result.

Other timed specimens may be used for determining peak and trough levels of certain drugs. Often, patients on drug therapy must be monitored to ensure that effective therapeutic levels are being given. If the trough level is too high, the drug may be discontinued for a period until blood drug level returns to lower and safer levels. Again, the timing of drawing blood from these patients can be critical and must be scheduled as close as possible to the time ordered. If a time delay is unavoidable, the actual time of the collection must be indicated on the requisition form.

Certain natural hormone levels, such as cortisol, increase and decrease with the time of day. For instance, a sample of blood taken at 8:00 AM shows the highest value for cortisol during the day, whereas a sample taken at 8:00 PM usually shows approximately two thirds the value of the morning sample. Therefore, if a health care worker has difficulty obtaining a blood specimen on a patient at 8:00 AM, someone else should try as soon as possible thereafter, or the test may be canceled until the following day at the discretion of the attending physician. Obtaining a specimen at noon for cortisol level determination may give the physician little information on which to base treatment.

Another hormone, aldosterone, requires another type of timing for blood collection and analysis. The patient must be in a recumbent position for at least 30 minutes prior to blood collection. Serum or plasma can be used in the analyte determination, but heparin or EDTA should be the anticoagulant if plasma is preferred. Because glass interferes in the aldosterone determination, the collecting container should be made of plastic.

✔ To collect blood for a renin-activity test, the health care worker must collect an anticoagulated blood specimen from the patient after a 3-day special diet. In addition, the health care worker must be sure to note whether the patient is in an upright position or **supine** (prone) position when blood is drawn. For this analyte, the blood should be collected from a peripheral vein (e.g., antecubital vein).

Fasting Specimens

✔ When a health care worker works at an institution where inpatients are treated, care should be taken that the patient is not unduly inconvenienced by an order for **fasting blood tests** (i.e., tests performed on blood taken from a patient who has abstained from eating and drinking [except water] for a particular period of time). Fasting levels of glucose, cholesterol, and triglycerides can be important in diagnosing patients and monitoring their progress during the hospital stay. If the health care worker finds that a patient has not been fasting, the health care worker should consult with a physician to determine whether a nonfasting level will be of benefit. The requisition should then indicate that the patient is nonfasting.

Stat Specimens

The term *stat,* which means "immediately," has come to indicate a patient whose medical condition suddenly may become critical and who must be treated or responded to as a medical emergency. When blood work is ordered stat, usually a specimen must be drawn and analyzed *immediately* so that a critically ill patient can be handled properly. Consequently, the health care team should be prepared for immediate response, employ effective technique, and have personnel constantly available for stat blood collections. The health care worker not only should draw the blood quickly and properly, but also should ensure its timely delivery to the laboratory for stat analysis. Regardless of the patient's physical state, the health care worker must adhere to the proper procedure for obtaining the best possible specimen from the patient. Despite the emergency situation that may be in progress, no shortcuts can be allowed. The health care worker has a responsibility to the patient to obtain a properly labeled, correct specimen for the test that is ordered; if this responsibility is not carried out, precious time for the patient who is being treated may be lost while a nonurgent specimen is collected.

SELF STUDY

KEY TERMS

Butterfly System

Decontaminate

Evacuated Tube System

Fasting Blood Tests

Hemoconcentration

Hemolysis

National Committee for Clinical
Laboratory Standards (NCCLS)

Stat

Supine

Syringe Method

Tourniquet

Winged Infusion System

STUDY QUESTIONS

The following questions may have *one* or *more* answers.

1. A patient may be identified by which of the following means?

   a. patient's chart

   b. nurse

   c. patient's armband

   d. ward clerk

2. Identification procedures for outpatients may include asking for which of the following?

   a. photo identification

   b. birth date

   c. address

   d. identification by a family member

3. The most common sites for venipuncture are in which of the following areas?

   a. the dorsal side of the wrist

   b. the antecubital area of the arm

   c. the middle finger

   d. the middle forearm

4. Palpating the venipuncture site serves what purpose(s)?

   a. provides an indication of the
   size of the vein

   b. distracts the patient from the
   discomfort of the procedure

   c. provides an indication of the depth
   of the vein

   d. helps the phlebotomist determine
   what angle to insert the needle

5. Using a butterfly needle is beneficial for which of the following:

   a. heel puncture

   b. veins in the wrist or hand

   c. geriatric patients

   d. patients who are burned

6. What effect does warming the site have on venipuncture?

   a. prevents veins from rolling
   b. makes veins stand out

   c. causes hemoconcentration
   d. increases localized blood flow

7. How long should the tourniquet be placed around the patient's arm?

   a. Approximately 4 minutes
   b. Until the needle is removed

   c. Until the entire venipuncture
      is completed
   d. No more than 1 minute

8. What is the best angle for needle insertion during venipuncture?

   a. 15 degrees
   b. 30 degrees

   c. 45 degrees
   d. 80 degrees

9. What is the suggested order of draw using the evacuated tube system for the following specimens?

   ①a. blood culture
   ④b. lavender-topped tube

   ③c. light blue–topped tube
   ②d. red-topped tube

10. Containers for the disposal of needles and syringes should have which of the following features?

   a. be puncture resistant
   b. be labeled with a "biohazard" sign

   c. have yellow and black markings
   d. contain antiseptic solution

References

1. College of American Pathologists (CAP): *So You're Going to Collect a Blood Specimen: An Introduction to Phlebotomy.* 6th ed. Northfield, IL: CAP; 1994.

2. National Committee for Clinical Laboratory Standards (NCCLS): *Procedures for the Collection of Diagnostic Blood Specimens by Venipuncture.* Approved Standard, H3-A4, Villanova, PA: NCCLS; June, 1998.

3. Becton-Dickinson Systems, Personal communication, July 1995.

4. Gottfried EL, Adachi MM: Prothrombin time and activated partial thromboplastin time can be performed on the first tube. *Am J Clin Pathol* 1997;107(6):681–683.

5. Yawn BP, Loge C, Dale J: Prothrombin time: one tube or two. *Am J Clin Pathol.* 1996;105(6):794–797.

6. Richael JL, Naples MF: Creating a workable specimen rejection policy. *Med Lab Observ.* March:37–42, 1995.

7. National Committee for Clinical Laboratory Standards (NCCLS): Procedures for the Handling and Processing of Blood Specimens. Approved Guideline, H18-A, Villanova, PA: NCCLS; 1990.

NINE

Skin Puncture Procedures

CHAPTER OUTLINE

CHAPTER OBJECTIVES

Upon completion of Chapter 9, the learner is responsible for the following:

1. Describe reasons for performing a skin puncture procedure.

2. Identify the proper sites for performing a skin puncture procedure.

3. Explain why controlling the depth of the puncture is necessary.

4. Describe the process of making a blood smear.

5. Explain why blood from a skin puncture procedure is different from blood taken by venipuncture.

■ INDICATIONS FOR SKIN PUNCTURE

Skin punctures are particularly useful for both adult and pediatric patients when small amounts of blood can be obtained and adequately tested. In contrast, venipuncture in children can be hazardous and difficult because of the risk of complications, such as anemia, cardiac arrest, hemorrhage, venous thrombosis, reflex arteriospasm, gangrene of an extremity, danger to surrounding tissues or organs, infections, and injuries from restraining the child during the procedure. It is particularly important to withdraw only the smallest amounts of blood necessary from neonates, infants, and children so that the effects of blood-volume reduction are minimal. A 10-mL blood sample, which could be tolerated by most adults, would represent 5 to 10 percent of the total blood volume in a neonate's body. Sample sizes and procedures for obtaining specimen collections from children are covered in Chapter 11, Pediatric Phlebotomy.

Skin punctures are also useful for the following adult patients:

- Patients with severe burns.
- Obese patients.
- Patients with thrombotic tendencies.
- Oncology patients whose veins are being "saved" for therapy.
- Geriatric patients.
- Those who have fragile veins.
- Patients doing home testing (e.g., blood glucose screening).

Sometimes a skin puncture cannot be used because testing may require larger amounts of blood, interstitial fluids dilute the blood to some extent, and/or a patient has poor peripheral circulation. Specific tests for which skin punctures are not recommended include coagulation studies (because of the interstitial fluid), blood cultures, and erythrocyte sedimentation rate (ESR) determinations.

■ COMPOSITION OF SKIN PUNCTURE BLOOD

The composition of skin puncture blood is significantly different from that of venous blood acquired by venipuncture. It is composed of blood from arterioles, venules, and capillaries, as well as some **tissue (interstitial) fluid,** which is released during the sticking process. The content of arterial blood is greater because the arterial pressure in the capillaries is stronger than the venous pressure. Therefore, skin puncture blood is actually more like arterial blood than venous blood.

■ BASIC TECHNIQUE FOR SKIN PUNCTURE

Many of the steps used for the venipuncture procedure also apply to skin puncture. Basic steps include the following:

1. Preparation for puncture—greeting, identification, handwashing.
2. Choosing supplies and equipment.
3. Site selection and warming, if necessary.
4. Cleaning the site.

5. Performing the puncture.
6. Obtaining the specimen.
7. Labeling the specimen.
8. Completing the interaction.

■ PREPARATION FOR SKIN PUNCTURE

Skin puncture procedures involve the same preparation steps as discussed for venipuncture procedures. Such steps include being prepared, exercising universal standard precautions, greeting the patient to put him or her at ease, ensuring proper patient identification, labeling procedures appropriately, and practicing the correct hand-washing techniques.

For additional discussion of these issues, see Chapter 8.

■ SUPPLIES FOR SKIN PUNCTURE

As mentioned in Chapter 7, Blood Collection Equipment, supplies for skin puncture include the following: disposable gloves, lancets or automatic puncture devices, micropipettes, disinfectant pads, cotton balls, sterile bandages or gauze pads, glass microscope slides, diluting fluids, microcollection tubes or plastic capillary tubes, capillary tube sealer, laboratory request slips or labels, a marking pen, and a biohazard discard bucket.

■ SKIN PUNCTURE SITES

Skin puncture in adults most often involves one of the fingers. The fleshy surface of the distal portion of the second, third, or fourth finger can be used for puncture. Patients generally prefer their nondominant hand. The fifth, or pinky, finger is not recommended because the tissue of this finger is considerably thinner than that of the others.[1] The middle (third) and ring (fourth) fingers are used most often.

The heels of infants and neonates are good sites for skin puncture if the procedure is performed properly. The most medial or lateral sections of the plantar, or bottom, surface of the heel should be used. (Refer to Chapter 11 for additional information regarding pediatric phlebotomies.) The thumb, great toe, and earlobe are rarely used as sites for skin puncture. Swollen or edematous areas should not be used for venipuncture or skin puncture because body fluids can contaminate the specimen. Fingers that are cyanotic, swollen, cold, or inflamed should also be avoided.

■ WARMING THE SKIN PUNCTURE SITE

Warming the skin puncture site helps facilitate phlebotomy by increasing arterial blood flow to the area. Although several easy-to-use methods of warming are available commercially, a surgical towel or a washcloth heated with warm water to 42°C will not burn the skin. When the towel or cloth is wrapped around the site for 3 to 10 minutes, the skin temperature can increase several degrees.[1]

■ CLEANING THE SKIN PUNCTURE SITE

The skin puncture site should be cleaned with 70 percent isopropanol and thoroughly dried before being punctured because residual alcohol causes rapid hemolysis and may contaminate glucose determinations. Furthermore, alcohol prevents round drops of blood, which are needed for blood smears, from forming. Povidone–iodine (Betadine) preparations are not recommended for use on skin puncture sites because these preparations can falsely elevate potassium, phosphorus, and uric acid determinations.[1]

■ SKIN PUNCTURE PROCEDURE

Microcollection by skin puncture involves many of the same steps used during venipuncture. If the phlebotomist is performing a heel stick, the infant's heel should be held firmly, with the forefinger at the arch of the foot and the thumb below and away from the puncture site (see Chapter 11). If a finger stick is being performed, the patient's finger should be held firmly, with the phlebotomist's thumb away from the puncture site (Box 9–1 and Figs. 9–1 and 9–2). Retractable safety puncture devices are currently available on the market and are widely used in place of the traditional sterile lancet (see Chapter 7). If a sterile lancet is used, the puncture should be in one sharp continuous movement, almost perpendicular

---

BOX 9–1.   SAMPLE PROCEDURE FOR PERFORMANCE OF A FINGER PUNCTURE

Procedure for Skin Puncture or Fingerstick

1. Remember the following supplies: gloves, sterile cotton balls or gauze sponges (2 × 2), alcohol swabs, commercial puncture-device, sterile lancets, pipettes, capillary tubes, microcollection tubes, glass tubes, diluting fluids, marking pen or pencil, and bandages. Exercise universal precautions, including the use of gloves.
2. Choose a finger that is not cold, cyanotic, or swollen. If possible, the stick should be at the tip of the fourth, or ring, finger of the nondominant hand.
3. *Gently* massage the finger five or six times from base to tip to aid blood flow.
4. With an alcohol swab, cleanse the ball of the finger. Allow to air dry.
5. Remove the lancet from its protective paper without touching the tip.
6. Hold the patient's finger firmly with one hand and make a swift, deep puncture with the retractable safety puncture device or the lancet halfway between the center of the ball of the finger and its side. The cut should be made across the fingerprints to produce a large, round drop of blood.
7. Wipe the first drop of blood away with clean gauze.
8. *Gently* massage the finger from base to tip to obtain the proper amount of blood for the tests required.
9. Each type of microsample has different collection tube and blood volume requirements. Follow the appropriate manufacturer's instructions. For containers with additives, they should be inverted gently 8–10 times to mix the blood with the additives.

Notes

If the patient's hands are cold, wrap one of them in a warm-to-hot towel 10 to 15 minutes before the puncture is performed. A free-flowing puncture is essential to obtain accurate test results. *Do not use excessive squeezing or massaging to obtain blood.*

Figure 9–1. The finger puncture should involve a quick, deep puncture across the fingerprints, not parallel to them.

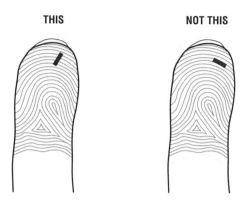

Figure 9–2. Skin puncture procedure. **A,B.** Decontamination of the site. **C.** A quick puncture is made with a retractable safety puncture device or sterile lancet, and the first drop of blood is wiped off with sterile gauze. **D.** Blood is collected into a Unopette capillary tube by capillary action. (*continued*)

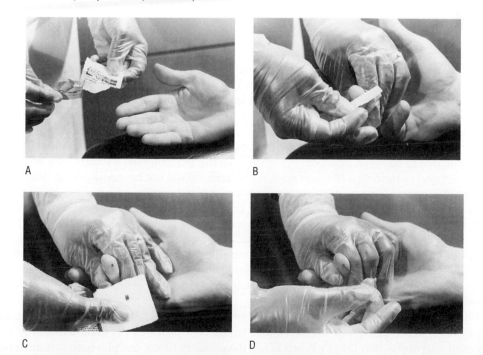

Figure 9–2. (*continued*)   **E.** Blood is collected into a microcollection tube. **F.** The patient presses sterile gauze on finger to stop the bleeding. **G.** The Unopette capillary tube is inserted into the vial, and the specimen is mixed gently by inverting 8–10 times.

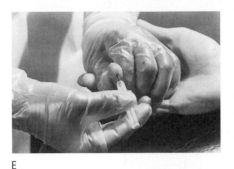

E

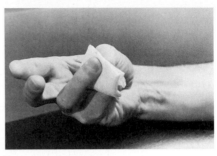

F

G

to the site and across the fingerprint. If the puncture is made along the lines of the fingerprint, the blood tends to run down the finger. The average depth of a skin puncture should be 2 to 3 mm to avoid hitting a bone. Special lancets that control the depth of the puncture are available commercially. New laser devices are also now being evaluated as skin puncture alternatives. They provide a smaller hole (about 250 μm wide and 1 to 2 mm deep). If the bone is repeatedly punctured, it can lead to **osteomyelitis,** which is an inflammation of the bone due to bacterial infection. Pressure from the phlebotomist's thumb may be eased and reapplied as the drops of blood appear. The area should not be massaged or milked excessively, however, because doing so causes hemolysis and contamination of the blood specimen with tissue and intracellular fluids. The first drop of blood should be removed with a dry, sterile pad, then capillary tubes (e.g., Unopette tubes [Becton-Dickinson VACUTAINER Systems, Franklin Lakes, NJ]) can be filled, and blood smears can be made from subsequent drops of blood. Capillary tubes are filled by **capillary action,** whereby blood flows freely into the tube on contact, without suction. (Refer to Chapter 7, Blood Collection Equipment.) If using a microcollection tube with additives, it is necessary to gently mix the blood in the tube by gentle inversion 8–10 times.

Figures 9–2 and 9–3 indicate methods for making blood dilutions and blood smears for performing white blood cell **differentials.** (Chapter 7 provides illustrations of different types of microcollection tubes.) When filling the capillary tubes, the phlebotomist must not allow air bubbles to enter the tubes because air bubbles can cause erroneous results in

Figure 9–3. The blood smear. Blood smears can be made from venous or capillary blood. In both cases, the smears should be made from fresh drops of blood. With the capillary method, the finger puncture should be made in the usual way, and the first drop of blood wiped away. The slide can be touched to the second drop. It should be touched approximately ½ to 1 in. (1.3 to 2.5 cm) from the end of the slide. **A.** A second (spreader) slide should be placed in front of the drop of blood. **B.** The blood collector should pull the spreader slide into the drop, allowing blood to spread along the width of the slide. When the blood spreads almost to the edges, the spreader slide should be quickly and evenly pushed forward at an angle of approximately 30 degrees. The only downward pressure should be the weight of the spreader slide. The slide should be allowed to air dry. It should *not* be blown on. If the venous method is being used, the needle should be touched to the slide immediately after it has been withdrawn. A drop about 1 to 2 mm in diameter will suffice. From this point on, the procedure is the same as for capillary blood smears. **C.** Good smears should have a **feathered edge** and should cover approximately half the surface of the glass slide. No ridges, lines, or holes should be visible in the smear. Errors are often the result of too large a drop, too long a delay in making the smear, or using a chipped slide. **D.** Blood smears should be allowed to air dry after they are labeled.

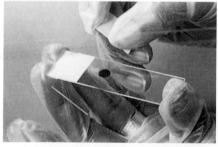

A

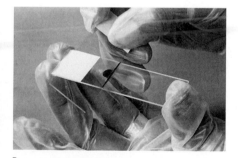

B

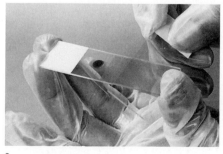

C

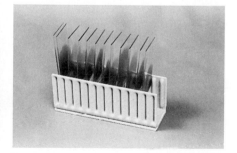

D

many laboratory tests. Blood flow is better and air bubbles are less likely if the puncture site is held downward and gentle pressure is applied. Scooping up blood from the skin surface is not advised.

■ LABELING AND COMPLETING THE INTERACTION

Hands should be washed after contact with each patient. *Before leaving the patient's side,* the phlebotomist must check the puncture site to make sure that the bleeding stopped. All tubes must be appropriately labeled, and the information on the labels confirmed. All supplies and equipment that were brought in should be removed or discarded appropriately, and the phlebotomist should thank the patient. An adhesive bandage may be applied. Such bandages are not recommended for infants or young children, however, because of possible irritation and the potential of swallowing or aspirating a bandage.

SELF STUDY

KEY TERMS

Capillary Action　　　　　　　**Osteomyelitis**
Differentials　　　　　　　　**Tissue (Interstitial) Fluid**
Feathered Edge

STUDY QUESTIONS

The following may have *one* or *more* answers.

1. Which of the following are *not* sites for skin puncture?
   a. wrist
   b. vein
   c. ankle
   d. heel

2. Controlling the depth of lancet insertion during skin puncture prevents which of the following?
   a. puncturing a vein
   b. bacterial contamination
   c. excessive bleeding
   d. osteomyelitis

3. A finger puncture should involve which of the following steps?
   a. puncturing parallel to fingerprint
   b. collecting the first drop
   c. puncturing across the fingerprint
   d. wiping away the first drop

4. Skin puncture is useful for patients who have which of the following conditions?
   a. obesity
   b. burns
   c. fragile veins
   d. thrombotic tendencies

5. Which fingers are used most often for skin puncture?
   a. thumb
   b. second, or index, finger
   c. third, or middle, finger
   d. fifth, or pinky, finger

6. Test(s) for which skin puncture cannot be used are
   a. routine hematology tests
   b. blood cultures
   c. coagulation studies
   d. erythrocyte sedimentation rate (ESR) determinations

7. Blood from skin puncture is more like arterial blood than venous blood for which of the following reasons?
   a. the skin has more arterioles
   b. arterial pressure is stronger in capillaries
   c. more arterial blood flows in capillaries
   d. venous pressure is greater in capillaries

271

8. Capillary or microcollection tubes should be filled with blood in which of the following ways?

   a. using a syringe to fill the tube
   b. allowing tube to fill by itself using capillary action
   c. using suction to pull blood into the tube
   d. using the tube to scoop droplets off the skin carefully

9. Alcohol should be allowed to dry completely prior to skin puncture

   a. to prevent stinging
   b. to prevent dilution of sample
   c. to prevent lysis of red blood cells
   d. to allow formation of a round drop of blood

10. The best angle for using two glass slides to make a blood smear is approximately

   a. 10 degrees
   b. 15 degrees
   c. 30 degrees
   d. 90 degrees

Reference

1. National Committee for Clinical Laboratory Standards (NCCLS). *Procedures for the Collection of Diagnostic Blood Specimens by Skin Puncture.* 3rd ed. NCCLS; Villanova, PA: 1991.

10

TEN

■

Complications in Blood Collection

CHAPTER OUTLINE

CHAPTER OBJECTIVES

Upon completion of Chapter 10, the learner is responsible for the following:

1. Describe physiologic and other complications related to phlebotomy procedures.
2. Explain how to prevent complications in blood collection and how to handle the complications that do occur.
3. List the effects of physical disposition on blood collection.
4. Discuss the types of substances that can interfere in clinical analysis of blood constituents and the methods used to prevent these occurrences.

Because complications can occur in blood collection, it is extremely important for the health care provider who is collecting the sample to know how to avoid complications if at all possible. If the complications are unavoidable, the health care worker must be knowledgeable of methods that will decrease the negative impact of the complication on the patient, on the quality of the blood sample, or on both.

■ COMPLICATIONS ASSOCIATED WITH BLOOD COLLECTION

FAINTING (SYNCOPE)

Many patients become dizzy and faint at the thought or sight of blood. Also, fasting patients sometimes become faint. Consequently, the health care worker should be aware of the patient's condition throughout the collection procedure. This can be done by asking ambulatory patients if they tend to faint or if they ever previously fainted during blood collections. If so, they should be moved from a seated position to a lying position. Even for an ambulatory patient without a history of fainting, it is still extremely important to use a blood collection chair with a "locked" arm rest to avoid the possibility of a fall if he or she faints. If a seated patient feels faint, the needle should be removed, the patient's head should be lowered between the legs, and the patient should breathe deeply. If possible, the health care worker should ask for help and move the patient to a lying position. Talking to patients can often reassure them and divert their attention from the collection procedure. Bed-bound patients also experience fainting, or **syncope,** during blood collection, although rarely. In any case, the health care worker should stay with the patient at least 15 minutes until he or she recovers. A wet towel gently applied to the forehead or a glass of juice or water may help the patient feel better.

Clinical Alert

If a patient faints during or after the procedure, the health care worker should try to terminate the venipuncture procedure immediately and make sure that the patient does not fall or become injured. Sometimes, controlling the situation is difficult because of the pa-

Clinical Alert (*cont.*)

tient's physical size; however, the health care worker should use common sense about the safest position for a patient. If a patient has fainted and is in a secure position, the health care worker should quickly request assistance from the nursing staff or a physician. A patient who has fainted should recover fully before being allowed to leave and should be instructed not to drive a vehicle for at least 30 minutes. An incident report must be filed with the health care facility regarding the fainting incident and the immediate precautions and instructions provided to the patient to prevent the possibility of long-term complications (e.g., car accident after fainting incident).

FAILURE TO DRAW BLOOD

Several factors may cause the health care worker to "miss the vein." These factors include not inserting the needle deep enough, inserting the needle all the way through the vein, holding the needle bevel against the vein wall, or losing the vacuum in the tube (Fig. 10–1). During needle insertion, the health care worker's index finger can be used to help locate the vein. The needle may need to be moved or withdrawn somewhat, and redirected. In the geriatric patient, the vein may be "tough" during needle entry and may roll; such rolling can cause the needle to slip to the side of the vein instead of properly puncturing it. Thus, the health care worker must securely anchor the vein prior to blood collection.

On occasion, a test tube will have no vacuum because of a manufacturer's error or tube leakage after a puncture. Consequently, the health care worker should carry an extra set of tubes in his or her pocket in case this happens during venipuncture. Also, needles for evacuated tube systems have been known to unscrew from the barrel during venipuncture. If this happens, the tourniquet should be released immediately, and the needle removed.

HEMATOMAS

Clinical Alert

When the area around the puncture site starts to swell, usually blood is leaking into the tissues and causing a **hematoma.** This complication can occur when the needle has gone completely through the vein, the bevel opening is partially in the vein, or not enough pressure is applied to the site after puncture. This swelling results in a large bruise after several days (Fig. 10–2). If a hematoma begins to form, the tourniquet and the needle should be *removed immediately,* and pressure should be applied to the area for approximately 2 minutes. If the bleeding continues, a nurse should be notified.

Figure 10–1.   Needle positioning and failure to draw blood. **A.** Correct insertion technique; blood flows freely into needle. **B.** Bevel on vein upper wall does not allow blood to flow. **C.** Bevel on vein lower wall does not allow blood to flow. **D.** Needle inserted too far. **E.** Needle partially inserted, which causes blood leakage into tissue. **F.** Collapsed vein

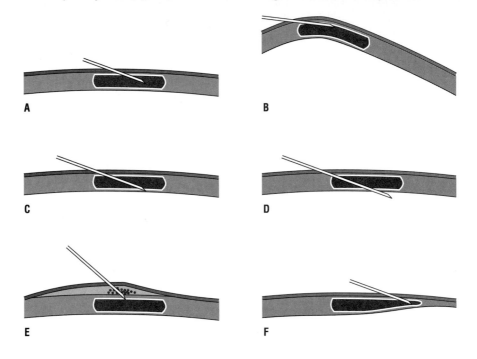

Figure 10–2.   Patient's hematoma several days after a venipuncture.

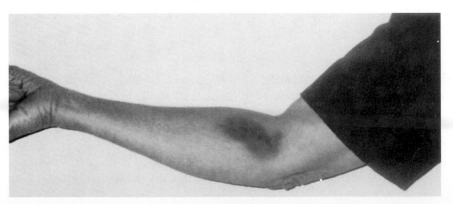

PETECHIAE

Petechiae, small red spots appearing on a patient's skin, indicate that minute amounts of blood have escaped into skin epithelium. This complication may be a result of a coagulation abnormality, such as platelet defects, and should be a warning to the health care worker that the patient's puncture site may bleed excessively.

EXCESSIVE BLEEDING

A patient usually stops bleeding at the venipuncture site within a few minutes. Patients on anticoagulant therapy, and/or those taking high dosages of arthritis medication or other medication, however, may bleed for a longer period. Thus, anytime a venipuncture is performed, pressure must be applied to the venipuncture site until the bleeding stops. The health care worker *must not* leave the patient until the bleeding stops or a nurse takes over to assess the patient's situation.

NEUROLOGIC COMPLICATIONS

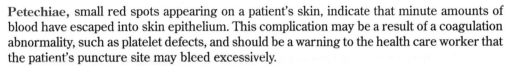

Clinical Alert

One rare complication that may occur during blood collection is seizures. If a patient begins to have a seizure, the health care worker should immediately release the tourniquet, remove the needle, attempt to hold pressure over the blood collection site, and call for help from the nursing station. No attempt should be made to place anything in the patient's mouth unless the health care worker is authorized to do so.

If the health care worker accidentally inserts the needle all the way through the vein, he or she may hit the nerve below the vein. If this happens, the patient will most likely have a sharp electric tingling sensation that radiates down the nerve. The health care worker should immediately release the tourniquet, remove the needle, and hold pressure over the blood collection site. An incident report on the occurrence should be completed and given to the supervisor.

MASTECTOMY

Clinical Alert

A woman who has had a **mastectomy** (removal of a breast) may also have **lymphosta-** **sis** (no lymph flow) due to lymph node removal adjacent to the breast. Without lymph flow on that particular side of the body, the patient is highly susceptible to infection and some chemical constituents may be altered. Also, the pressure from the tourniquet could lead to injuries in a patient who has had this type of surgery. Thus, venipuncture should *not* be performed on the same side as that of a mastectomy.

EDEMA

Some patients develop an abnormal accumulation of fluid in the intercellular spaces of the body. This swelling can be localized or diffused over a larger area of the body. The health care worker should avoid collecting blood from these sites because veins in these areas are difficult to palpate or stick, and the specimen may become contaminated with fluid.

OBESITY

Obese patients generally have veins that are difficult to visualize and palpate. If the vein is missed, the health care worker must be careful not to probe excessively with the needle because doing so ruptures red blood cells (RBCs), increases the concentration of intracellular contents, and releases some tissue clotting factors.

INTRAVENOUS THERAPY

Every time a catheter is used, vein damage occurs. Circulatory blood is rerouted to collateral veins and can result in hemoconcentration. Consequently, patients on intravenous (IV) therapy for extended periods often have veins that are palpable and visible but damaged or occluded (blocked). Whenever a patient has an IV line, the arm with the IV line should not be used for venipuncture because the specimen will be diluted with IV fluid. Instead, the other arm or another site should be considered. Alternatively, sometimes the nurse or the physician can disconnect the IV line and draw blood from the needle that is already inserted. In this situation, the first few milliliters of the specimen should be discarded to remove the IV fluid, and a note should be made on the laboratory requisition form that this step was performed. (Refer to Chapter 12 for more detailed information about blood collection from intravenous lines.)

DAMAGED, SCLEROSED, OR OCCLUDED VEINS

Obstructed or **occluded veins,** do not allow blood to flow through them; **sclerosed,** or hardened veins are a result of inflammation and disease of the interstitial substances; and patients' veins that have been repeatedly punctured often become scarred and feel hard when palpated. Because blood is not easily collected from these sites, they should be avoided.

HEMOCONCENTRATION

An increased concentration of larger molecules and formed elements in the blood is called **hemoconcentration**. Several factors can cause this complication, including prolonged tourniquet application; massaging, squeezing, or probing a site; long-term IV therapy; and sclerosed or occluded veins.

HEMOLYSIS

When RBCs are lysed, hemoglobin is released and serum, which is normally straw colored, becomes tinged with pink or red. If a specimen is grossly hemolyzed, the serum appears very dark red. **Hemolysis** can be caused by improper phlebotomy techniques, such as using a needle that is too small, pulling a syringe plunger back too fast, expelling the blood vigorously into a tube, and shaking or mixing tubes vigorously. Hemolysis causes falsely increased results for many analytes, including potassium, magnesium, iron, lactate dehydro-genase, phosphorus, ammonia, and total protein.[1] These problems can easily be prevented with appropriate handling. Hemolysis may also be the result of physiological abnormalities. The health care worker should make a note on the requisition form whenever he or she notices that a specimen is hemolyzed.

COLLAPSED VEINS

If a syringe plunger is withdrawn too quickly during venipuncture or the vacuum draw of a tube is too great, the vein may collapse, especially when blood is being collected from smaller veins (see Fig. 10–1F) and veins in geriatric patients. Thus, the blood collector should pull slowly on the syringe plunger or use an evacuated tube with a smaller volume during the collection process on patients with smaller veins and geriatric patients. A collapsed vein should *not* be probed with the needle.

ALLERGIES

Clinical Alert

Some patients are allergic to iodine or other solutions used to disinfect a puncture site. If a patient indicates that he or she is allergic to a solution, all efforts should be made to use an alternative method.

THROMBOSIS

Thrombi are solid masses derived from blood constituents that reside in the blood vessels. A thrombus may partially or fully occlude a vein (or artery), and such occlusion will make venipuncture more difficult.

BURNED OR SCARRED AREAS

Clinical Alert

Areas that have been burned or scarred should be avoided during phlebotomy. Burned areas are very sensitive and susceptible to infection, whereas veins under scarred areas are difficult to palpate.

INFECTIONS

The health care worker should remember at all times that many patients have transmittable diseases (e.g., hepatitis) and that likewise, he or she can pass an infection to a patient. (For precautionary techniques, refer to Chapter 4, Infection Control, and Chapter 5, Safety and First Aid.)

■ EFFECTS OF PHYSICAL DISPOSITION ON BLOOD COLLECTION

BASAL STATE

Blood specimens that will be used to determine the concentrations of body constituents, such as glucose, cholesterol, triglycerides, electrolytes, and proteins, should be collected when the patient is in a **basal state**—that is, in the early morning, approximately 12 hours after the last ingestion of food. The results of laboratory tests on basal state specimens are more reliable because normal values are most often determined from specimens collected during this time. Several factors, such as diet, exercise, emotional stress, obesity, menstrual cycle, pregnancy, *diurnal variations*, posture, tourniquet application, and chemical constituents (alcohol or drugs), cause changes in the basal state.

DIET

To ensure that the patient is in the basal state, the physician must require the patient to fast overnight. The term **fasting** refers to abstinence from food and beverages (except water). The required time period necessary for abstaining varies with the test procedures to be performed. Before collecting a specimen, the health care worker should ask the patient if he or she has eaten. Blood composition is significantly altered after meals and consequently is unsuitable for many clinical chemistry tests. If the patient has eaten, and the physician still needs the test, the word *nonfasting* must be written on the requisition form, noted directly on the specimen, or indicated in the organization's computer system.[2]

Inadequate patient instructions are often the cause of mistakes in specimen collection. The health care worker may be asked to explain fasting restrictions to a patient. In such cases, these restrictions must be explained clearly and in detail. Some patients assume that the term *fasting* refers to abstaining from food *and* water. Abstaining from water can result in dehydration, which can alter test results. Thus, the health care worker must ensure that the patient understands what is required of him or her. Written instructions can be given, if available.

Gaining the patient's understanding and cooperation is important and is determined by the professional behavior and the degree of confidence displayed by the health care worker. Casual instructions are apt to be taken lightly by the patient or even forgotten. A health care worker who is organized, attentive, and skilled and who emphasizes important points of the procedure is more likely to get patient cooperation and an accurate test result, and to make the patient more comfortable.

If a procedure involves some discomfort or inconvenience, the patient should be informed. For example, if blood is to be drawn for a timed blood glucose level determination, the patient needs to fast for 8 to 12 hours. Prolonged fasting, however, has been shown to falsely alter blood test results.[2] The health care worker can inform the patient that several specimens will be collected at timed intervals and that he or she may drink water, but that coffee and tea should be avoided because they cause a transitory fluctuation in the blood sugar level.

Normally, serum is clear, light yellow, or straw colored. **Turbid** serum appears cloudy or "milky" and can be a result of bacterial contamination or high lipid levels in the blood. Turbidity is caused primarily by ingestion of fatty substances, such as meat, butter, cream, and cheese, or can occur when an intralipid supplement is included in parenteral nutrition preparations. If a patient has recently eaten fatty substances, he or she may have a temporarily elevated lipid level, and the serum will appear **lipemic,** or cloudy. Because lipemic serum does not represent a basal state and may indicate some chemical abnormalities,[2] a note on the requisition form about the appearance of the serum may be useful to the physician.

EXERCISE

Muscular activity, as a result of moderate or excessive exercise, has a marked effect on laboratory test results, especially when the levels of lactic acid, creatinine, fatty acids, some amino acids, proteins, and some enzymes are being tested. Most of these values, except certain enzyme levels, return to baseline shortly after the exercise stops. The levels of enzymes, such as creatine phosphokinase (CPK), aspartate aminotransferase (AST), and lactate dehydrogenase (LD), can, however, remain elevated as long as 24 hours after a person engages in 1 hour of moderate-to-strenuous exercise.[2]

Research suggests that exercise also has some effects on hemostasis. Some reports indicate that physical exercise activates coagulation, fibrinolysis, and platelet formation. Because different types of exercise were studied, other reports cite conflicting results or no changes in measured hemostatic parameters. Nevertheless, most researchers conclude that some hemostatic changes do occur after strenuous exercise.[3]

STRESS

Patients are often frightened, nervous, and overly anxious, especially prior to blood collection. These emotional stresses can cause a transient elevation in the white blood cell (WBC) count, a transient decrease in serum iron levels, and abnormal hormone (e.g., cortisol, aldosterone, renin, thyroid-stimulating hormone [TSH], prolactin) values.[3,4] Also, mental anxiety can increase blood concentrations of albumin, fibrinogen, glucose, cholesterol, and insulin.[4] Newborns who have been crying violently will have WBC counts that are 140 percent above resting baseline counts. Even mild crying has been shown to increase WBC counts 113 percent. These elevated counts return to baseline values within 1 hour. Consequently, blood samples for WBC counts should be taken approximately 1 hour after a crying episode.[5] Anxiety that results in hyperventilation also causes acid–base imbalances, increased lactate levels, and increased fatty acid levels.[2]

DIURNAL RHYTHMS AND POSTURE

Diurnal rhythms are body fluid fluctuations during the day. Certain hormone levels decrease in the afternoon (e.g., cortisol, adrenocorticotropic hormone [ACTH] TSH, T_4, iron), whereas eosinophil counts and serum iron levels increase. Thus, collecting specimens during the designated time periods is important for proper clinical evaluation.

Posture changes are also known to vary laboratory test results of some chemical constituents (e.g., aldosterone). This consideration is important when inpatient and outpatient results are being compared. Thus, blood collection should be performed under standardized posture conditions. Changing from a **supine** (or lying) position to a sitting or standing position causes body water to shift from intravascular to interstitial compartments (in tissues). Certain larger molecules cannot filter into the tissue; therefore, they concentrate in the blood. Enzyme, protein, lipid, iron, and calcium levels are significantly increased with changes in position.[6] These effects can be more pronounced in patients with congestive heart failure, hepatic disorders, and other, edematous disorders.

AGE

Laboratory test results vary considerably during the stages of life: infancy, childhood (pediatric population), adulthood, and older adulthood (geriatric population). For example, blood cholesterol and triglyceride values increase as a person ages. Various hormone levels, such as estrogen and growth hormone (GH) levels, decrease in geriatric women. GH levels are also decreased in geriatric men.

TESTING INTERFERENCE FROM TOURNIQUET PRESSURE

Laboratory test results can be falsely elevated or decreased if the tourniquet pressure is too tight or is maintained too long. The pressure from the tourniquet causes biological analytes to leak from the tissue cells into the blood, or vice versa. For example, plasma cholesterol, iron, lipid, protein, and potassium levels will be falsely elevated if the tourniquet pressure is too tight or prolonged. Significant elevations may be seen with as short as a 3-minute application of the tourniquet.[6] In addition, some enzyme levels can be falsely elevated or decreased because of tourniquet pressure that is too tight or prolonged.

OTHER FACTORS AFFECTING THE PATIENT

Many other factors can affect laboratory test results. Gender and pregnancy have an influence on laboratory testing; thus, reference ranges are often noted according to gender. Geographic factors, such as altitude, temperature, and humidity, also affect normal baseline values. Collecting blood during home health care visits may entail traveling to different regions than the location of the laboratory. Thus, geographic information of this type should be provided on the laboratory requisition slip in order to be considered in the patient's tests results.

Medications may also alter laboratory test results significantly. Consequently, physicians must work closely with pharmacy and laboratory staff to rule out laboratory test results that are altered because the patient is taking medication.

■ INTERFERENCE OF DRUGS AND OTHER SUBSTANCES IN BLOOD

Many prescribed drugs can interfere with clinical laboratory determinations or can physiologically alter the levels of blood constituents measured in the clinical laboratory. The interference of drugs and other substances is so complicated and dependent on the chemical procedures used that only general recommendations are described in this section.

The direct analytic interference of drugs is decreasing with the advent of more specific and sensitive chemical procedures. The physiologically induced abnormalities from various types of drugs, however, are the major causes of interference from medications. Drugs administered to alleviate an illness can induce physiologic abnormalities in one or more of the following systems: hepatic, hematologic, hemostatic, muscular, pancreatic, and renal. The erroneous results may obscure the clinical diagnosis.

Prior to laboratory measurement of chemical constituents, the attending physician should take the necessary precautions in prescribing drugs to the patient. If the patient must be maintained on medication that may cause interferences in laboratory assays, the medication name should be written on the laboratory request form. Unless interference of medications can be avoided by ordering different laboratory assays, medications should be discontinued if possible, and assays should be repeated when false laboratory values are suspected.

Direct analytic interference in laboratory determinations is least likely to occur in blood assays because drug concentrations are usually low. Some drugs or drug metabolites in blood can, however, directly cause falsely decreased or falsely elevated values in laboratory analyses.

A more complete list of such drugs can be found in Young's *Effects of Drugs on Clinical Laboratory Test Results.*[7]

Interference from medications usually causes falsely elevated values rather than falsely decreased values. Some drugs, such as acetaminophen (Tylenol) and erythromycin, can increase serum AST and bilirubin levels and, thus, falsely create a clinical interpretation of hepatic dysfunction without the true presence of hepatic abnormality.[8] Drug-induced elevations of blood constituents can be mistakenly interpreted as falsely increased or normal, when the true values are in the normal range or the subnormal range, respectively.

In addition to prescribed oral medications, intravenous injections of medications and dyes can interfere with laboratory test results. For example, the results of laboratory tests performed after fluorescein angiography may be erroneous owing to interference by the intravenous fluorescein.[9] The results for blood creatinine, cortisol, and digoxin determinations are altered by this dye. Consequently, if the health care worker, nurse, or clinical assistant collects blood in a cardiology section or a specialized health care institution for heart patients, he or she needs to be alert to this potential for laboratory test interference. If he or she is aware of collecting blood from a patient who just had a dye injection, this information must be communicated promptly to the specimen collection supervisor.

Physiologically, drugs can alter blood analytes through various metabolic reactions; the production of blood cells and platelets, as well as their survival times, can be changed. Chemotherapeutic drugs can lead to a decrease in all forms of blood cellular elements and, thus, their metabolic and immunologic processes.

A variety of medications are toxic to the liver (Table 10–1) and, thus, can lead to acute hepatic necrosis.[8] In turn, the hepatic dysfunction leads to an increase in the concentration of blood liver enzymes, such as alanine aminotransferase (ALT), alkaline phosphatase (ALP), and LD. Also, the production of globulins and clotting factors is decreased in patients with drug-induced hepatotoxicity.

Patients receiving medications that may result in renal impairment should be monitored for a possible electrolyte imbalance and elevation of blood urea nitrogen (BUN) levels. Antihypertensive agents given for a long period to lower high blood pressure can lead to kidney damage if the patient is not monitored closely.

Pancreatitis can be caused by corticosteroids, estrogens, and diuretics and causes elevations of serum amylase and lipase values. Aspirin causes **hypobilirubinemia** (a decrease in bilirubin) by expelling bilirubin from the plasma to the surrounding tissue cells.[10]

The health care worker collecting the blood specimen is the link between the clinical lab-

Table 10–1.   Drugs Toxic to the Liver

Salicylates	Penicillin	Acetaminophen
Mitomycin	Isoniazid	Chlorpromazine
Actinomycin	Halothane	Methyldopa
Thiazides	Chloramphenicol	Acetohexamide
Trifluoperazine	Sulfamethoxazole	Chlorpropamide
Sulfachlorpyridazine	Tetracycline	Paramethadione
Phenytoin		

Adapted from Sher PP. Drug interferences with clinical laboratory tests. *Drugs*. 1982; 24:24; and Sherlock S. Progress report: Hepatic reaction to drugs. *Gut*. 1979; 20:634

oratory and the patient. Laboratory tests are often ordered without knowledge of the drugs taken by a person. Yet, as discussed previously, these drugs will lead to falsely elevated or decreased values. Sometimes during blood collection, a patient will mention that he or she has taken over-the-counter drugs, such as Tylenol. It is important for the health care worker to communicate the patient's name and the possible drug interference to the clinical laboratory supervisor in charge of specimen collection. The supervisor can then communicate with the attending physician and determine whether the medication will interfere in the laboratory assays. The follow-up communication can lead to better patient care by preventing the presence of interfering substances in laboratory specimens.

■ SPECIMEN REJECTION

Each department or section in the clinical laboratory should establish its own guidelines for specimen rejection. In general, the factors shown in Table 10–2 should be considered.

When a problem arises, the appropriate investigational channels should be followed. The health care provider who drew the specimen and his or her supervisor should try to solve the problem initially. Other personnel may be involved as needed. Communication and honesty are the keys to an efficient and reliable health care environment.

Table 10–2.   Complications Leading to Blood Specimen Rejection

Hemolyzed specimen (except for tests in which hemolysis does not interfere)
Nonfasting specimen
Anticoagulated blood containing clots
Improper specimen transportation (e.g., blood gas specimen not transported in slurry of ice water)
Improper blood collection tube
Variation in patient's posture (e.g., aldosterone level changes depending on patient sitting or lying for blood collection)
Lipemic specimen
Insufficient quantity of blood in collection tube
Discrepancies between requisition form and labeled tube (e.g., names, dates, times)
Unlabelled tube
Outdated equipment, supplies, or reagents
Contaminated specimen

SELF STUDY

KEY TERMS

Basal State
Diurnal Rhythms
Fasting
Hematoma
Hemoconcentration
Hemolysis
Hypobilirubinemia
Lipemic
Lymphostasis

Mastectomy
Occluded Veins
Petechiae
Sclerosed Veins
Supine
Syncope
Thrombi
Turbid

STUDY QUESTIONS

The following questions may have *one* or *more* answers.

1. Which of the following factors result in failure to draw blood during venipuncture?

   a. losing the vacuum in the tube
   b. tying the tourniquet too tightly
   c. inserting the needle through the vein
   d. puncturing a sclerosed vein

2. Hematomas during venipuncture result from which of the following?

   a. needle bevel is against vein wall
   b. needle bevel is partially inserted in the vein
   c. needle is occluded
   d. patient has coagulation problems

3. Hemoconcentration can be caused by which of the following?

   a. long-term IV therapy
   b. lengthy tourniquet application
   c. excessive needle probing
   d. sclerosed or occluded veins

4. Which of the following is a solid mass derived from blood constituents and can occlude a vein (or an artery)?

   a. hemolyzed RBC
   b. hemolyzed WBC
   c. thrombus
   d. triglyceride

5. If blood is to be drawn for a timed blood glucose level determination, the patient must fast for how long?

   a. 4 to 6 hours
   b. 6 to 8 hours
   c. 8 to 12 hours
   d. 14 to 16 hours

6. Which of the following laboratory test results are affected most if the patient is not fasting?

   a. AST and CPK

   b. triglycerides and glucose

   c. cortisol and testosterone

   d. complete blood cell (CBC) count and prothrombin time

7. An abnormal accumulation of fluid in the intercellular spaces of the body that is localized or diffused is referred to as which of the following?

   a. hemoconcentration

   b. edema

   c. atherosclerosis

   d. hemolysis

8. If a patient is taking high doses of Tylenol, which of the following analyte results is most likely to be affected?

   a. serum bilirubin

   b. CPK

   c. blood glucose

   d. blood cholesterol

9. If the tourniquet is applied for longer than 3 minutes, which of the following analytes will most likely become falsely elevated?

   a. potassium

   b. bilirubin

   c. GGT

   d. parathyroid hormone

10. Emotional stress, such as anxiety or fear, can lead to alterations of which of the following analytes?

   a. serum iron

   b. WBCs

   c. cortisol

   d. RBCs

References

1. Meites S, ed. *Pediatric Clinical Chemistry, Reference (Normal) Values.* 3rd ed. Washington, DC: AACC Press; 1989.

2. Statland BE, Winkel P: Preparing patients and specimens for laboratory testing. In: Henry JB, ed. *Clinical Diagnosis and Management by Laboratory Methods.* Philadelphia; WB Saunders; 1991.

3. Rudmann SV: The effects of exercise on hemostasis: a review of the literature and implications for research. *Am J Med Technol.* 1987;4(5):215.

4. Guder WG, Narayanan S, Wisser H, et al. *Samples: From the Patient to the Laboratory.* Germany: Git Verlag Pub; 1996.

5. Becton-Dickinson and Company: *Blood Specimen Collection by Skin Puncture in Infants.* East Rutherford, NJ: Becton-Dickinson and Company; 1982.

6. Statland BE, Winkle P, Bokelund H: Factors contributing to intra-individual variation of serum constituents: Effects of posture and tourniquet application on variation of serum constituents in healthy subjects. *Clin Chem.* 1974;20:1513.

7. Young DS: *Effects of Drugs on Clinical Laboratory Tests.* 4th ed. Washington, DC: AACC Press; 1995.

8. Sherlock S: Progress report: hepatic reaction to drugs. *Gut.* 1979;20:634.

9. Elin RJ, Bloom JN, Herman DC, et al. interference by intravenous fluorescein with laboratory tests. *Clin Chem.* 1989;35(6):1159.

10. Routh J, Paul W: Assessment of interference by aspirin with some assays commonly done in the clinical laboratory. *Clin Chem.* 1976;22:837.

PHLEBOTOMY CASE STUDY

■

Ambulatory Health Care Collections

Ms. Jeanne Peterson is a health care provider who contracts with two community hospitals to make home health care visits. This morning as she arrived at Lake Mountain Hospital late due to an early winter snowstorm, she noticed she had seven home visits. She quickly threw blood collection equipment in her lockable container and hurried to her first patient, Ms. Verle Ragsdale, an 82-year-old African American woman, who has type II diabetes with myocardial complications. Her physician had requested a complete chemistry profile and protime, in addition to a physical examination. After Ms. Peterson checked Ms. Ragsdale's vital signs, she decided to collect Ms. Ragsdale's blood with a winged infusion blood collection set due to the fragility of her veins. She prepared the site for blood collection and after opening a 25-gauge safety winged infusion needle set, she inserted the needle into the patient's vein in her hand and first collected blood in a light blue–topped tube for the protime, followed by blood collection into a red speckled–topped vacuum tube. After completing the physical exam and blood collection, she labeled the tubes, discarded the biohazardous blood collection items in her biohazardous disposal container, and left Ms. Ragsdale's home with the collected blood and health care equipment, including the blood collection items.

Next, she traveled over the slippery, snow-covered roads to Mr. Ben Sadler's home, a 32-year-old white hemophiliac who had acquired hepatitis C from a blood transfusion. His physician had requested a liver profile. Ms. Peterson introduced herself to Mr. Sadler and prepared her blood collection supplies and equipment for blood collection for Mr. Sadler. As she checked Mr. Sadler's veins, she decided to use a butterfly needle in Mr. Sadler's lower arm due to the sclerosed veins in the antecubital fossa area on both arms. She looked for a blood collection set in her supplies but only found a 23-gauge needle, separate tubing, and a separate luer lok. She put the pieces together and found a needle holder assembly and red-speckled collection tube. After attaching the various pieces, hoping they would work together, she prepared Mr. Sadler's arm for blood collection. She inserted the needle into his vein and as she pushed the tube onto the needle holder assembly, the luer lok became disengaged and splattered blood over Ms. Peterson's laboratory coat and into her face. She immediately pulled the tourniquet off of Mr. Sadler's arm, pulled the needle out of his vein, cleaned the area around him, and ran to his bathroom to wash the blood from her face and eyes.

QUESTIONS:

1. Did the health care provider use the proper order of draw for Ms. Ragsdale's laboratory tests? Explain.

2. Was the proper blood collection procedure used for obtaining blood from Ms. Ragsdale? Explain.

3. Was the proper blood collection procedure used for obtaining blood from Mr. Sadler? Explain.

See Answers in Appendix.

PHLEBOTOMY CASE STUDY

■

Venipuncture Site Selection

The medical laboratory technician, Sara Wong went to collect blood from a 65-year-old hospitalized patient, Mary McDonald. Mrs. McDonald was a diabetic. She had recently undergone a partial mastectomy on her right side. The area around the mastectomy appeared swollen. She had an IV going just below the antecubital area of her left arm. The ordered tests were CBC, differential, and electrolytes. Sara carefully selected a site and was successful on the first attempt to collect the blood samples.

QUESTIONS:

1. What would be the preferred site and method of choice for the phlebotomy procedure for this patient?
2. Explain why other sites were eliminated.
3. What special documentation (if any) might be helpful for this phlebotomy procedure.
4. List several techniques that can facilitate the selection of a suitable site.

See Answers in Appendix.

SPECIAL PROCEDURES AND POINT-OF-CARE TESTING

T HE PRACTICE OF PHLEBOTOMY INVOLVES specialized duties and functions in certain circumstances. Part IV describes the special procedures and work settings that are becoming part of the expanding role of health care workers. Each new activity can be learned alone or along with other, more routine duties. For some phlebotomists, a procedure that was previously "special" and off limits is now routine. Moreover, specimen collections occur in a variety of settings and in circumstances that may require new knowledge about special groups of patients.

Chapter 11, Pediatric Procedures, focuses on the special attention and technical skills necessary for dealing with infants and children. The chapter describes effective communication with children and parents; different procedures for blood collection, including heel sticks, neonatal screening procedures, and the dorsal hand vein technique; and special concerns regarding diagnostic testing for children.

Chapter 12, Arterial, Intravenous (IV), and Special Collection Procedures, covers site selection and puncture procedures for blood collection for arterial blood gas determinations; the Allen test; bleeding-time tests; blood cultures; glucose, lactose, and other tolerance tests; and therapeutic drug monitoring (TDM) tests. Also discussed are blood collections through intravenous lines, central venous catheters, blood donor room collections, and emergency room blood collections.

Chapter 13, Elderly, Home, and Long-term Care Collections, highlights procedures that are becoming more routine in the care and monitoring of patients in these settings. Emphasis is on point-of-care testing, such as glucose monitoring, blood gas and electrolyte analysis, and cholesterol screening.

Chapter 14, Urinalysis and Body Fluid Collections, describes the various alternative procedures for urine and other body fluid collections, including cerebrospinal fluid, seminal fluid, amniotic fluid, and specimens for microbiological cultures. Emphasis is on proper collection and safe handling of the specimens.

Chapter 15, Specimen Collection for Forensic Toxicology, Workplace Testing, Sports Medicine, and Related Areas, describes specimen collections related to drug testing in forensic toxicology and workplace testing. Emphasis is on the role of the health care worker in appropriate sample collection, handling various types of samples, detecting altered specimens, securing the chain of custody, and transporting the specimen.

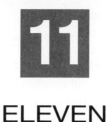

ELEVEN

■

Pediatric Procedures

CHAPTER OUTLINE

CHAPTER OBJECTIVES

Upon completion of Chapter 11, the learner is responsible for the following:

1. Describe fears or concerns that children in different developmental stages might have toward the blood collection process.

2. List suggestions that might be appropriate for parental behavior during a venipuncture or skin puncture.

3. Identify puncture sites for a heel stick on an infant and demonstrate the procedure.

4. Describe the venipuncture sites for infants and young children.

5. Discuss the types of equipment and supplies that must be used during microcollection and venipuncture of infants and children.

6. Describe the procedure for screening neonates for phenylketonuria (PKU).

Drawing blood from a pediatric patient requires much expertise and knowledge. Not all **pediatric phlebotomies** are fingersticks, so the novice health care worker must study anatomy and physiology, be familiar with special types of equipment that are available, observe the various techniques as they are performed by an experienced health care worker, and practice the techniques to develop the necessary skills.

Performing venipunctures on young patients is technically and emotionally challenging for the health care worker because of these patients' small size and because children are less emotionally and psychologically prepared to cope with pain. Therefore, a successful outcome requires the use of good interpersonal skills in dealing with children and their concerned, apprehensive parents.[1]

With proper training in technique and an understanding of pediatric psychological development, the delicate task of drawing blood from a frightened child need not strike fear or dread in the heart of the health care worker. Skills should be perfected on older children first, then, when confidence is attained, venipunctures can be attempted on younger children. When learning the techniques, the health care worker should remember to ask for help if needed and to allow adequate time to develop the necessary skills.

■ AGE-SPECIFIC CARE CONSIDERATIONS

Age-specific care considerations are shown in Table 11–1. It describes not only the fears and concerns of the pediatric patient at various ages, but also suggests parental involvement at each stage, and provides competencies and tips for the phlebotomist.

■ PREPARING CHILD AND PARENT

Preparing the child and the parent for the blood collection procedure involves the following steps:

1. Introduce yourself. Be warm, friendly, establish eye contact, and show that you are concerned about the child's health and comfort. When you interact with a pediatric patient and his or her parent, you should instill a sense of trust and confidence in the parent and the child. A calm, confident approach is the first step in limiting their anxiety and obtaining their cooperation.

2. Correctly identify the patient. A hospitalized infant usually has an identification bracelet on his or her ankle. Newborns who are not yet named are usually referred to by their last names (e.g., Baby Boy Smith, Baby Girl Jones) and are identified by a unique identification number. If the mother is still in the hospital after delivery, the baby may wear a bracelet that is cross-referenced to the mother for breastfeeding times and so forth. Keeping identifications straight is always crucial, but especially so when specimens from twin babies must be collected and labeled.

Table 11-1. Age-specific care considerations and competencies for phlebotomists

AGE	FEARS AND CONCERNS	COMMUNICATION	COMFORT	SAFETY	PARENT BEHAVIOR
0–6 months	• Totally dependent on and trusts parents and other adults	• Introduce yourself to caregiver • Explain procedures	• Keep patient warm • Warm site of puncture if needed • Parent may hold child • Use very gentle approach • Use of a distraction, such as light pen, key ring, or bell, may minimize fear	• Keep side rails up during procedure • Do not leave any supplies or discarded items on bed • Encourage parent to hold or cuddle infant after procedure • Use appropriate microcollection supplies and equipment	• Parent may hold child as an aid to the phlebotomist and to provide comfort
6–12 months	• Fear of strangers • Fear of separation from parent • Limited language use	• Introduce yourself to caregiver • Talk slowly to infant • Try to make eye contact with infant	• Keep patient warm • Warm site of puncture if needed • Allow familiar health care worker to perform procedure • Allow parent to be in close proximity • Allow child to use pacifier, hold teddy, blanket, or other comforting items	• Do not separate from caregiver unless absolutely necessary • Keep side rails up • Do not leave any supplies or discarded items on bed • Encourage parent to hold or cuddle infant after procedure • Use appropriate microcollection supplies and equipment	• Parent may assist by holding, explaining to, and comforting the child • Parent may help identify comforting toy

(continued)

Table 11-1 (continued).

AGE	FEARS AND CONCERNS	COMMUNICATION	COMFORT	SAFETY	PARENT BEHAVIOR
1–3 years	• Self-centered • Fear of injury • Fear of long separation from parent	• Introduce yourself to both child and caregiver • Child will understand simple commands and may choose to cooperate • Take it slowly, do not rush patient, he or she needs time to think about your requests • Allow child to touch supplies but dispose if they become contaminated • Ask parent to also explain procedure in familiar terms	• Keep patient warm • Warm site of puncture if needed • Allow familiar health care worker to perform procedure • Allow parent to be in close proximity • Allow child to use pacifier, hold teddy, blanket, or other comforting items	• Try not to separate from parent unless absolutely necessary. If needed, reinforce that it is only for a short period of time • Keep side rails up • Do not leave supplies or discarded items on bed • Use appropriate microcollection supplies and equipment	• Parent may assist by holding, explaining to, and comforting the child • Parent may help identify comforting toy • Encourage parent to praise child after procedure
3–5 years	• Self-centered • Fear of injury • Enjoys pretending and role playing	• Introduce yourself • Talk to child in simple terms • Allow child to touch equipment • Try using familiar cartoon characters (Disney, Sesame Street) in the explanation • Perhaps use toys to demonstrate procedure • Child may pretend he or she is the doctor and will "help" with the procedure • Provide tokens for bravery	• Allow child to have familiar things or people near by • Give them time to verbalize their fears	• May tolerate separation from parent • Able to recognize danger and obey simple commands • Needs close supervision • Keep side rails up • Do not leave supplies or discarded items on bed • Use appropriate microcollection supplies and equipment	• Parent may be present to provide emotional support and to assist in obtaining the child's cooperation • Encourage praise for bravery

(continued)

Table 11–1 (continued).

AGE	FEARS AND CONCERNS	COMMUNICATION	COMFORT	SAFETY	PARENT BEHAVIOR
6–12 years	• Less dependent on parents • Fear losing self-control • More willing to participate • Tries to be independent • Curious	• Introduce yourself • Child may be interested in health concepts, "why" and "how" • Explain "why" the blood is needed • Involve child in the procedure	• Try not to embarrass the child but offer them a comforting toy or familiar object • May want parent to hold their hand • Take it slowly, allow time for repeat questions • Allow child some input on decisions (e.g., color of bandage, etc.)	• Side rails should be left up after procedure • Do not leave supplies or discarded items on bed • Use appropriate microcollection supplies and equipment	• Child may ask parent to leave room
13–17 years	• Actively involved in anything concerning the body • More independent • Embarrassed to show fear • Needs privacy • May act hostile to mask fear	• Introduce yourself • Use adult vocabulary, do not "talk down" • Explain procedure thoroughly • Ask if he or she would like to help with the procedure • Ask what might make them more comfortable • Allow time for questions or to handle supplies	• Maintain privacy • Take extra time for explanations and or preparation • Offer them the opportunity to have parent close by • Give them time to recover after the procedure if they have cried	• Use same strategies as adult • Use appropriate collection supplies and equipment depending on the size of the individual and the physical and emotional tolerance to procedure	• Child may not want parent to be present
Children with special problems or mental disabilities	• Fears are similar to the behaviors of the developmental level • Need relaxed, gentle approach	• Use strategies that are appropriate for the developmental stage	• Use strategies that are appropriate for the developmental stage	• Use strategies that are appropriate for the developmental stage	• Use strategies that are appropriate for the developmental stage

3. Find out about the child's past experience with blood drawing. This can be accomplished easily by asking whether the child has ever had blood collected. The child and the parent can then tell about their experiences with past procedures and provide you with valuable information about the approaches that worked effectively for them and those that were not as successful.

4. Develop a plan. Asking the parent how cooperative his or her child will be is a simple and accurate means of predicting the level of the child's distress. Usually, the younger child with poor venous access will experience more distress. A successful plan involves not only the parent's ability to make educated choices about what will be most helpful, but also one's knowledge of pediatric phlebotomy techniques. If possible, allow the child to have some control by asking him or her from which arm or finger he or she prefers blood to be taken. After assessing the experiences, anxiety, and fears of the parent and the child, tailor the procedure for optimal success.

5. Explain and demonstrate the procedure at their eye level. When explaining what you will be doing, use words appropriate for the child's age. Children interpret words literally, so be careful of your choice of words. Use of a doll, puppet, or stuffed animal in the demonstration can help you relate to the child in a nonthreatening manner. If the child has a favorite doll, blanket, or toy, he or she should be encouraged to hug it for comfort and support.

6. Establish guidelines. Tell the child and the parent that the procedure will most likely be successful on the first attempt, but if not, it will be attempted only once more. Then another health care worker will be called in to complete the procedure.

7. Be honest with the child who asks whether the puncture will hurt. Some children cannot separate pain from fear. Instructing the child to say when he or she feels pain will help the child to make this distinction. The child should be told that saying "ouch" or making faces is acceptable, but that he or she must make an effort to keep the arm absolutely still. Also tell the child that if the procedure hurts too much, it can be momentarily stopped; but that the quicker the procedure is performed the less painful it will be. Tell the child it is okay to cry if it does hurt and remind them that it will only be for a short time. Reassure the child that the blood will be drawn as quickly as possible so that the pain will be brief.[2]

8. Encourage parent involvement. Most recent research demonstrates that **parental involvement**—the parent's presence and support—has the most beneficial effect on the child's anxiety.[3] Some parents, however, may be reluctant to be present because they do not understand how they can assist or because they do not want to be a part of a procedure that will cause their children pain. Each parent's ability to assist must be assessed, and if after discussing his or her role, the parent is still reluctant to participate, his or her wishes should be respected.

Studies have shown that parental behavior influences the child's behavior during the procedure. The following parental behaviors and examples will have a positive effect on relieving the child's distress.[3,4]

Behaviors:	*Examples:*
Distraction	"Look at Mommy"; "Tell the nurse about your doll"
Emotional support	Hugging, stroking hair, patting, and saying soothing words
Explanation	"We need to take a tiny bit of blood from your finger"; "Mommy will help you hold your arm so that we can finish quickly"

PSYCHOLOGICAL RESPONSE TO NEEDLES AND PAIN

Children especially fear needles, and an emotionally distraught child has difficulty separating fear from actual pain. Many children perceive that a "shot," or needle, hurts more than anything else that has ever happened to them. Children's drawings of hospital procedures often depict huge needles that go entirely through the limb.[2] Nevertheless, with proper preparation, the child and the parent can develop coping skills to help alleviate the fear and thereby diminish the "hurt."

ROOM LOCATION

For psychological reasons, the best room location for a painful procedure is a treatment room away from the child's bed or playroom. For a hospitalized child, the bed should be a safe, secure place to rest and sleep, not a place associated with pain. If the child shares a room with another child, performing the procedure at the bedside can upset the roommate as well. If the child cannot be moved to a treatment room, privacy should be maintained by drawing a curtain between the beds and speaking in a calm, quiet manner.

EQUIPMENT PREPARATION FOR A FRIENDLIER ENVIRONMENT

Just the sight of needles, syringes, and a person in a white laboratory coat can be frightening to a child. Nurses and other health care providers working with children frequently wear bright, colorfully printed uniforms or smocks to create a friendlier environment. Equipment, too, can be modified to appear less threatening. As an example, prepare the phlebotomy equipment and supplies prior to entering the room in which the child is located so that the child does not become even more anxious in the health care environment. Use shorter needles if possible, and keep threatening-looking supplies (e.g., needles) covered and out of sight. If the hospital policy requires goggles or face shields for blood-exposure precautions, put this equipment on after greeting the child. At the completion of the procedure, reward the child with praise, a special Band-Aid with cartoon characters, a sticker, an age-appropriate toy, or, with parental permission, a lollipop. If no parent is present to assist in relieving the child's anxiety, you or the nurse in charge may cuddle and offer a pacifier to an infant, gently stroke, or talk softly to sooth a small child.

POSITIONS FOR RESTRAINING A CHILD

To ensure that a child does not move the limb during venous access, physical restraint may be required. A supportive parent can assist with restraining while providing comfort to the child.

Two preferred methods of restraining a child to immobilize the arm are the vertical position and the horizontal, or supine, position.[2,5] In both cases, the mother's face is in close proximity to the child's, thereby providing a comforting and secure feeling. The vertical technique, which works well for toddlers, requires the parent to hold the child on the lap. As the parent hugs and holds the child's body and the arm not being used, the health care worker can firmly hold the other arm to perform the procedure (Fig. 11–1).

In the horizontal position, the child lies supine, with the health care worker on one side of the bed and the parent on the opposite side. The parent gently but firmly leans over the child, restraining the near arm and the body while holding the opposite extended arm securely for the health care worker (Fig. 11–2).

Figure 11–1. Vertical position for restraining a child to perform a phlebotomy.

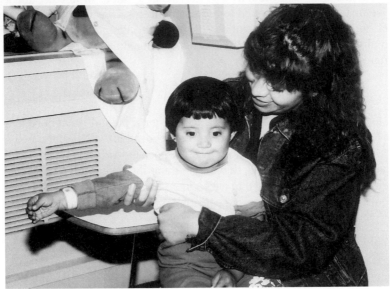

Figure 11–2. Horizontal, or supine, position for restraining a child to perform a phlebotomy.

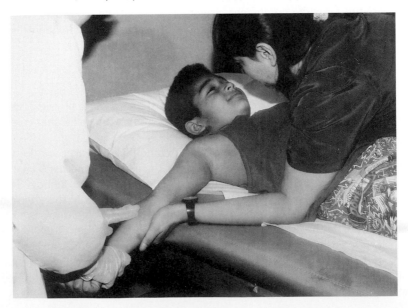

Neonates and infants younger than 3 months usually do not require restraint. Consequently, they can be managed by the health care worker alone.

COMBATIVE PATIENTS

At times, a child will become uncooperative even after the proper steps have been followed to elicit cooperation. Children may become combative—kicking and thrashing—if force is used. Because sharps are involved in blood collection, the health care worker must be certain that the procedure can be performed safely. Using force to the point of potential physical injury is unethical and unprofessional. Therefore, if the risk of injury to the health care worker or the child is likely, the blood collection attempt should be discontinued, and the nurse or the physician notified.[6] In such instances, alternative coping measures or pharmacological intervention may be necessary prior to the next attempt.

INTERVENTIONS TO ALLEVIATE PAIN

Depending on the anticipated duration of the procedure, the severity of the child's illness, and the anxiety of the child, pharmacological intervention may be used to alleviate pain and anxiety. A topical anesthetic, **EMLA (eutectic mixture of local anesthetics),** which is an emulsion of lidocaine and prilocaine can be applied to intact skin. This local anesthetic is ideal for use on children prior to venipuncture or starting intravenous (IV) therapy because it does not require a needle. EMLA penetrates both the epidermal and dermal layers, anesthetizing to a depth of 5 mm. It is applied to the skin as a patch or a cream that is then covered with a transparent occlusive dressing. Optimal anesthesia occurs after 60 minutes and may last as long as 2 to 3 hours. Drawbacks to the use of EMLA are cost, the need to apply it 60 minutes prior to the procedure, and having to know in advance the location of the vein to be used. Two separate locations may be anesthetized if the child has difficult venous access. EMLA has minimal side effects but may cause pallor at the application site or erythema due to the adhesive covering; however, EMLA should not be used if the child is allergic to local anesthetics or is younger than 1 month.[2,7]

SUCROSE NIPPLE OR PACIFIER

Giving an infant a **sucrose nipple or pacifier** to suck during and immediately after phlebotomy offers some degree of comfort, although it does not alleviate the pain. Once the infant is crying vigorously and the heart and respiratory rates have increased, a pacifier has no significant effect on changing the rates. Infants given pacifiers or sucrose nipples have, however, been shown to be more alert following the procedure and to be less fussy and to cry for a shorter duration.[8]

■ PREVENTION OF DISEASE TRANSMISSION

If a child is in isolation, a sign posted on the door will describe the type of isolation and the personal protective equipment (PPE) to be worn. Isolation categories are based on the mode of transmission (see Chapter 4, Infection Control).[9] All necessary supplies—a gown, gloves, and a mask—should be available at the room. Hands should be washed according to policy before and after gloving. Usually, an anteroom is available before the isolation room, where you may wash and put on the protective equipment.

Universal standard precautions should be followed throughout pediatric phlebotomy procedures. All children should be treated as if they could be potentially infectious. To prevent transmission of blood-borne pathogens, standard precautions should always be used in addition to transmission category isolation precautions.[9] (See Chapter 4, Infection Control, and Chapter 5, Safety and First Aid.)

PRECAUTIONS TO PROTECT THE CHILD

Premature babies, newborns, infants, and children who are chronically ill, immunocompromised, or have extensive burns are more likely to be susceptible to environmental microorganisms. To protect these children, some hospitals may require PPE, gowns, gloves, and masks to be worn as indicated before entering the room. Remove the PPE according to policy and dispose of them in the appropriately marked container. Hands should be washed and a clean gown and gloves put on before attending to the next child or infant.

LATEX ALLERGY OR ALERT

 Some children and health care workers may be allergic to latex. Usually, a sign posted on the door will note the child's allergy, or the child may wear a bracelet indicating a **latex allergy** or a latex alert. Several brands of nonlatex gloves should be available for use with children who have this allergy. Children with spina bifida and those with congenital urinary tract abnormalities or neurogenic bladders are particularly sensitive to latex.[10,11]

■ PEDIATRIC PHLEBOTOMY PROCEDURES

Two methods are used to obtain blood from infants and children: microcapillary skin puncture and venipuncture. The previously described steps for preparing the child and the parent should be taken before the procedure is performed.

MICROCAPILLARY SKIN PUNCTURE

Skin punctures are useful for pediatric phlebotomy when only small amounts of blood need to be obtained and can be adequately tested. It is particularly important to withdraw only the smallest amounts of blood necessary from neonates, infants, and children so that the effects of **blood volume** reduction are minimal.

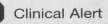 Clinical Alert

Small infants can become anemic if too much blood is taken in the course of a day.

A 10-mL sample taken from a premature or newborn infant is equivalent to 5 to 10 percent of the infant's total blood volume. Calculation of blood volume is based on weight. It can be calculated for any size person if the weight (in kilograms) of the individual is known. The total blood volume of a person is calculated by multiplying weight (kg) by the following blood volumes:

115 mL/kg	Premature infants
80–110 mL/kg	Newborns
75–100 mL/kg	Infants and children
70 mL/kg	Adults

Clinical Alert

A 3-kg infant (approximately 6.6 pounds) will have a total blood volume between 225 to 300 mL. It is important to monitor how much of this is withdrawn each day.[12] Table 8–1 provides the maximum amounts of blood to be drawn from infants and children.

When performing skin punctures, the hematology specimens are collected first to minimize platelet clumping, then chemistry and blood bank specimens. Each laboratory has approved procedures for phlebotomy; these procedures should always be followed.

Sites

The heel of the infant or neonate is the most desirable site for skin puncture to obtain capillary blood. The most medial or lateral section of the plantar, or bottom, surface of the heel should be used (Fig. 11–3). For children older than 1 year, the palmar surface of the tip of the third or fourth finger may be used instead (see Chapter 9, Skin Puncture Procedures). The plantar surface of the great toe is rarely used and only in children older than 1 year.

Equipment for Microcapillary Sampling

(See Chapter 7, Blood Collection Equipment for additional information.) The following equipment is necessary for pediatric skin puncture procedures:

1. Sterile automatic disposable pediatric safety lancet devices.
2. Seventy percent isopropyl alcohol swabs in sterile packages.
3. Sterile cotton balls or gauze sponges.
4. Plastic capillary collection tubes and sealer.
5. Microcollection containers and Unopettes.
6. Glass slides for smears.
7. Puncture-resistant sharps container.
8. Disposable gloves (nonlatex if child is allergic).
9. Compress (towel or washcloth) to warm heel if necessary.
10. Marking pen.
11. Laboratory request slips or labels.

Figure 11–3. Sites for heel stick on an infant.

(From Ball J, Bindler R. *Pediatric Nursing: Caring for Children*. Norwalk, CT: Appleton & Lange; 1995, p 814, with permission.)

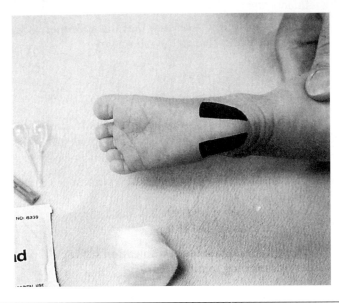

Special Equipment for Capillary Blood Gas Collection

See Chapter 12, Arterial and Special Collection Procedures, for details on capillary blood gas collection. The following supplies are needed for this procedure:

1. Heparinized plastic capillary tube and caps or sealer.
2. Metal filing and magnet.
3. Container of ice water.
4. Warm compress (towel or washcloth).
5. Clean, dry towel.
6. Sterile gauze sponge.

HEEL STICK

 Clinical Alert

Microsamples from the heel are preferred for routine laboratory, platelet count, blood chemistry, and drug level determinations for **neonates** and infants who have not begun to stand. If an infant has compromised circulation to the extremity, is in shock, or has edema or infection at the heel, another site should be used. Avoid **heel stick** in an area that has many previous puncture sites because such a stick could cause an infection.

The lancet should be of proper pediatric size, making an incision that is less than 2.4-mm deep (see Fig. 11–4). Major blood vessels lie 0.3 to 1.6 mm beneath the skin at the dermal–subcutaneous junction in newborns. If an incision goes deeper, the **calcaneus** or heel bone may be hit and may lead to **osteomyelitis.**

Clinical Alert

Commercially available heel-incision devices are designed specifically for use on infants and premature babies. As an example, the Tenderfoot (International Technidyne Corp., Edison, NJ) heel incision device (Fig. 11–4) can be obtained in different calibrations for heel sticks on infants, premature infants, and toddlers. The standard size makes an incision 1.0 mm in depth. The size of incision for premature infants is 40 percent smaller to ensure safety for these infants.

Specific guidelines for performing a heel stick include the following:

- Do not puncture the anteromedial aspect or the posterior curve of the heel because a puncture at either site could injure the underlying calcaneus. Figure 11–3 shows the proper sites for a heel puncture.
- When holding the infant's foot, be firm but gentle. A **premature infant** in particular, has delicate tissue that may bruise easily. Holding the foot too tightly also restricts blood flow.
- Avoid excessive milking or squeezing, which causes **hemolysis** and dilutes the blood with interstitial and intracellular fluid.
- Avoid covering puncture sites with adhesive bandages because newborn skin is fragile and may macerate under the bandage.

Heel Warming

The amount of blood that can be obtained from a single heel stick is limited, so to obtain an adequate sample, prewarming the heel may be indicated. Prewarming the heel increases blood flow dramatically and arterializes the specimen. This step is essential for drawing specimens for capillary blood gas analysis.

There are several methods of warming the heel; however, a surgical towel or a washcloth heated with warm water to 39 to 42°C works well. If the temperature of the towel exceeds 44°C, it may burn the infant. Wrap the warm, wet towel around the infant's foot, and encase the wrap in a plastic bag to help retain heat and to keep the patient's bed dry. Prewarming the site for 3 to 5 minutes is effective in raising the skin temperature several degrees. Chemical heel-warming packs are also available commercially for this purpose. Caution should be used if the towel is heated in a microwave oven because heating is uneven, and the towel may have hot spots. Depending on the institution's policy, the nurse may be called in advance to prewarm the infant's heel, or one may apply the warm wrap, attend to another patient, then return in a few minutes to perform the heel stick.[13]

Figure 11–4. Tenderfoot heel incision device.

(International Technedyne Corporation, Edison, NJ)

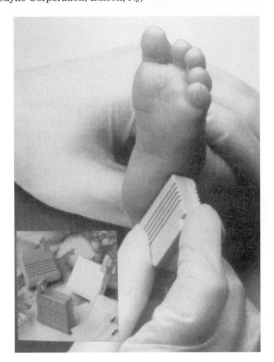

Procedure

Hands should be washed and then gloves put on. Also, if required, the health care worker may don a gown and a mask. The infant must be identified properly. If the infant is not wearing an identification bracelet, the nurse must identify the infant. The heel area should be inspected and assessed for proper warmth. If it is cool or a blood gas specimen is to be collected, prewarm the foot with a warm, wet towel or a chemical heel-warming pack, according to policy. When the heel has been warmed and dried, the side of the heel should be disinfected with the alcohol swab, using firm circular motions, starting at the center of the area and working outward. Allow the alcohol to dry. Blowing on the area to hasten drying is not advised because doing so will contaminate the area. To ensure that the site is dry and free of alcohol, it should be wiped with a sterile cotton ball or gauze sponge.

The nondominant hand should hold the infant's ankle "tennis racket" style: forefinger across the arch and thumb supporting the heel. The infant's foot should be gripped firmly but carefully to prevent bruising or injury and to avoid restricting blood flow. Using the dominant hand, the pediatric lancing device should be held perpendicular to the heel. As mentioned previously, an automatic lancing device will control the incision depth, which should not exceed 2.4 mm. The skin should be pierced with the lancet. The first drop of blood should be wiped away with the sterile gauze sponge because this drop of blood contains excess tissue fluid. As the drops form, blood is drawn into the capillary tubes and the microcollection containers, both of which should be held at a downward angle, not horizontally. Intermittent, gentle pressure with the forefinger may facilitate the blood flow. Massaging or milking the area is not advisable, however, because doing so causes hemolysis or dilution of the blood with tissue fluids.

Clinical Alert

If the blood flow is inadequate for collection of all required specimens, a second puncture may be needed at another heel site. In such cases, the skin is prepared as before. A puncture device should *never* be reused, and no more than two punctures should be attempted. Box 11–1 provides a sample nursery procedure for performing a heel stick on an infant.

Care of the Heel After Collection

When collection is complete, the heel should be evaluated, a sterile gauze sponge placed over the puncture site, and pressure applied until the bleeding stops. An adhesive strip should not be used because, as mentioned before, infants have delicate skin that may macerate under the Band-Aid or may be damaged when the strip is removed.

Clean Up

Used lancing devices are disposed of in a sharps container. The infant's bed is checked for any equipment or trash left behind. Used gauze sponges, gloves, and gowns should be disposed in a biohazardous waste container. Hands should be washed after removing the gloves.

Complications From Heel Stick

Clinical Alert

Some complications associated with neonatal heel sticks include cellulitis, osteomyelitis of the calcaneus, abscess formation, tissue loss, scarring of the heel, and calcified nodules. Calcified nodules occur most commonly in infants who, as preemies (premature babies) or neonates, received multiple heel sticks. In neonates, these nodules appear as small depressions, which progress to firm nodular lesions that appear 4 to 12 months later, migrate to the skin surface, and disappear by 18 to 20 months.[14]

NEONATAL SCREENING

In the United States, **neonatal screening** for **phenylketonuria (PKU)** and **hypothyroidism** is mandatory by law. These diseases can result in severe abnormalities, including mental retardation, if not discovered and treated early. Blood spot testing for these and

BOX 11–1.   SAMPLE NURSERY PROCEDURE FOR PERFORMING A HEEL STICK ON AN INFANT

Principle:

To obtain blood specimens from infants with the least amount of trauma while maintaining good isolation techniques.

Procedure:

1. Locate the entrance to the nurseries (intensive care, intermediate care, and low risk). It is located on _____.
2. Place blood collection tray on the table near the scrub sinks outside the nurseries.
3. Remove rings, watch, and laboratory coat.
4. Wash hands with regular soap. Control the water with foot pedals.
5. Put on a gown with ties in the back.
6. Wear sterile gloves.
7. Pick up tray with two clean paper towels and enter nursery area.
8. Find the small metal cart and place tray on a clean diaper on the cart.
9. Discard paper towels.
10. Identify the baby by making sure that the information on the request slip is identical to that on the baby's armband.
11. After ensuring that the skin is warm, perform a heel puncture to obtain the proper blood specimens for the tests requested.
12. Hold clean cotton gauze over the puncture site until bleeding stops. Do not put adhesive strips on the baby's feet.
13. Remove all collection equipment from the crib to avoid harming the baby.
14. Before collecting blood from the next baby, wash hands at the sink inside the nursery proper and change gloves.
15. Initial the log book for all work completed.
16. Remove gown and gloves and discard in proper receptacle.
17. Wash hands.
18. When moving from one nursery area to the other, repeat the complete procedure and put on a clean gown and gloves.

Notes:

1. The baby's heel may be punctured a maximum of two times. Do not stick a baby more than twice to obtain a specimen at any given time. If a particular baby must always be punctured the maximum number of times, notify the phlebotomy supervisor and the baby's primary nurse.
2. Do not puncture a foot if bruises, abrasions, or sloughing skin is present. Call the situation to the attention of the baby's nurse.
3. To help obtain a free-flowing puncture wound from a baby who does not bleed freely, have a nurse wrap the baby's heel in a warm towel 10 to 15 minutes before the puncture is made. Prewarming the site is also necessary for collection of all specimens for capillary blood gas analysis.
4. Use only a gentle massage when obtaining blood. Excessive massaging dilutes the blood with tissue fluids and may cause hemolysis. It is sufficient to massage with your thumb and forefinger.
5. Never repuncture old puncture wounds.
6. Never remove a baby from its crib or change its position in any way without the approval of a nurse.

other diseases is performed before the newborn is 72 hours old. If blood is collected before the newborn is 24 hours of age, the screening must be repeated before the infant is 14 days old.[5]

The heel is the most frequently used site for collection of blood for screening. Appropriate collection cards are kept in the hospital laboratory or the nursery. Circles are printed on the filter paper portion of the card; one blood drop is to be placed in each circle. It is important not to touch or contaminate the circle areas with substances other than the newborn's blood. Wash hands and put on gloves. Then, positively identify the newborn and prepare the infant in the same manner as for a heel stick. Once the puncture is made and the blood drop appears, the circle area is touched on the filter paper with the blood until the circle is filled. If the circle does not fill entirely, the heel is wiped and another, larger drop is expressed to a different circle. Do not add a second drop of blood to a previously used circle. Only one side of the filter paper should be used. Allow the paper to air dry thoroughly in the horizontal position. Direct application of blood from the heel to the card is the technique of choice; however, blood from a heparinized capillary tube may be applied if care is taken not to scratch or dent the filter paper. Make sure all the information on the screening card is completed correctly so that follow up can be done if the results are abnormal. The screening card should be placed in an appropriate envelope and sent to the laboratory within 24 hours (Box 11–2).

FINGER STICK

Clinical Alert

A finger stick to obtain blood for routine laboratory analysis is usually preferred for children older than 1 year. Also, a finger stick may be necessary if a child has damaged veins from repeated venipuncture or if the veins are covered with bandages or casts. Do not perform a finger stick if the extremity has compromised circulation, is edematous, or is infected.

Precautions

Use a proper-sized pediatric safety lancet designed for the age and size of the child. An automatic lancet controls the puncture depth, which should not exceed 2.4 mm in small children. The distance from the skin surface to bone or cartilage in the middle, or third, finger is between 1.5 and 2.4 mm. Automatic incision devices are available in sizes that incise to depths of 1.75 mm, 1.25 mm, and 0.85 mm for toddlers. For a detailed description of the blood collection procedure and supplies, refer to Chapter 9, Skin Puncture Procedures and Chapter 7, Blood Collection Equipment.

VENIPUNCTURE

Venipuncture in children is used when larger quantities of blood are needed for sampling. The veins of the antecubital fossa or the forearm are most accessible and are chosen for

BOX 11–2.   PKU COLLECTION PROCEDURE

Principle:

It is a state requirement that a PKU screening be performed on all newborn patients. The test determines the level of phenylketonuria in the blood.

Procedure:

1. Pick up completed PKU slips at nursing unit or PKU health department forms in a physician's office.
2. Properly identify patient, and explain the procedure to the parent(s).
3. Place patient's foot (limb) in dependent position.
4. Sterilize skin with alcohol; allow to *dry* and puncture with disposable lancet.
5. Allow drops to form and apply *directly* to filter paper. Apply blood to only one side of paper while viewing from other side to ensure *complete saturation* of entire circle. All five circles *must* be completely filled.
6. Allow card to dry thoroughly in a horizontal position (minimum of 3 hours). *Do not* stack wet samples.
7. Reference laboratory personnel will mail the newborn screen in an envelope provided by the State Health Department within 24 hours to the State Health Department. In a physician's office, the health care worker may be responsible for placing the card in a mailer to the Health Department.

Notes:

Specimens may be considered unsatisfactory if

1. All circles are not completely filled.
2. All filled circles are not thoroughly saturated.
3. Uneven saturation is present because of multiple-sample application or the use of capillaries.
4. The specimens appear to be contaminated.
5. Clotted or caked blood is present on the filter paper.
6. Elution of blood from the filter paper is incomplete.
7. The filter paper is separated from the form.
8. The specimen is received more than 5 days following the date of collection.

(Courtesy of Hermann Hospital Clinical Laboratories, Houston, TX, with permission.)

most toddlers and children. Dorsal hand veins are preferred sites for venous access in neonates and well newborns. Other sites for venipuncture are the medial wrist, the dorsum of the foot, the scalp, and the medial ankle. If the neonate or child is receiving fluid or medication intravenously, the distal veins should be avoided for phlebotomy and preserved for IV therapy. Venipuncture is indicated for blood sampling for routine laboratory tests, sedimentation rate, blood cultures, cross-matching, coagulation studies, and drug and ammonia levels. Do not use veins in an extremity or area if there is edema or infection or if an IV line is present. Avoid deep veins in a child with hemophilia or other bleeding disorders.

Precautions

Remove the tourniquet before withdrawing the needle. Do not use alcohol preparation pads to apply pressure because they sting and prevent hemostasis. Instead, apply pressure with the gauze sponge or a cotton ball for 3 minutes to prevent a hematoma. For neonates, use small, winged safety (butterfly) needles. If feasible, use winged safety needles for small children as well.

Equipment for Venipuncture

The equipment necessary for a pediatric venipuncture includes the following:

1. Winged safety infusion needle (23 or 25 gauge) or transparent hub needle (21 gauge × 1 in. or 23 gauge × ¾ in.).
2. Syringes slightly larger than the volume of blood needed.
3. Large-bore or 19-gauge needle.
4. Seventy percent isopropyl alcohol swab in a sterile package.
5. Cotton balls or gauze sponges.
6. Appropriate specimen containers.
7. Tourniquet (nonlatex if child is allergic).
8. Sterile disposable gloves (nonlatex if child is allergic).
9. Blood culture:
    a. bottles, aerobic and anaerobic.
    b. povidone–iodine swabs.
10. Paper tape and adhesive strip (only for use with older children).
11. Marking pens.
12. Biohazardous waste container.

Dorsal Hand Vein Technique

The dorsal hand vein technique is appropriate for neonates and infants who are younger than 2 years old. Although the neonate will not need restraint, an older infant can be wrapped snuggly in a receiving blanket or restrained by an assistant to minimize movement. As for all procedures, the infant should be positively identified before beginning. Select the hand that has easily visible veins (Fig. 11–5). No tourniquet is necessary. The phlebotomist's middle finger and forefinger should encircle the wrist and are used to apply pressure to distend the dorsal veins (Fig. 11–6). Placing one's thumb against the infant's fingers, the infant's wrist can be flexed downward as the dorsum of the infant's hand is examined. Be careful not to bend the wrist too much or the vein may collapse. Lightly brushing a finger across the back of the infant's hand as it is palpated helps select the best vein and determine its direction. Never attempt the venipuncture if one cannot see or feel the vein. Once the optimal vein has been chosen, the finger tourniquet should be released to allow blood to recirculate. Disinfect the back of the infant's hand with the alcohol swab. Take time and allow the area to air dry, then wipe with sterile gauze. Select the appropriate needle according to the size of the vein. Next, the phlebotomist should reposition fingers on the infant's wrist as a tourniquet and flex the infant's hand with his or her thumb. The transparent hubbed needle should be bevel up, parallel to the vein. The needle should be angled about 15 degrees to the skin. The skin should be pierced 3 to 5 mm distal to the vein, then advanced slowly and carefully until the vein is punctured. As soon as blood appears in the hub, the needle should stop advancing. The blood may flow slowly as the venous pressure is very low. A few seconds should pass, then if no blood appears, it may be necessary to reposition the needle gently. The needle need not be held because the surrounding skin will hold it in place.

As soon as the blood begins to flow, the microcollection tubes should be filled *directly*

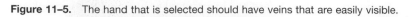

Figure 11–5.   The hand that is selected should have veins that are easily visible.

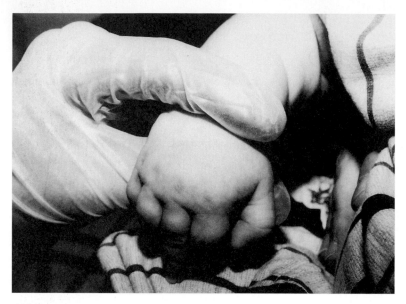

Figure 11–6.   Positioning of health care worker's fingers for dorsal hand vein technique.

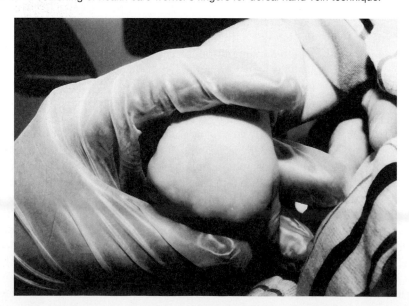

from the hub. Caution is advised to avoid bumping the hub and pushing the needle through the vein. The finger tourniquet should be released intermittently to allow the vein to refill. If the blood flow slows or stops, gently rotating the needle without advancing it may reestablish the flow. Once the necessary tubes are filled, a dry gauze sponge should be placed over the puncture site, while applying pressure as the needle is quickly withdrawn. Pressure should be maintained for 2 to 3 minutes or until the bleeding stops. An adhesive strip may be used to cover the puncture site on well babies and older infants. Tape should not be used on ill neonates because their skin is fragile. The infant may be comforted by offering a sucrose nipple, if permitted. All used supplies should be discarded in the appropriate biohazardous containers. Gloves and the gown should be discarded, and hands washed.

Dorsal hand vein venipuncture has several advantages over skin puncture: it is less stressful for the infant and the health care worker, there is less dilution of the specimen with tissue fluids and less hemolysis, and fewer punctures are required.[13,15]

Venipuncture at Other Sites

The procedure for performing venipuncture on children is similar to that for adults (see Chapter 8). The differences include the necessary preparation of the child and the parent, assistance in restraining the child, and the use of special pediatric-sized needles or safety winged infusion sets. After the child is securely positioned, place the tourniquet proximal to the selected vein to distend it. If necessary, the limb may be lowered, rubbed gently, or even warmed to promote dilation of the vein. Disinfect the site thoroughly. Allow the alcohol to dry completely. Then, hold the two wings of the infusion set together in the dominant hand as the other hand pulls the skin below the puncture site taut. When inserting the needle in children, it is best to insert 3 to 5 mm below the vein. When blood appears in the tubing, release the wings of the infusion set. The skin will hold the needle in place, or paper tape can be used to secure it. Gently aspirate the syringe until the required amount of blood is withdrawn. Release the tourniquet, apply pressure over the puncture site with a gauze pad as the infusion set is quickly removed. Ask the parent or the nurse to hold pressure on the site until the bleeding stops, then apply the adhesive strip. Remove the syringe from the infusion set, attach the large-bore needle, and insert it into the collecting tubes to be filled.

Scalp Vein Venipuncture

Scalp veins may be used on infants when access to other veins is difficult or undesirable. Figure 11–7 shows the scalp veins used for peripheral vascular access.

Additional equipment required for this procedure includes a disposable razor and a large, flat rubber band. A 23- or 25-gauge safety winged infusion set (butterfly needle) is used for the venipuncture. The appropriate procedures should be followed: hand washing and gloving, preparing the infant, and positioning with an assistant to provide restraint. If the scalp veins are not readily visible through the hair, a disposable razor may be used to shave the hair carefully in the frontal or parietal scalp area. A prominent vein may be occluded proximally with a finger as in the dorsal hand vein technique. Feel for a pulse to prevent hitting an artery. If a vein cannot be distended with the finger, a large, flat rubber band may be placed around the upper head as a tourniquet.[5] (Placing a gauze pad under an area of the band helps in removing it after the procedure.) Disinfect the scalp with a povidone–iodine (Betadine) preparation or with alcohol, allow the scalp to dry, and then wipe it with sterile gauze. After the scalp is inspected for the desired vein, release the tourniquet to permit refilling of

Figure 11–7.   Scalp veins frequently used for peripheral vascular access in infants.

(From Ball J, Bindler R. *Pediatric Nursing: Caring for Children.* Norwalk, CT: Appleton & Lange; 1995, p 823, with permission.)

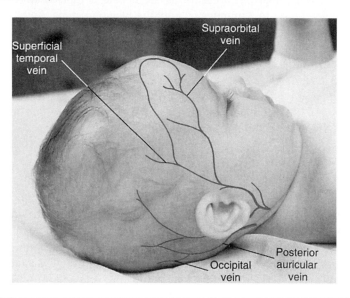

the veins. Reapply finger pressure or the rubber band. Hold the skin taut with the non-dominant hand distal to the site to be punctured. Hold the infusion set with the two wings folded together and the bevel of the needle up. Position the needle at a 15-degree angle over the vein in the direction of the blood flow. Puncture the skin, and slowly advance the needle until blood begins to flow into the tubing of the needle set. Attach the syringe. Gently and slowly aspirate the blood to prevent hemolysis or occlusion by the vein wall. When sufficient blood is collected, release the finger tourniquet or rubber band. Place the sterile gauze pad over the puncture site, and apply pressure before quickly removing the needle. Apply additional pressure for several minutes to ensure that the bleeding has stopped. Fill the collecting tubes in the usual fashion. Comfort the infant by stroking him or her softly, or by offering a pacifier if permitted. Be sure all used supplies are removed from the bed area.

Withdrawing Blood From IV Lines

Hospitalized children who are undergoing IV therapy, whether for total parenteral nutrition (TPN), administration of an antibiotic, or chemotherapy, often have poor veins. They may have a heparin or saline lock or a central venous catheter when long-term access is required. Some blood tests can be performed with blood drawn from these lines; however, one must check with the nurse in charge or the doctor and verify the policy because some hospitals limit the number of times that a line can be accessed. Also, confirm the amount of blood that can be drawn on the basis of the child's weight (see Table 8–1).

Equipment

The equipment required for blood withdrawal from IV lines includes the following:

1. Syringe filled with 5 mL of normal saline.
2. Syringe filled with 5 mL of heparinized flush solution (1 mL for heparin lock).
3. Five-mL syringe for discard.
4. Syringe for blood specimen.
5. Small blood collection tubes.
6. Large-bore needle for transferring blood to tubes.
7. Nineteen- to 25-gauge needles for gaining access to heparin lock.
8. Isopropyl alcohol or povidone–iodine (Betadine) swabs.
9. Double stopcock for central line.
10. Luer-Lok (Becton-Dickinson, Franklin Lakes, NJ) catheter cap.
11. Sterile 4 × 4 in. gauze sponge.
12. Mask.
13. Gloves (nonlatex if child is allergic).

Procedure for Heparin or Saline Lock

When drawing blood from a heparin or saline lock, disinfect the catheter cap with an alcohol or a povidone–iodine (Betadine) swab. Check patency of the line by flushing with a small amount of normal saline. Attach a needle to the discard syringe, and insert it into the cap of the lock. Gently withdraw approximately 2 to 3 mL of fluid and blood, remove the syringe and needle, and discard in a sharps container. Insert another needle and syringe to collect the blood sample. When a sufficient amount of blood has been obtained, withdraw the needle and fill the collection tubes. Clean the cap of the heparin lock, then insert the syringe with the heparinized flush solution, slowly injecting the solution.

Procedure for Central Venous Catheter

Wash hands, put on a mask and gloves, open a sterile 4 × 4 in. gauze sponge, and place it under the catheter port to serve as a sterile field. Open the sterile stopcock and attach the discard syringe to the access port closest to the child. Attach the blood-collecting syringe to the next port and the normal saline–filled syringe to the distal port, all with sterile technique. Clean the connection site with alcohol swabs. Two or three swabs must be used to clean the site for 2 minutes. Then, allow the connection to dry. Clamp the catheter, then remove the catheter cap. Connect the preassembled stopcock setup, ensuring a tight seal. Unclamp the catheter, open the stopcock to the discard syringe, and withdraw 3 to 5 mL of fluid. Close that port, then open the stopcock port to the collection syringe and aspirate the required amount of blood. Close that port, and remove the syringe. An assistant can attach the large-gauge needle and fill the collection tubes. Attach the syringe with the heparinized solution to that port. Open the distal port. Gently aspirate to clear the stopcock of air, holding the syringe vertically to allow bubbles to rise. Tap the syringe to free any bubbles sticking to its side. Flush the catheter with 5 mL of saline, close that port, and then open the port to the heparinized solution and flush with 5 mL. Reclamp the catheter and remove the stopcocks. Clean the connection site of the catheter with a new alcohol preparation pad, then attach a new Luer-Lok cap.[5] Discard used items in the appropriate containers. Remove gloves and mask, and wash hands.

SELF STUDY

KEY TERMS

Age-Specific Care Considerations
Blood Volume
Calcaneus
Eutectic Mixture of
    Local Anesthetics (EMLA)
Heel Stick
Hemolysis
Hypothyroidism
Latex Allergy

Neonatal Screening
Neonates
Osteomyelitis
Parental Involvement
Pediatric Phlebotomies
Phenylketonuria (PKU)
Premature Infant
Sucrose Nipple or Pacifier

STUDY QUESTIONS

The following questions may have *one* or *more* answers.

1. Performing a phlebotomy on a child is challenging because of which facts?

   a. a child is less emotionally mature than an adult

   b. a child is small

   c. smaller equipment must be used

   d. a child's blood clots more quickly

2. Which of the following describe the behavior of an adolescent undergoing a painful procedure?

   a. fears separation from parent

   b. embarrassed to show fear

   c. fears injury to body

   d. may not want parent present in room

3. Which of the following are important steps in preparing the child and the parent for a pediatric phlebotomy?

   a. assess their past experience with blood drawing

   b. perform the phlebotomy as quickly as possible

   c. ask the parent to leave the room

   d. use a doll or a puppet to demonstrate the procedure

4. Which is the *best* location for performing a phlebotomy on a hospitalized child?

   a. bedside in a chair

   b. playroom

   c. treatment room

   d. in his or her bed

5. The preferred technique(s) for restraining a child is/are which of the following?

   a. vertical—child sitting in
      parent's lap
   b. total sedation

   c. mechanical restraint
   d. supine with parent leaning
      over child

6. Which of the following are acceptable interventions to alleviate pain?

   a. xylocaine injection
   b. sucrose nipple

   c. ice pack
   d. EMLA cream

7. Which is the preferred site for a heel stick?

   a. anteromedial aspect
   b. medial or lateral aspect

   c. posterior curve
   d. a previous puncture site

8. Warming the heel provides which of the following benefits?

   a. arterializes blood
   b. dramatically increases
      blood flow

   c. prevents hemolysis
   d. hastens hemostasis

9. Complications of heel sticks may include which of the following?

   a. osteomyelitis
   b. abscess formation

   c. paralysis of the foot
   d. calcified nodules

10. What is the optimal depth of a finger stick in a child?

    a. greater than 3.0 mm
    b. less than 0.5 mm

    c. less than 2.4 mm

11. What is/are the preferred technique(s) for obtaining blood in neonates?

    a. finger stick
    b. heel stick

    c. dorsal hand vein technique
    d. antecubital fossa venipuncture

12. Neonatal blood screening is used to identify which disease(s)?

    a. syphilis
    b. hypothyroidism

    c. cystic fibrosis
    d. PKU (phenylketonuria)

References

1. Mehne C: Cultivating a tender touch: *MT Today.* September:12–16, 1992.
2. Colaizzo D, Tesler M. Children's pain: 4. *Nurseweek.* 1994; March:14–15.
3. Jacobson PB, Manne S, Gorfinkle K, et al: Analysis of child and parent behavior during painful medical procedures. *Health Psychol.* 1990; 9(5):559–576.
4. Manne S, Bakeman R: Adult–child interaction during invasive medical procedures. *Health Psychol.* 1992;11(4):241–249.
5. Ball J, Bindler R: *Pediatric Nursing: Caring for Children.* Norwalk, CT: Appleton & Lange; 1995.
6. Kelly S: Pediatric blood collection made easy. *Lab Med.* 1993; 24(4):247–248.
7. Robieux I, Eliopoulos C, Hwang P, et al: Pain perception and effectiveness of the eutectic mixture of local anesthetics in children undergoing venipuncture. *Pediatr Res.* 1992;32(5):520–523.
8. Marshall RE: Neonatal pain associated with caregiving procedures. *Pediatr Clin North Am.* 1989;36(4):885–903.

9. Department of Health and Human Services, Centers for Disease Control and Prevention. Guidelines for isolation precautions in hospitals—Part I, Evolution of isolation practices; Part II, Recommendations for isolation precautions in hospitals. *Federal Register.* Fall 1994.

10. Centers for Disease Control and Prevention. Anaphylactic reactions during general anesthesia among pediatric patients. *MMWR.* 1991; 40(28):437–443.

11. Food and Drug Administration (FDA). Allergic reactions to latex-containing medical devices. *FDA Med Alert.* Mar 29, 1991.

12. National Committee for Clinical Laboratory Standards (NCCLS). *Procedures for the Collection of Diagnostic Blood Specimens by Skin Puncture.* 3rd ed. Villanova, PA: NCCLS; 1991.

13. Clagg ME, Jamieson B: *Pediatric Phlebotomy.* American Society of Clinical Pathologists (ASCP) Fall Teleconference Series, No 9434, Chicago: ASCP; Sept 6, 1990.

14. Sell EJ, Hansen MD, Struck-Pierce S: Calcified nodules on the heel: A complication of neonatal intensive care. *J Pediatr.* 1980; 96(3).

15. Clagg ME: Venous sample collection from neonates using dorsal hand veins. *Lab Med.* 1989;20(4): 248–250.

12

TWELVE

■

Arterial, Intravenous (IV), and Special Collection Procedures

CHAPTER OUTLINE

CHAPTER OBJECTIVES

Upon completion of Chapter 12, the learner is responsible for the following:

1. Explain the special precautions and types of equipment needed to collect capillary or arterial blood gases.

2. Describe the equipment that is used to perform the bleeding-time test.

3. Discuss the requirements for the glucose and lactose tolerance tests.

4. Differentiate cannulas from fistulas.

5. List the steps and equipment in blood culture collections.

6. List the special requirements for collecting blood through central venous catheters (CVCs).

7. Differentiate therapeutic phlebotomy from autologous transfusion.

8. Describe the special precautions needed to collect blood in therapeutic drug monitoring (TDM) procedures.

9. List the types of patient specimens that are needed for trace metal analyses.

Depending on the specific needs of individual clinical settings, health care workers may be required to perform a variety of special tests or procedures in addition to routine skin test and venipunctures. This chapter presents the basic techniques and precautions for various special tests. Extensive training sessions and supervision should accompany the student in these procedures because they can harm the patient if performed incorrectly.

■ ARTERIAL BLOOD GASES

Arterial blood gases (ABGs) provide useful information about the respiratory status and the acid–base balance of patients with pulmonary (lung) disease or disorders. In addition, critically ill patients with other diseases, such as diabetes mellitus, benefit from ABG measurement, which is used to help manage their electrolyte and acid–base balance. Arterial blood is used rather than venous blood because arterial blood has the same composition throughout the body tissues, whereas venous blood has various compositions relative to metabolic activities in body tissues.

Arterial puncture to obtain arterial blood for blood gas evaluation requires skill and knowledge of technique. A health care provider must undergo extensive training on arterial punctures, including demonstration of the procedure, observation, and, under the supervision of a qualified instructor, several performances on patients.

RADIAL ARTERY PUNCTURE SITE

When an ABG analysis is ordered, the experienced health care worker, nurse, medical technologist, or physician should palpate the areas of the forearm where the artery is typically close to the surface. The **radial artery,** located on the thumb side of the wrist (Fig. 12–1), is the artery most frequently used for blood collection for ABG analysis.[1] This artery has widespread collateral flow, which means that the hand area is supplied with blood from more than one artery. Arterial blood flows into the hand from both the radial and the ulnar arteries. In addition, the radial artery lies over ligaments and bones of the wrist and can be easily compressed to lessen the chance of a hematoma during the procedure. A drawback to using the radial artery is its small size.

To use the radial artery for blood collection for ABG analysis, the health care provider must first perform the **Allen test** to make certain that the ulnar and radial arteries are providing collateral circulation. The Allen test is performed as follows: (1) The health care provider compresses both arteries with the index and middle fingers, and the patient is asked to tightly clench his or her fist repetitively in order to squeeze the blood out of the

Figure 12–1. Technique of radial artery puncture.

(From Saunders CE, Ho MT, eds. *Current Emergency Diagnosis and Treatment.* Norwalk, CT: Appleton & Lange; 1992, p 922, with permission.)

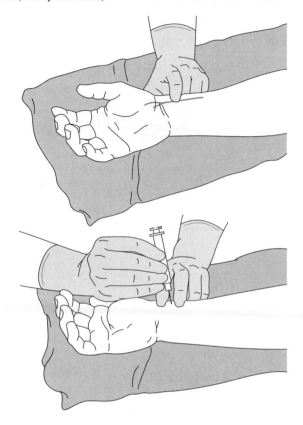

hand (Fig. 12–2A). (2) The patient is then asked to open his or her hand (Fig. 12–2B), and the health care provider releases the pressure on the ulnar artery. (3) The hand should fill with blood within 5 to 10 seconds (Fig. 12–1C); if so, the Allen test is positive. If color returns to the hand after 5 to 10 seconds, the Allen test is negative. A negative Allen test indicates the inability of the ulnar artery to supply blood to the hand adequately and shows a lack of collateral circulation. Thus, the radial artery should not be used in a negative Allen test since this artery might be accidentally damaged during puncture, resulting in total lack of blood flow to the hand.

BRACHIAL AND FEMORAL ARTERY PUNCTURE SITES

The **brachial artery** is an alternative site for blood collection for ABG analysis. The brachial artery is in the cubital fossa of the arm, as shown in Figure 12–3. Another choice, the **femoral artery,** is the largest artery used in ABG collections. It is located in the groin

Figure 12–2.   Allen test. **A.** Using the index and middle fingers, the health care worker compresses the patient's ulnar and radial arteries. The patient tightly clenches his or her fist repetitively. **B.** The patient opens the hand, and the health care worker releases the pressure. **C.** If the patient's hand refills with blood (i.e., color returns) within 5 to 10 seconds, the test is positive; if not, the test is negative.

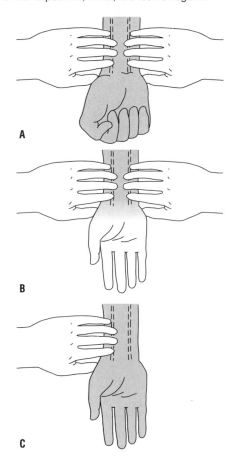

area of the leg, lateral to the femur bone, as shown in Figure 12–4. Even though the brachial and femoral arteries are larger than the radial artery, they are used less frequently because they lack collateral circulation. In addition, the branchial artery lies close to the median nerve, which can be accidentally punctured. The femoral artery is a site sometimes used on patients with cardiovascular disorders. The possibility of releasing plaque from the inner wall of the artery in geriatric patients, however, is a definite disadvantage of using the femoral artery as a puncture site. Usually, the femoral artery is the last choice for an arterial puncture site, and the health care provider must have expertise in obtaining blood from this artery.

Figure 12–3.   Arteries in the arm.

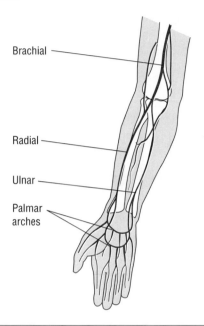

Brachial

Radial

Ulnar

Palmar
arches

PREPARATION OF SUPPLIES AND PATIENT

The necessary equipment and supplies, as listed in Table 12–1, should be gathered and organized for a successful arterial puncture. The patient must be properly identified and informed of the arterial puncture procedure. It should be determined that the patient has been in a stable state for at least the previous 30 minutes (i.e., no respirator changes). The health care provider should attempt to calm the patient before drawing the specimen if the patient appears anxious. The anxiety can lead to hyperventilation, which will falsely alter the ABG levels. Before proceeding, the health care provider must also determine whether the patient is on anticoagulant therapy or is allergic to iodine or lidocaine, and the patient's temperature, oxygen concentration from the respirator (if applicable), and respiratory rate must be recorded.

RADIAL ABG PROCEDURE

When an ABG analysis is ordered, the experienced phlebotomist, nurse, or physician should wash his or her hands, put on gloves, a facial mask, and a protective laboratory coat, and palpate the radial artery in the radial sulcus of the forearm. The radial artery in the patient's nondominant hand is usually the best choice. With the forefinger or first two fingers, the health care worker should press at these sites to find the artery. The thumb should never be used for palpating because there is a pulse in the thumb that may be confused with the patient's pulse. Any site that has a hematoma or that was previously used for an arterial

Figure 12–4. Arteries in the leg.

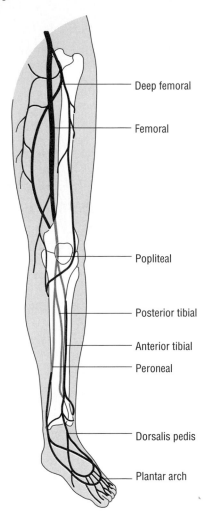

Deep femoral

Femoral

Popliteal

Posterior tibial

Anterior tibial

Peroneal

Dorsalis pedis

Plantar arch

puncture should be avoided. The patient's arm should be positioned with the wrist slightly extended and rotated. Check for adequate collateral circulation using the Allen test.

The syringe should be quickly capped, mixed with the anticoagulant, labeled, and placed in ice water immediately in an effort to prevent the blood gases from escaping into the atmosphere. Ideally, the specimen should be analyzed within 10 minutes of collection. Therefore, the specimen should immediately be labeled and transported to the laboratory. Before

Clinical Alert

Once the radial artery site is chosen, the area should be cleaned well with povidone–iodine (Betadine) solution. No tourniquet is required because the artery has its own strong blood pressure. As in venipuncture, a syringe with a needle can be used to withdraw the sample. The syringe, however, should be small (1 or 5 mL). The addition of liquid lithium heparin to coat the syringe barrel will anticoagulate the blood. Using too much liquid heparin is probably the most common preanalytic error in blood gas measurements.[2] Therefore, the amount of anticoagulant should be 0.05 mL of liquid heparin (1000 IU/mL) for each milliliter of blood. The health care worker should pull the skin taut and pierce the pulsating artery at a high angle, usually no less than 45 degrees. Little or no suction is needed because the blood pulsates and flows quickly into the syringe under its own pressure. When enough sample has been drawn (usually about 1 mL), the health care worker withdraws the needle carefully to avoid introducing bubbles into the syringe and applies gauze and direct manual pressure on the site for at least 5 minutes.

Table 12–1. Equipment and Supplies for an Arterial Puncture

Povidone–iodine (Betadine) solution or chlorhexidine
One-half to 1 percent lidocaine to numb site
Prefilled heparinized syringe, 1 to 5 mL (especially designed plastic syringe for collections for ABG analysis)
Stopper for syringe
Needles (20 to 22 gauge, for collections for ABG analysis)
Needles (25 to 26 gauge, for lidocaine administration)
Syringe for lidocaine administration (1- or 2-mL plastic syringe)
Gauze squares to be held on site after puncture
Plastic bag or cup with crushed ice and water
Patient identification label
Laboratory requisition slip
Waterproof ink pen
Alcohol pad
Adhesive bandage strip
Oxygen-measuring device to record on laboratory requisition slip the oxygen concentration on patient receiving oxygen
Thermometer to record patient's temperature on laboratory requisition slip
Mask
Gloves (nonlatex if patient is allergic)
Protective laboratory coat or smock
Biohazardous waste containers for sharps

leaving the patient, the health care worker should clean the puncture site with an alcohol pad to remove the excess Betadine solution, and a pressure bandage should be left on. If bleeding from the site persists, the health care worker should apply more manual pressure and ring for assistance from the patient's primary nurse. The health care worker should never leave a patient who is bleeding, particularly after an arterial puncture. The primary nurse should be notified after an arterial puncture is performed so that the area may be checked frequently for deep or superficial bleeding.

Arterial blood results for some analytes (e.g., ammonia, glucose, lactic acid, alcohol) may differ from venous blood results because of metabolic activities. Therefore, arterial blood samples should be collected for the blood gas measurements only when specifically requested by the attending physician. In such situations, the request slip must indicate that arterial blood was collected for the analytes.

■ CAPILLARY BLOOD GASES

Arterial blood is the specimen of choice for testing the pH, oxygen (O_2) content, and carbon dioxide (CO_2) content of the blood. Skin puncture blood is less desirable as a specimen source because it contains blood from capillaries, venules, arterioles, and fluids from the surrounding tissue. In addition, common collection methods for capillary blood gas specimens employ an open collection system in which the specimen is temporarily exposed to room air, theoretically allowing for a brief exchange of gases (both O_2 and CO_2) before sealing the specimen from the air.

Blood for **capillary blood gas analysis** is often collected from small children and babies for whom arterial punctures can be too dangerous. They are collected from the same areas of the body as other capillary samples, such as the lateral posterior area of the heel, the great toe, or the ball of the finger. (See Chapter 11, Pediatric Procedures.)

When a capillary blood gas analysis is ordered, the health care worker should choose a site and prewarm the area to ensure that good blood flow is obtained and that blood can be quickly collected, anticoagulated, and sealed from contact with room air. To prewarm the site, the health care worker must wrap a cloth or towel that is saturated with warm water around the foot or hand for 3 to 10 minutes. Care should be taken that the warming cloth is not too hot; if the warmed cloth can be held comfortably in the hand, it is not too warm for the patient. When the health care worker is prepared to collect the blood gas specimen, the towel should be removed and the area dried. The puncture site should be cleaned and entered in the usual manner for skin punctures (as discussed in Chapter 9). A heparinized capillary tube (Fig. 12–5) with a volume of at least 100 μL should be used to collect the specimen. A metal filing may be inserted into the tube before collecting to help mix the specimen while it is entering the tube. It is extremely important that the specimen be collected with *no air bubbles,* which can distort the values obtained from the specimen. When the tube is full, the ends should be sealed with plastic caps or clay (according to individual laboratory protocol), and a magnet should be used to draw the metal filing back and forth across the length of the tube to mix the specimen completely. The tube should then be labeled and submerged in a slurry of ice water for transfer to the laboratory. The sample

Figure 12–5.   Capillary blood gas tube.

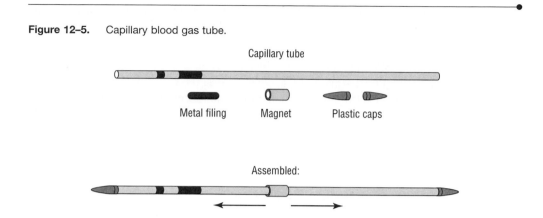

should be analyzed immediately in the laboratory; however, if the specimen is stored horizontally, capped, and in the slurry of ice water, it can be kept as long as 2 hours without serious degradation. The skin puncture site should be pressed with a clean gauze sponge until the bleeding stops.

■ BLEEDING-TIME TEST

The **bleeding-time test** is a useful tool for testing platelet plug formation in the capillaries. It is generally used along with other coagulation tests for diagnosing coagulopathies or problems in hemostasis, such as thrombocytopenia, qualitative platelet defects, vascular abnormalities, and von Willebrand's disease. This diagnostic tool is most frequently used as a preoperative screening test.

The test is performed by making a minor standardized incision in either the earlobe or the forearm and recording the length of time required for bleeding to cease. The duration of bleeding from a punctured capillary depends on the quantity and quality of platelets and the ability of the blood vessel wall to constrict.

Many methods have been used to measure bleeding time, the oldest dating to 1910 when Duke originally described a method in which a lancet was used to make a puncture wound in the earlobe. This test was difficult to standardize, did not allow space for repeat testing, and often caused undue apprehension in the patient. Ivy improved the bleeding-time test in 1941 by using a lancet to make puncture wounds on the forearm while maintaining a constant venous pressure with a blood pressure cuff. Both methods are difficult to reproduce because of several variables (e.g., depth of puncture, length of puncture).

Clinical research has led to the development of automated incision-making instruments for bleeding-time tests. One is called Surgicutt.[3] It is a sterile, standardized, easy-to-use, disposable instrument that makes a uniform, surgical incision. This instrument is a spring-activated surgical steel blade housed in a self-containing plastic unit from which the blade protracts and retracts automatically, eliminating the variable of blade incision. The following steps provide the procedure for the Surgicutt Bleeding Time Test.[4]

1. Prior to beginning the procedure, patients should be advised that there is an occasional scarring problem inherent in the bleeding time test. Butterfly-type bandages can reduce the potential scarring by applying one to the incision area for a 24-hour period. If there is ooze from the incision, as may be encountered in severe primary hemostatic disorders, then a pressure-type dressing should be used in conjunction with the butterfly-type bandage. If the puncture site is still bleeding beyond 15 minutes, the test should be discontinued by applying pressure to the area. A physician should be notified. The patient can also be asked if he or she has taken aspirin or other salicylates within the previous 2 weeks; these drugs interfere with the test.

2. Materials and supplies should be prepared before beginning the procedure. The following items are needed:

   - Surgicutt instrument. Each self-containing unit is sufficient for a single bleeding time determination. If package has been broken, do not use.
   - Gloves.
   - Antiseptic swab.
   - Blood pressure cuff (sphygmomanometer).
   - Filter paper disk (one to two Whatman's no. 1 filter paper disks per bleeding time test).
   - Butterfly-type bandage.

3. Place the patient's arm on a steady support with the volar surface exposed. The incision is best performed over the lateral aspect, volar surface of the forearm, approximately 5 cm below the antecubital crease. Avoid surface veins, scars, bruises, and edematous areas. Lightly shave the area if body hair will interfere with the test.

4. Place the blood pressure cuff on the upper arm. Inflate the cuff to 40 mm Hg. The time between inflation of the cuff and the incision should be 30 to 60 seconds. Hold at this exact pressure for the duration of the test.

5. Cleanse the area with an antiseptic swab and allow to air dry. Remove the Surgicutt device from the package, being careful not to contaminate the instrument by touching or resting the blade-slot end on any unsterile surface.

6. Remove the safety clip. (Safety clip may be replaced if the test is momentarily delayed; however, prolonged exposure of Surgicutt to uncontrolled environmental conditions prior to use may affect its sterility.) Once safety clip is removed, DO NOT push the trigger or touch the blade slot.

7. Hold the device securely between the thumb and the middle finger. Gently rest it on the patient's forearm and apply minimal pressure so that both ends of the instrument are lightly touching the skin. A horizontal incision parallel to the antecubital crease is the most sensitive technique for the bleeding time.

8. Gently push the trigger, starting the stopwatch simultaneously. The blade will make an incision 5 mm long by 1 mm deep. Remove the device from the patient's forearm immediately after triggering. After 30 seconds, wick the flow of blood with filter paper. Bring the filter paper close to the incision, but DO NOT touch the paper directly to the incision, so as not to disturb the formation of a platelet plug.

9. Wick the blood every 30 seconds thereafter until blood no longer stains the paper. Stop the timer. Bleeding time is determined to the nearest 30 seconds. Reference ranges vary from one health care facility to another. Most, however, are in the approximate range of 2.0 to 8.0 minutes.
10. Remove the blood pressure cuff and cleanse the incision site with an antiseptic swab. Apply the nonallergenic butterfly-type bandage for 24 hours.

The Simplate R (Retractable) and Simplate II R are sterile, disposable devices (Fig. 12–6) used to make uniform incisions for the bleeding-time test. The spring-loaded blades are contained in a plastic housing. When triggered on the forearm, Simplate R and Simplate II R provide one and two incisions, respectively, 5-mm long by 1-mm deep. Simplate II R is used for duplicate determinations. These devices standardize bleeding-time testing by producing uniform incisions that provide reliable and reproducible results.

POSSIBLE INTERFERING FACTORS

The bleeding-time test is only a screening test, so the results of this test alone are insufficient to diagnose a specific condition. A prolonged bleeding time may indicate the need for further testing (e.g., platelet count). In addition, the following items should be considered:

- The ingestion of aspirin-containing products up to 7 to 10 days prior to testing may affect results.
- Other drugs (e.g., dextran, streptokinase, streptodornase, ethyl alcohol, mithramycin) may cause a prolonged bleeding time.

Figure 12–6.   Simplate R (retractable) bleeding device.

(Courtesy of Organon Teknika Corp., Durham, NC.)

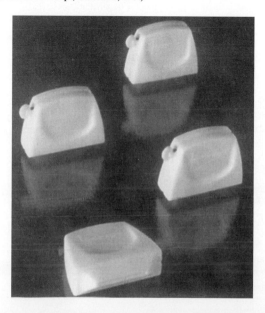

There are other variations of this same procedure using different devices. For reproducible results, it is important to follow the manufacturer's instructions and to teach all health care workers in the same manner.

■ BLOOD CULTURES

Blood cultures are often collected from patients who have **fevers of unknown origin (FUO).** Sometimes during the course of a bacterial infection in one location of the body, **bacteremia** or **septicemia** (presence of bacteria or toxins in the blood) may result and become the dominant clinical feature. Blood cultures aid in identifying the specific bacterial organism causing the infections, and when combined with antibiotic sensitivity tests can provide information to the physician about which antibiotic works best against that particular species of bacteria. In the case of a patient who experiences fever spikes, it is generally recommended that blood cultures be drawn before and after the spike, when bacteria may be most likely present in the peripheral circulation. It is best to draw one set (two bottles) of aerobic and anaerobic cultures at the time the order is given. Thirty minutes later, a second set of anaerobic and aerobic cultures should be obtained. A request for "second site" blood cultures that are obtained concurrently on opposite arms, is useful when the physician suspects bacteremia due to a local internal infection. A "second site" culture, however, is *not* a very effective tool for *routine* blood culture orders and provides relatively little information that properly spaced, timed blood cultures cannot provide.[5]

Prior to beginning the procedure, the health care provider should briefly explain the test to the patient. Then, the following steps should be taken for blood culture collection:

1. The necessary equipment and supplies should be gathered and prepared next to the patient as listed in Table 12–2.

Table 12–2. Equipment and Supplies for Blood Culture Collections

Gloves (recommended sterile gloves for aseptic technique)
Three alcohol/acetone or alcohol preps
Two iodine scrub swabsticks (10 percent povidone–iodine solution)
Two blood culture vials (one for anaerobic microorganisms and one for aerobic microorganisms)
   or
SPS evacuated tubes
Needles (22 or 20 gauge) or blood collection set
Syringe or evacuated tube assembly
Sterile gauze pads
Nonlatex bandages
Nonlatex tourniquet
Patient identification labels
Laboratory requisition slip and pen
Biohazard waste container

2. After donning gloves (nonlatex if patient has latex allergy), scrub the site of the venipuncture with an alcohol pad to rid the site of excess dirt, and then scrub with the iodine scrub swab stick for at least 2 minutes. The excess foam should be removed with the acetone–alcohol swab stick. The phlebotomist's gloved forefinger should also be cleaned in the same manner. If the patient is known to be hypersensitive to iodine, omit the iodine scrub and clean the site twice with alcohol. A blood culture preparation kit is available commercially from Medi-Flex Hospital Products, Inc. (Overland Park, KS) (Fig. 12–7). This kit, the Blood Culture Prep Kit II, provides another method for preparing to collect blood culture specimens. It is a two-step prep system without pads or swab sticks.

3. Prep the area of the venipuncture with the iodine swab stick by beginning in the center and rubbing the swab outward in concentric circles covering an area approximately 4 inches in diameter. Do not go back over any area that has been prepped (Figs. 12–8 and 12–9). Allow the area to dry for 1 minute in order for the antiseptic to be effective against skin bacteria.

   As the venipuncture site dries, prep the tops of the blood culture vials or SPS evacuated tubes with a new iodine swab stick, then wipe the tops of the vials with a new alcohol prep. This wipes the iodine away and decreases the likelihood of iodine entering with the blood into the vial. For some manufacturers of blood culture vials, it is recommended to clean the vial top with *only* alcohol after removing the cap from the vial. *The prepping of the vials should occur IMMEDIATELY prior to the blood collection.*

Figure 12–7.   Blood Culture Prep Kits.

(Courtesy of Medi-Flex Hospital Products, Inc., Overland Park, KS.)

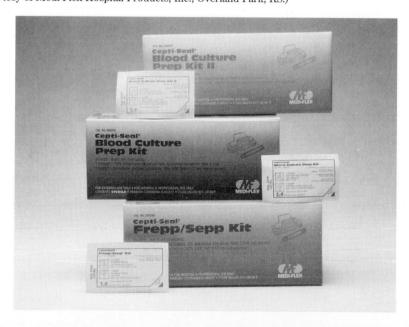

Figure 12–8.   Arm preparation for collection of blood culture specimens.

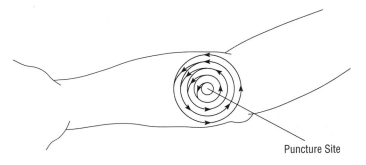

Puncture Site

Figure 12-9.   Scrubbing a blood culture venipuncture site with the povidone–iodine prep system.

(Courtesy of Medi-Flex Hospital Products, Inc., Overland Park, KS.)

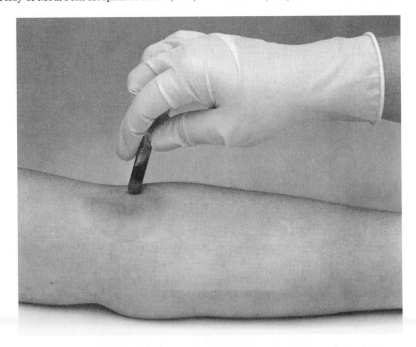

Removal of the entire metal ring on some manufacturer's bottles introduces air into the vials and can cause contamination. *Read* the manufacturer's directions on blood culture vials before using them because they may vary as to size of blood sample needed and preparation requirements.

4. The venipuncture procedure can be performed four different ways. These include:

- Using a syringe and then transferring the blood from the syringe into the blood culture vials. If the blood culture specimen from an adult is collected with a syringe, it is commonly recommended to have a 20-mL collection and transfer the first 10 mL to the anaerobic vial and then 10 mL to the aerobic vial. If the blood collector can only collect 3 mL or less, the entire amount should be placed in the aerobic vial. For pediatric patients younger than 10 years old, it is recommended to collect 1 mL of blood for each year of life for the blood culture workup.[6]
- Using a butterfly assembly (blood collection set) and transferring the blood via a direct draw adapter that fits directly over the blood culture vial (Fig. 12–10) for a safe method to collect blood. Using this method, blood is transferred to the aerobic vial first since the assembly tubing contains air.
- Using a winged infusion set (blood collection set) with a syringe attached to the end of the tubing, and then transferring the blood from the syringe to the blood culture vials. This procedure is recommended for patients with fragile veins (i.e., oncology, geriatric), since the direct adapter technique may lead to collapsed veins. Thus, after the blood collection, the 20-mL syringe must be removed from

Figure 12-10.   BACTEC Direct Draw Adapter.

(Courtesy of Becton-Dickinson Diagnostic Instrument Systems, Sparks, MD.)

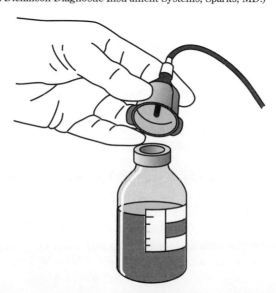

the luer adapter of the blood collection set tubing, and then a new sterile needle is attached to the syringe for insertion into each blood culture vial to pull the 10 mL of blood for each vial. *It is extremely important for the health care worker to be very careful in this transfer technique to avoid a possible needle-stick injury.*

- Using a holder/needle apparatus to collect blood in the yellow-topped evacuated tubes containing **sodium polyanethole sulfonate (SPS)** or in bottles, such as the BACTEC VACUTAINER culture vials (Becton-Dickinson Diagnostic Instrument Systems, Sparks, MD), that are shaped to fit into the barrel apparatus just as an evacuated tube would, thereby eliminating one step (see Fig. 7–8).

POSSIBLE INTERFERING FACTORS

! Clinical Alert

For any of these blood culture collection procedures, the venipuncture site MUST NOT be repalpated after the venipuncture site is prepared for blood collection.
Exceptions: It can be repalpated if

1. The health care worker is wearing sterile gloves and has not contaminated the finger used for palpating the site.
2. The health care worker has cleaned the gloved palpating finger with the iodine scrub.

If blood culture collections are ordered with other laboratory tests, blood culture specimens *must* be collected *first.* If an evacuated blood collection tube is used prior to the blood culture vials or SPS evacuated tubes, the needle can become contaminated.

When entering the needle into the venipuncture site, do not scrape the needle across the skin since this can contaminate the needle, and thus, blood cultures.

Also, the anaerobic blood culture vial *must* be inoculated first in all procedures because injection of air into the anaerobic bottle can cause the death of some anaerobic microorganisms and result in a false-negative culture.

Some culture vials contain resin beads that neutralize antibiotics in the patient's blood specimen. If not neutralized, the antibiotics can inhibit bacterial growth and cause false-negative results.

The blood should always be delivered gently to the vials and/or the tubes to prevent hemolysis of the cells. This is performed by directing the flow from the needle or the syringe hub along the side of the tube without foaming or extra pressure on the plunger. Evacuated tubes fill themselves, and therefore, the blood does *not* need to be forcefully ejected from the syringe. Then, invert the vials and/or tubes gently. After collecting the blood, remove the iodine from the patient's skin with an alcohol prep. The health care provider must initial the patient identification labels, indicate the time of collection on the labels, and attach a label to each vial or tube. Indicate on the request form and on the vials which culture (number) was collected if a series of blood cultures have been ordered.

Two studies have shown that the practice of changing needles after collecting blood for culture and inoculating the blood specimen into culture vials has little if any effect on the contamination of blood collected for culture.[7,8] In addition, changing needles after collecting blood for culture can lead to a needlestick injury to the phlebotomist. Careful skin cleansing was shown to be a more important factor in minimizing the specimen contamination rate than is the common practice of replacing the needle used for venipuncture with a fresh, sterile needle before inoculating the blood into culture media. If a laboratory decides to discontinue the practice of changing needles during blood culture collection, the contamination rate of blood cultures should be compared before and after the procedural change to confirm that the contamination rate has not increased.

Clinical Alert

Blood collected for culture must not be obtained through **central venous catheter (CVC)** lines if it cannot be obtained by venipuncture. Contamination rates may increase if the indwelling catheter is used to obtain culture specimens.[9] The only exception is if blood culture specimens are collected to determine if bacterial contamination is in the line. In this case, blood culture specimens need to be collected both from the IV line and by venipuncture for determination of the bacterial source. If using a syringe, a 20-mL size is the largest syringe that should be used with a CVC because larger sizes may collapse the catheter wall. Also, if possible, blood should be collected below an existing intravenous (IV) line because blood above the line will be diluted with the IV fluid.

Another source of error may involve failure to follow the sterile procedure, which results in contamination of the blood culture and misinformation for the clinician. For instance, palpating the venipuncture site after the site has been prepared without first cleaning the gloved finger can result in contamination of the culture. Likewise, failure to wipe the iodine from the tops of the vials with alcohol or using too little blood for the culture can result in a false-negative culture.

The Isostat system (Isolator microbial tubes) manufactured by Wampole Laboratories (Cranbury, NJ) is a special blood culture tube system (Figs. 12–11 and 12–12). The Isolator microbial tube has (1) a stopper that fits standard blood collection vacuum holders, (2) lysing and anticoagulating agents, (3) reagents in the tube that inactivate human immunodeficiency virus (HIV) within the normal 60-minute transport and processing time, and (4) containment adapters that help protect health care workers and laboratorians against infection due to aerosol spray or breakage during centrifugation. Using this tube affords the advantage of faster microbial test results. It also helps safeguard the laboratorian since the reagents in the Isolator tube inactivate HIV within the normal 60-minute transport and

Figure 12-11.   Wampole Isolator adult and microbial tube.

(Courtesy of Wampole Laboratories, Cranbury, NJ.)

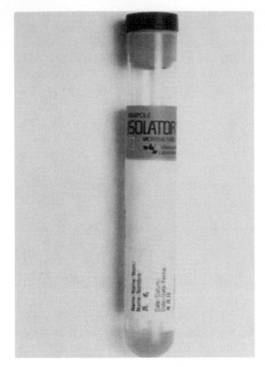

Figure 12-12.   Wampole Isolator pediatric microbial tube.

(Courtesy of Wampole Laboratories, Cranbury, NJ.)

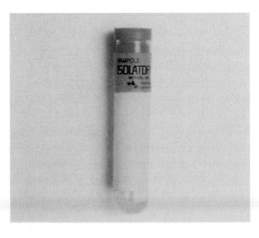

processing time. Also, the tube decreases the many procedural manipulations required during conventional blood culture collections.

■ GLUCOSE TOLERANCE TEST

For patients who have symptoms suggesting problems in carbohydrate metabolism, such as diabetes mellitus, the **glucose tolerance test** can be an effective diagnostic tool. The test is performed by first obtaining fasting blood and urine specimens, giving the fasting patient a standard load of glucose, and obtaining subsequent blood and urine samples at intervals, usually during a 5-hour period. Each specimen is then analyzed for its glucose content. In general, glucose levels should return to normal within 2 hours after ingestion of the glucose. With diabetic patients, the test must be carried out for 4 to 5 hours to observe how the patient metabolizes the glucose.

Clinical Alert

When a glucose tolerance test is to be performed, the patient should be given complete instructions about the procedure so that his or her cooperation can be ensured (Box 12–1). For best results, the patient should eat normal, balanced meals for at least 3 days prior to the test. Twelve hours prior to the beginning of the test, the patient should fast completely. Water intake is strongly encouraged because frequent urine specimens are required throughout the procedure. Other beverages, including unsweetened tea or coffee, are not allowed. Smoking, tobacco chewing, and gum chewing (including sugarless gum) should be discouraged until the completion of the test because they may stimulate digestion and interfere with the interpretation of the results. If a patient is chewing gum prior to or during the test, note this on the requisition slip.[10]

During the test, the patient drinks a standard dose of glucose, 75 g for adults or approximately 1 g/kg of body weight for children and small adults. A dose of 75 g is recommended for diagnosis of gestational diabetes.[10] Commercial preparations are available as flavored drinks to make the glucose more palatable. The patient must start and finish the drink within 5 minutes. Water intake is encouraged throughout the procedure. If the patient should vomit at any point in the procedure, the physician should be notified immediately to decide whether the test should be continued or stopped.[10]

When the patient finishes drinking the solution, the time is noted, and 30-, 60-, 120-, and 180-minute blood and urine specimens are obtained. Thus, if the glucose is administered to the patient at 7:30 AM, at 8:00 AM the 30-minute blood and urine specimens are obtained from the patient. This collection is followed by collections of blood and urine specimens at 8:30 AM (60 minutes), 9:30 AM (120 minutes), and 10:30 AM (180 minutes) (Fig. 12–13). The tubes should be labeled with the time, as well as "30 minutes," "1st hour," and so on. If blood is obtained initially by venipuncture, all succeeding specimens must also be venous blood. Similarly, if capillary blood is used, all specimens should be collected by microtechnique because the values and methods of analysis may vary between the two types of samples. Venous blood is the preferred specimen since glucose normal values are determined on

BOX 12–1.   SAMPLE PATIENT INFORMATION CARD

Patient Information Card Glucose Tolerance Test

Introduction

A glucose tolerance test (GTT) has been ordered by your physician. The purpose of a GTT is to test the efficiency of your body's insulin-releasing mechanism and glucose-disposing system.

You must prepare your body for the GTT by changing your eating and medication routines slightly for 3 days before the test. It is very important that you follow the instructions below in order for accurate results to be obtained.

Basically, you will need to follow these three guidelines to prepare for your GTT test:

1. Your carbohydrate intake must be at least 150 g per day for 3 days prior to the GTT.
2. Do not eat anything for 12 hours before the GTT, but do not fast for more than 14 hours before the test.
3. Do not exercise for 12 hours before the GTT.

Preparation: Medication

Before proceeding with the GTT, you must tell your physician if you are currently using any of the following medications because they may interfere with test results:

- Alcohol.
- Anticonvulsants (seizure medication).
- Blood pressure medication.
- Clofibrate.
- Corticosteroids.
- Diuretics (fluid pills).
- Estrogens (birth control pills or estrogen replacement pills).
- Salicylates (aspirin, pain killers)—only if taken in high doses, such as for rheumatoid arthritis.

Preparation: Diet and Exercise

Remember that for 3 days prior to your test, your diet must contain at least 150 g of carbohydrates per day. The following is a list of high carbohydrate foods:

- *Milk and milk products*—12 g of carbohydrates per serving. One serving is equal to 8 oz of milk (whole, skim, or buttermilk), 4 oz of evaporated milk, or 1 cup of plain yogurt.
- *Vegetables*—5 g of carbohydrates per serving. One serving is equal to 1/2 cup of any vegetable, excluding starches (e.g., potatoes, corn, or peas).
- *Fruits and fruit juices*—10 g of carbohydrates per serving. One serving is equal to 1/2 cup of juice, 1 small piece of fresh fruit, or 1/2 cup of unsweetened canned fruit, with the following exceptions:

Apple juice	$1/3$ cup
Grape juice	$1/4$ cup
Raisins	2 tbsp
Watermelon	1 cup
Prunes	2 medium
Banana	$1/2$ small
Dates	2
Cantaloupe	$1/4$ 6-in. melon
Honeydew melon	$1/8$ 7-in. melon

(continued)

BOX 12–1.   *(continued)*

- *Breads and starches*—15 g of carbohydrates per serving. One serving is equal to 1 slice of bread or 1 small roll. Other one-serving sizes are:

Bagel, English muffin	$1/2$
Tortilla	1
Cooked cereal	$1/2$ cup
Dry cereal	$3/4$ cup
Cooked rice, noodles, pasta	$1/2$ cup
White potatoes, dried beans, and peas	$1/2$ cup
Yams	$1/4$ cup
Corn	$1/3$ cup
Crackers	5–6

- *Meats, cheeses, and fats*—These foods contain few or no carbohydrates.
- *Miscellaneous*

Ice cream	$1/2$ cup	15 g of carbohydrates
Sherbet	$1/2$ cup	30 g of carbohydrates
Gelatin	$1/2$ cup	30 g of carbohydrates
Jams, jellies	1 tbsp	15 g of carbohydrates
Sugar	1 tsp	4 g of carbohydrates
Carbonated beverage	6 oz	20 g of carbohydrates
Hard candy	2 pcs	10 g of carbohydrates
Fruit pie	$1/6$	60 g of carbohydrates
Cream pie	$1/6$	50 g of carbohydrates
Plain cake	$1/10$	30 g of carbohydrates
Frosted cake	$1/10$	38 g of carbohydrates

Preparation: General Health

The following physical conditions should be reported to your doctor because they too may affect the results of your test:

- Acute pancreatitis.
- Adrenal insufficiency.
- Diabetes mellitus.
- Hyperinsulinism (excess insulin secretion, resulting in hypoglycemia).
- Hyperthyroidism.
- Hypopituitarism (decreased function of pituitary gland).
- Pregnancy.
- Stress.

If you have any difficulty making the necessary alterations in your diet or medication schedule, please inform your doctor. For accurate test results, the instructions on this card must be followed.

(Courtesy of Division of Laboratory Medicine, M D Anderson Hospital and Tumor Institute, Houston, TX.)

Figure 12-13. Graph of glucose tolerance test results.

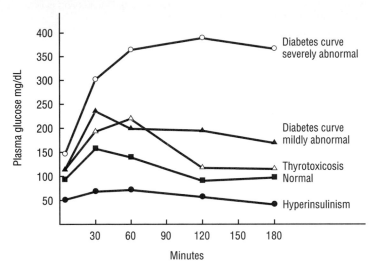

venous blood. If serum samples are used instead of plasma samples with a preservative, the tubes should be centrifuged immediately after collection, then the serum should be separated from the blood cells and placed in the refrigerator to inhibit glucose use by the blood cells.

■ POSTPRANDIAL GLUCOSE TEST

The 2-hour **postprandial glucose test** can be used to screen patients for diabetes because glucose levels in serum specimens drawn 2 hours after a meal are rarely elevated in normal patients. In contrast, diabetic patients usually have increased values 2 hours after a meal.

For this test, the patient should be placed on a high carbohydrate diet 2 to 3 days before the test. The day of the test, the patient should eat a breakfast of orange juice, cereal with sugar, toast, and milk to provide an approximate equivalent of 100 g of glucose. A blood specimen is taken 2 hours after the patient finishes eating breakfast. The glucose level of this specimen is then determined, and the physician can decide whether further carbohydrate metabolism tests (such as a glucose tolerance test) are needed.

■ LACTOSE TOLERANCE TEST

Some otherwise healthy adults experience difficulty in digesting lactose, a milk sugar. They appear to lack a mucosal lactase enzyme that breaks down the lactose into the simple sugars glucose and galactose. Instead, gastrointestinal discomfort may result, followed by diarrhea. These patients usually show no further symptoms if milk is removed from their diet.

To determine if a patient suffers from lactose intolerance, a physician may order a **lactose tolerance test.** A 3-hour glucose tolerance test should be performed 1 day in advance to determine the patient's normal glucose curve. A lactose tolerance test should be performed the next day in the same manner as the glucose tolerance, substituting the same amount of lactose for the glucose given the previous day. Fasting, 1-hour, 2-hour, and 3-hour blood samples are drawn and tested for glucose. When the results are graphed, the curve should be similar to that obtained from the glucose tolerance test, if the patient has the mucosal lactase enzyme and digests the sugar properly. If the patient is intolerant to lactose, his or her blood glucose level will increase by no more than 20 mg/dL from the fasting sample level.

The health care worker should be sure that a bathroom is located near the patient testing area because patients who are lactose intolerant may experience severe discomfort during the testing.

False-positive lactose tolerance test results have been known to occur in 25 to 33 percent of the patients tested who had normal lactase activity in small intestine biopsy specimens. Such results have been attributed to slow gastric emptying, not to the absence of the lactase enzyme.

■ THERAPEUTIC DRUG MONITORING (TDM)

Therapeutic drug monitoring (TDM), is used to monitor the serum concentration of certain drugs. It is an important laboratory assessment tool in the following circumstances:

- If the drug is highly toxic.
- When underdosing or overdosing can have serious consequences.
- If use of multiple drugs may alter the action of the drug being measured.
- If individual patients metabolize drugs at different rates.
- If the effectiveness of the drug is questionable.

TDM is often used for patients taking anticonvulsant drugs, tricyclic antidepressants, digoxin, theophylline, lithium, chemotherapeutic agents, such as methotrexate, or antibiotics, such as gentamicin.

Laboratory drug monitoring of therapeutic agents is a complex endeavor that requires much coordination among laboratory, nursing, and pharmacy personnel. A basic understanding of the variables, information needed, and definitions of terms is important to obtain accurate laboratory results. For most drugs, either plasma, serum, or whole blood are used to determine circulating levels of the drug.[11]

To evaluate the appropriate dosage levels adequately of many drugs, the collection and evaluation of specimens for trough and peak levels is necessary. The trough level is the lowest concentration in the patient's serum; that is, the specimen should be collected immediately prior to administration of the drug to ensure that the medication level stays within the therapeutic (effective dosage) range. The peak level is the highest concentration of a drug in the patient's serum. The time required to reach the highest concentration varies with the mode of administration (intramuscular injection v. IV infusion) and the rate at which the drug is infused. In addition, random levels may be appropriate for monitoring the drug dosage if the drug is administered by continuous infusion and if enough time has elapsed for the drug to reach equilibrium.

As a result of all these factors, laboratory personnel must acquire and document additional information when performing these tests. A health care worker may be asked to acquire the following information: patient's name; patient's identification number; patient's location; test ordered; requesting physician; collection time and date; mode of collection

> **⚠ Clinical Alert**
>
> The time of collection is much more critical for drugs with shorter half-lives (e.g., gentamicin, tobramycin, and procainamide) than for those with longer half-lives (e.g., phenobarbital and digoxin). Certain drug levels (e.g., aminoglycosides) in the blood can be falsely altered if collected through a central venous catheter.[12] Also, blood should not be taken from the arm into which drugs or other fluids are being infused.[13]

(venipuncture, central venous catheter collection) whether the order is for a peak level, a trough level, or a continuous-infusion random level determination; time and date of last dose; time and date of next dose; and a unit nurse's verification that the dose was administered. Specific specimen guidelines for each drug should be established by pharmacy and laboratory staff and strictly adhered to.

Blood specimens for TDM should be maintained in an upright position during transportation. In addition, because falsely low levels of lidocaine, phenytoin, and pentobarbital occur with the use of gel serum separator tubes, this type of evacuated blood collection tube should be avoided in TDM unless the gel serum separator tube has been evaluated and determined not to cause interferences.[14]

Most TDM assays should be performed on clotted blood. The National Committee for Clinical Laboratory Standards (NCCLS) has devised toxicology and drug-monitoring requirements for blood collection containers; these requirements can be helpful to the pharmacy and laboratory personnel who are responsible for establishing specific specimen guidelines for each drug.

■ COLLECTION FOR TRACE METALS (ELEMENTS)

Testing for **trace metals** involves the use of specially prepared trace metal evacuated blood collection tubes. Also, special acid-washed plastic syringes are usually suitable for trace metal testing. For aluminum level determinations, a needle that is free of aluminum must be used. For lead level determinations, lead-free heparinized evacuated blood tubes equipped with sterilized stainless steel needles should be used for blood collection.[15] Specific specimen collection guidelines should be established as part of the clinical laboratory's technical procedures for trace metal testing. The NCCLS guidelines entitled *Control of Preanalytical Variation in Trace Element Determinations* are very helpful in the preparation of procedures to collect trace elements.[16]

■ IV LINE COLLECTIONS

Drawing blood specimens through intravenous (IV) or central venous catheter (CVC) lines requires special techniques, training, and experience. A CVC, also called a **central intravenous line,** is one of numerous **vascular access devices (VADs).** The CVC is usually inserted into the: (1) subclavian vein, which is in the chest area below the clavicle; (2) jugular vein; or (3) superior vena cava at or above the junction of the right atrium. A dressing covers the tubing that extends above the skin. Another type of VAD is a **peripherally inserted central catheter (PICC),** which is inserted into the peripheral venous system with a lead into the central venous system. A PICC is usually placed in the arm in the basilic or cephalic vein. The PICC should not be used for blood collection because it may collapse during aspiration. An **implanted port** is another VAD that is a small chamber attached to an indwelling line. This port is surgically implanted beneath the skin. Ports must only be accessed with specially designed noncoring needles called Huber needles.

A **heparin or saline lock,** a device that can be inserted into a VAD, is used for medication administration and blood collection. This device is flushed with a heparin solution (Fig. 12–14) on a scheduled basis to prevent blood clots from developing in the line. If a heparin solution is used in this device, coagulation specimens must not be collected from it, otherwise, the solution will falsely alter coagulation test results. Many facilities have shifted to the use of saline in lieu of heparin.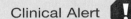

Clinical Alert

Usually, managers of health care facilities require nursing or laboratory personnel to take specialized training courses prior to allowing them to collect blood from a central venous line. The IV line is a direct pathway into the patient's bloodstream. Each time the IV system is entered, the possibility of contamination and infection exists. If aseptic technique is strictly adhered to, this procedure can provide a relatively safe means of access to the VAD and can save the patient some of the trauma of undergoing frequent venipunctures for laboratory studies. It has been determined, however, that hemolysis of blood samples obtained by an IV collection is significantly higher than when blood is obtained through venipuncture with the evacuated blood collection tube system. A lower incidence of hemolysis occurred with larger catheter diameters (i.e., 20 gauge, 18 gauge, 16 gauge, 14 gauge).[17] In regard to the CVC line, its use should be limited to once daily unless other instructions are received from a physician. Specific criteria must be established at each health care facility for obtaining blood through a CVC line.

DRAWING BLOOD THROUGH A CVC

Clinical Alert

To draw blood through a CVC, a 20-mL syringe is the largest syringe recommended for use with a soft-wall catheter because larger sizes may collapse the catheter wall. The patient should be positioned with the catheter hub at or below the level of the patient's

Clinical Alert (cont.)

heart to prevent possible air emboli when the CVC is entered. Nursing or medical staff should be consulted before opening the CVC line to avoid interrupting medication, which is extremely vital to the maintenance of the patient's care. When drawing blood from multilumen catheters, the lumen(s) not being drawn should be clamped during the procedure to prevent dilution of the blood sample being drawn. With multilumen catheters, blood specimens should be obtained from the most proximal lumen whenever possible.

The following equipment and supplies should be prepared prior to the procedure: laboratory requisition forms, tubes, and labels for the specimen; sterile gloves; two or three 20-mL disposable syringes; one 10-mL disposable syringe; one 10-mL syringe filled with injectable normal saline used for flushing the catheter; two or three sterile needles; a 4 × 4-in. piece of sterile gauze; a linen protector to provide a clean work area; a plastic or paper container for wastes or soiled items; adhesive tape; a sterile heparin cap; alcohol wipes; and 100 U/mL heparin (optional).

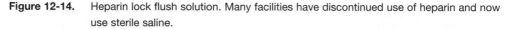

Figure 12-14.   Heparin lock flush solution. Many facilities have discontinued use of heparin and now use sterile saline.

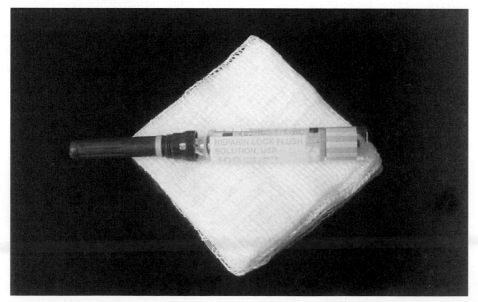

The procedure may involve the following steps but is subject to differences among hospitals and must be performed by *authorized personnel only.*[18]

1. Check patient's chart for physician's order to draw blood through CVC.
2. Obtain laboratory requisitions and labels that reflect patient location and tests for which blood is needed.
3. Check labels against slips and patient's identification bracelet as described in Chapter 8.
4. Determine amount of blood to be drawn so that correct size of syringe(s) can be used.
5. Assemble equipment, wash hands, and put sterile gloves on.
6. Aseptically draw up to 10 mL injectable normal saline and cap with sterile needle cover to maintain sterility. Take all supplies to bedside in a tray or other enclosed container to avoid a needle stick.
   Note: Take *only* tubes for the patient, no others.
7. Identify patient by armband ID, noting full name and hospital number. Check against preprinted labels.
8. Explain procedure to patient.
9. Provide adequate room and light for procedure.
10. Position patient by elevating the bed to a comfortable working level and making the bed flat, and have catheter hub at or below the level of the patient's heart.
11. After placing linen protector on bed, place tray of supplies on protector. Place sterile 4 × 4-in. gauze under connection site.
12. If IV is infusing, clamp off mainline IV tubing. Close slide clamp on short microbore tubing.
13. Loosen IV tubing connection or heparin cap. Aseptically disconnect IV tubing or injection cap from short microbore tubing, holding short microbore tubing and IV tubing "up" to avoid contamination.
14. Aseptically disconnect IV tubing and cap with sterile needle cover, and aseptically insert 10-mL syringe in short microbore tubing.
15. Unclamp short microbore tubing. Aspirate (slowly and steadily) the following amount of blood for discard:

   - Pediatrics, 2 mL; adults, 5 to 7 mL.
   - Coagulation studies: withdraw 20 mL of blood (13 mL may be used for testing after discarding 7 mL); collect 3 mL in a separate syringe. This process is only required when the CVC has been used to infuse heparin or has been heparin locked.

   Close clamp, remove syringe with blood, and place in tray in order to discard later.

Clinical Alert

Since the possibility exists for transferring an infectious agent or causing a blood clot in the CVC line, most health care facilities do *not* allow reinfusion of the discarded blood.

An alternative to collecting a discard sample is to flush the catheter with 0.9 percent sodium chloride (saline) and then aspirate/flush back and forth several times to clear the catheter. Blood specimens may be obtained for most laboratory tests.

16. Aseptically insert syringe of correct size for needed blood specimen into short microbore tubing.
17. Open the slide clamp on short microbore tubing and slowly aspirate blood in the quantity needed.
18. Close slide clamp on short microbore tubing. Remove syringe and place sterile needle on syringe.
19. Quickly and aseptically insert the 10-mL syringe with normal saline into the short microbore tubing. Open slide clamp on short microbore tubing.
20. Gently irrigate catheter with 5 mL normal saline.
21. Close slide clamp on short microbore tubing; temporarily leave syringe with 5 mL normal saline in place.
22. Place blood into blood collection tubes using the correct order of draw.
23. Open slide clamp on short microbore tubing. Complete irrigation of catheter with remaining 5 mL normal saline. Close slide clamp on short microbore tubing.
24. Aseptically reconnect IV tubing to short microbore tubing. Open clamp on IV tubing and slide clamp on short microbore tubing.
25. Determine that IV fluids are infusing properly at rate set by unit nurse.
    Note: If pump is being used, make certain pump is ON and alarm is ON. If the rate of IV flow appears altered, the unit nurse should be notified *immediately.* Retape connection between short microbore tubing and IV tubing.
26. Make sure the patient is in a safe and comfortable position with the bed down, siderails up, and bedside table and call light accessible to patient. Place used equipment and supplies in appropriate discard containers. The needles should NOT be recapped before discarding.
27. Write the date, time, and initial labels on blood specimens and place tubes of blood with the correct lab requisitions. Dispatch to laboratory in usual manner.
28. Document completion of procedure and any problems in the patient's medical record.
    Note: The uncapped used needles should NOT be placed on the patient's bed, but rather in an appropriate container until they can be properly discarded.

POSSIBLE INTERFERING FACTORS

 Clinical Alert

Heparin Interference

If possible, protime (PT) and partial thromboplastin time (PTT) levels should not be performed on blood specimens obtained from CVCs that have been heparin locked or into which heparin is infusing. If a successful venipuncture is improbable, however, coagula-

Clinical Alert (cont.)

tion studies may be collected from a heparinized catheter as explained earlier in the procedure. The description of the collection process and possible heparin contamination needs to be documented via computer, laboratory requisition slip, or medical record forms dependent on the documentation requirements of the health care facility.[19]

Catheter Interference in Blood Collection

The position of the catheter tip within the vein can lead to interference in blood collection. As two examples, if the tip of the catheter is against the wall of the vein or if the tip is positioned within a valve, the aspiration of blood from the IV line will be affected. If possible, attempt to reposition the catheter or extremity and try the blood collection procedure again.

Vein Interference in Blood Collection

Excessive vacuum pressure from the blood collection syringe or blood collection tubes can cause enough negative pressure to collapse the vein around the tip of the catheter and decrease or cut off blood flow through the catheter line. Complications associated with long-term indwelling lines may also result in the inability to collect blood specimens from the line. Examples of these complications include: (1) thrombus development preventing a free flow of blood within the vein and limiting the amount of blood for collection; (2) phlebitis, which is the swelling of the tissues due to an inflammatory process, preventing a free flow of blood within the vein; (3) a fibrin sheath can develop over the tip of the catheter that results in less blood flow to the syringe or blood collection tubes; and (4) sclerosis can occur in which the lumen of the vein narrows and slows venous blood return and blood flow for collection.

Patient Interference in Blood Collection

If the patient has a cold external temperature, then he or she may have vasoconstriction that can lead to poor blood flow through the IV line for collection. Another possible complication can be low venous pressure in a patient. This low pressure increases the tendency of the vein to collapse during the collection procedure and lowers the amount of blood collected. Most likely, the tubes will be partially filled, increasing the likelihood of poor sample quality and bad laboratory results.

■ CANNULAS AND FISTULAS

A **cannula** is a tubular instrument that is used in patients with kidney disease to gain access to venous blood for dialysis or blood collection. Blood should be drawn from the cannula of these patients only by specially trained personnel because the procedure requires special techniques and experience.

A **fistula** is an artificial shunt in which the vein and artery have been fused through surgery. It is a permanent connection tube located in the arm of the patients undergoing kidney dialysis. The health care worker should use extreme caution when collecting a blood specimen from these patients and avoid using the arm with the fistula as the site for venipuncture. If no other location can be found for the venipuncture site, the patient's arm must be cleaned *thoroughly* prior to blood collection. If the venipuncture site in this arm becomes infected, the inflammation in the blood vessels of the arm may shut down all the veins, requiring surgery to place a new shunt in the patient.

■ DONOR ROOM COLLECTIONS

Properly trained health care providers may be employed in a regional blood center or a hospital blood donor center to screen and collect blood from donors. This section summarizes the procedure outlined by the American Association of Blood Banks (AABB).[20] Only an experienced, properly trained health care worker or technologist should be considered for this function because a physical, emotional, or traumatic experience may keep a donor from volunteering in the future.

DONOR INTERVIEW AND SELECTION

Not everyone who wants to donate blood is eligible, so the interviewer must determine the eligibility of each potential donor. Carefully determining donor eligibility not only helps prevent the spread of disease to blood product recipients, but also prevents untoward effects on the potential donor.

The following information should be kept on file on every donor indefinitely and is initially obtained from every prospective donor, regardless of the acceptability[20] of his or her donation:

1. Date of donation.
2. Name: last, first, and middle initial.
3. Address.
4. Telephone number.
5. Gender.
6. Age and birth date. (Donors should be at least 17 years of age; however, minors may be accepted if written consent is obtained in accordance with applicable state law. Elderly prospective donors may be accepted at the discretion of the blood bank physician.)
7. Written consent form signed by the donor: (1) allowing the donor to defer from being a donor if he or she has risk factors for HIV, the causative agent of acquired immunodeficiency syndrome (AIDS), or (2) authorizing the blood bank to take and use his or her blood.
8. A record of reasons for deferrals, if any.
9. Social security number or driver's license number (may be used for additional identification but is not mandatory).
10. Name of patient or group to be credited, if a credit system is used.
11. Race (not mandatory, but this information can be useful in screening patients for a specific phenotype [chromosomal makeup]).
12. Unique characteristics about a donor's blood. (Donated blood that is negative for cytomegalovirus or that is Rh-negative group O blood is used for neonatal patients.)

To help minimize the incidence of dizziness, fainting, or other reactions to blood loss, donors are encouraged to eat within 4 to 6 hours of donating blood. Eating a light snack just before the phlebotomy may help prevent these reactions, but a donor should not be required to eat if he or she does not want to do so.

Blood bank records must link each component of a donor unit (red blood cells [RBCs], white blood cells [WBCs], platelets, etc.) to its disposition. If the donation is a "replacement for credit" for a particular patient, the donor must supply the patient's name or the group name that is to be credited.

A brief physical examination is required to determine whether the donor is in general good condition on the day that he or she is to donate blood. The physical examination entails a few simple procedures easily mastered by the health care worker:

1. *Weight.* Donors must weigh at least 110 lb (50 kg); if the weight is less, the volume of blood donated must be carefully monitored and care taken that not too much blood is collected. Also, the anticoagulant in the bag must be modified for the lesser donation. Most blood banks will not routinely accept donors who weigh less than 110 lb.
2. *Temperature.* The donor's oral temperature must not exceed 37.5°C (99.5°F).
3. *Pulse.* The donor's pulse should be regular and strong, between 50 and 100 beats per minute. The pulse should be taken for at least 30 seconds.
4. *Blood pressure.* The systolic blood pressure should measure no higher than 180 mm Hg, and the diastolic blood pressure should be no higher than 100 mm Hg. People with blood pressure outside these limits should be deferred as donors and referred to their physicians for evaluation of a possible health problem.
5. *Skin lesions.* Both arms should be examined for signs of drug abuse, such as needle marks or sclerotic veins. The presence of mild skin disorders, such as psoriasis, acne, or a poison ivy rash, does not necessarily prohibit an individual from donating unless the lesions are in the antecubital area or the rash is particularly extensive. Donors with purulent skin lesions, wounds, or severe skin infections should be deferred, as should anyone with purplish-red or hemorrhagic nodules suggestive of Kaposi's sarcoma (an HIV-associated clinical sign). The skin at the site of the venipuncture must be free of lesions.
6. *General appearance.* If the donor looks ill, excessively nervous, or under the influence of alcohol or drugs, he or she should be deferred.
7. *Hematocrit or hemoglobin values.* The hematocrit value must be no less than 38 percent for donors. The hemoglobin value must be no less than 12.5 g/dL. A finger stick is commonly used to draw blood for such determinations. The health care worker may either collect blood in a hematocrit tube for centrifuging and reading, measure hemoglobin spectrophotometrically, or use the copper sulfate method, in which the hemoglobin is qualitatively determined. (For further details on the copper sulfate method, please refer to the AABB technical manual.)[20]

An extensive medical history must be taken on all potential donors, regardless of the number of previous donations on record. Most blood bank donor rooms have a simple card listing all the questions to be asked and "yes" or "no" columns that are used to indicate the donor's responses. The health care provider should refer to the protocol of the donor room at the institution's blood bank or the AABB technical manual, which sets guidelines for donor screening and acceptance.

COLLECTION OF DONOR'S BLOOD

The health care worker in a donor room must operate under the supervision of a qualified, licensed physician. Blood should be collected by using aseptic technique; a sterile, closed system; and a single venipuncture. If a second venipuncture is needed, an entirely new, sterile donor set is necessary; the first is discarded according to the contaminated material disposal protocol of the institution.

A donor should never be left alone either during or immediately after blood collection. The health care worker should be well versed in donor reactions, equipment safety precautions, first-aid techniques, and location of first-aid equipment in case it is needed in the course of donation.

The health care worker should prepare the antecubital portion of the donor's arm in the same manner as for collection of a blood culture specimen (Boxes 12–2 and 12–3). The blood-collecting bag should be placed conveniently, and the tubing should be extended to ensure that it has no kinks that would prevent a free flow. After the arm is properly prepared, the tourniquet should be replaced and the donor given instructions to open and close the hand during the course of the phlebotomy (Box 12–4). A 15-gauge regular or 17-gauge thin-walled needle is used most often. The 17-gauge thin-walled needle is preferable because it has the internal diameter of a 15-gauge needle and the outside diameter of a 17-gauge needle; that is, it has the large-bore size of a 15-gauge needle, but the smaller total size of the 17-gauge needle. The sterile needle is uncapped, and with a quick, sure motion, the needle is slipped under the skin and into the vein. As the draw begins, the needle and tubing should be taped in place and a dry, sterile gauze sponge laid on top. The health care worker should encourage the donor to continue to open and close the hand slowly and to report any discomfort or dizziness that occurs.

The health care worker should make sure that the blood in the bag mixes the anticoagulant during the collection, either manually or by placing it on a mechanical agitator. If the collection process takes more than 8 minutes to complete, platelet concentrates or antihemophilic factor preparations may not be possible. As long as the flow is constant and the bag contents continue to be mixed well, however, no time constraints are necessary.

Once the proper amount of blood is collected (405 to 495 mL), the phlebotomy should be stopped, the tubing clamped off with a hemostat or some other temporary clamp, the tourniquet or blood pressure cuff released, the needle removed, and pressure placed over the site for several minutes. It is advisable that the donor be instructed to raise his or her arm over the head while holding the gauze with pressure over the puncture site. This method minimizes bleeding into the site and surrounding tissues, but also helps restore the integrity of the vascular tissue. The donor should not be allowed to bend the arm until the bleeding stops; otherwise, the tissue may be further traumatized by bleeding into the area below the skin, as well as encouraging the vascular tissue to overlap and form scar tissue on the site during the healing process. A pressure bandage may be placed over the site once the bleed-

BOX 12–2. PRE-PHLEBOTOMY PROCEDURES FOR WHOLE BLOOD DONATIONS

Preparation for Phlebotomy

Purpose

To provide instructions for the procedures that must be performed in preparation for phlebotomy, such as confirmation of donor's identity, final phlebotomy check of the donor record, and vein selection.

Scope

This procedure is to be performed by the phlebotomist for each donor that has been determined to be acceptable for donation.

Procedure

Materials needed:

Donor record.

Pen with blue or black ink (do not use pencil, felt-tip or fountain pen).

Blood pressure cuff or tourniquet.

Hand gripper.

Permanent marker.

1. Greet the donor as he or she enters the phlebotomy area and show him or her to a donor chair or bed.
2. Ask the donor, "What is your name?" and verify that the name is the same as the one on the donor card. If you cannot understand the donor's pronunciation, ask him or her to spell the name.
3. Review the following parts of the donor record for completeness, accuracy, and legibility: donor demographics, Donor Disqualification Directory or computer check, medical history interview, physical examination, and confidential unit exclusion and blood unit ID number. Ensure that the donor has signed the informed consent statement and that interviewer has signed.
   a. If any section is incomplete, ask the donor for the appropriate information or send him or her back to the screening area.
   b. If any reason for deferral is identified that was not identified by the screener, document this in the deferral section and defer the donor according to the appropriate deferral SOP.
4. Once the review is done, place the donor record near the donor and keep the record with the donor throughout the entire procedure.
5. Inspect both of the donor's arms for a good vein, as well as the presence of skin disease, tattoos, or scars suggestive of intravenous drug use. If these are observed, defer the donor according to SOP 313.00.04, "Deferral Based on Physical Examination."
6. If it is documented in the Medical History section that the donor has taken aspirin, piroxicam, or medications containing either of these drugs, write "ASA" on the upper right side of the primary label. Do not write over the bar code on the base label. Write the blood type, if known, on the upper right side of the primary bag base label. Do not write over the bar code on the base label.
7. Verify that all bar coded and eye-readable labels on the donor record, blood bags, and vacutubes are identical and have been appropriately placed on the vacutubes.
8. Record the following information in the appropriate areas of the donor record below the informed consent statement: type of collection bag (single, double, triple, quad), and lot number of the blood bag pack.

(continued)

BOX 12–2.   *(continued)*

9. Tie a tourniquet snugly around the donor's arm or wrap and inflate a blood pressure cuff around the arm to make the veins more prominent.

10. Place a gripper in the donor's hand, and ask him or her to squeeze it several times.

11. Select a site for venipuncture.

12. If you are not able to find an adequate vein, ask another phlebotomist to look. If no veins can be found, defer the donor and document the deferral. Record in the Comments section that the donor did not have good veins for phlebotomy.

Procedure Notes

1. Blood donors shall be interviewed and their blood collected and hematroned by trained individuals. One employee should not perform all the procedures involved in the collection of a unit of whole blood (screen, collect, and hematron). In circumstances when it is necessary for one employee to perform all of these procedures, however, another employee must be available to review the donor record, the unit of blood, and the test samples for potential discrepancies or errors.

2. It is the responsibility of the phlebotomist to ensure that the bar codes have been placed properly on the bags and vacutubes.

References

1. Walker RH, ed. *Technical Manual.* 11th ed. Bethesda, MD: American Association of Blood Banks; 1993.

2. *Code of Federal Regulation.* Current ed. 21 CFR. Washington, DC: U.S. Government Printing Office.

Records or Reports

Donor record.

Appendices

None.

(Courtesy of Gulf Coast Regional Blood Center, Houston, TX.)

ing stops. The blood in the bag and tubing should be mixed well, properly labeled, and stored in accordance with blood bank standards.

If the donor complains of dizziness or other discomfort, he or she should be encouraged to remain seated or prostrate for 10 to 15 minutes or longer. If the donor appears to be well, he or she should be encouraged not only to drink more fluids than usual to replace the volume loss, but also to refrain from strenuous exercise or work until after a full meal. Refreshments should be offered to the donor as a courtesy and as an opportunity for the donor to restore some of the lost body fluids. Any adverse reactions experienced by the donor should be recorded on the donor card. If the donor leaves before staff members recommend that he or she does so, this fact should also be noted on the donor's medical record.

BOX 12–3.   VENIPUNCTURE SITE PREPARATION FOR BLOOD DONATIONS

Purpose

To provide instructions on the correct procedure for cleaning the venipuncture site on the arm prior to phlebotomy.

Scope

This procedure will be performed by the phlebotomist for each donor prior to phlebotomy.

Procedure

Materials needed:

Tourniquet.

Hand gripper.

Sterile gauze.

0.75 percent PVP-iodine scrub solution and 1% PVP-iodine solution swabs or

Green soap and acetone alcohol swabs.

1. Tie a tourniquet snugly around the donor's arm and have the donor squeeze a hand gripper intermittently. Select a vein for venipuncture. Avoid scarred or pitted spots for venipuncture. (See Procedure Note 2.) You may mark the location of the vein with the stick end of an iodine scrub, so that the vein can be easily located. Release the tourniquet.

2. Ask the donor if he or she is allergic to iodine. If the donor is not allergic to iodine, use 0.75 percent PVP-iodine scrub solution and 1 percent PVP-iodine solution swabs for cleaning the arm. If the donor is allergic to iodine, use green soap and acetone alcohol swabs to clean the arm.

3. Using the 0.75 percent PVP-iodine scrub swab or the green soap swab, scrub the intended phlebotomy site and approximately a 3-inch-diameter area all around the site. Scrub continuously and randomly for *at least* 30 seconds (iodine scrub) or *at least* 2 minutes (green soap scrub).

4. Using the 1 percent PVP-iodine solution swab or the acetone alcohol swab, start at the intended venipuncture site and move the swab in an outward spiral. Cover the entire 3-inch-diameter area that was initially scrubbed, and DO NOT reswab any area that has already been swabbed.

5. If iodine was used, allow it to stand for at least 30 seconds; the iodine need not be dry in order to proceed. If acetone alcohol was used, allow it to stand for 7 minutes or until dry, then cover the area with a sterile gauze if the venipuncture is not going to be performed immediately.

6. DO NOT touch or repalpate the area after it has been cleaned. Do not wipe the iodine off the scrubbed area. If the area is touched or otherwise compromised, repeat the entire arm prep procedure.

Procedure Notes

1. Proper preparation of the venipuncture site helps to assure that the phlebotomy procedure will be as aseptic as possible. The first scrub debrides the area of dead skin cells and bacteria. The second solution removes these possible contaminates, leaving an aseptic area.

2. Phlebotomists should pay careful attention to selecting and cleansing the phlebotomy site. Avoid areas that are scarred or have pits or dimples associated with prior phlebotomies since these areas are difficult to clean and bacteria are harder to remove. (See Reference 3.)

(continued)

BOX 12–3.   *(continued)*

References

1. Walker RH, ed. *Technical Manual.* 12th ed. Bethesda, MD: American Association of Blood Banks; 1996.
2. Code of Federal Regulation. Current ed. 21 CFR. Washington, DC: U.S. Government Printing Office.
3. American Association of Blood Banks Association Bulletin #96-6, regarding "Bacterial Contamination of Blood Components," August 7, 1996.

Records or Reports

None.

Appendices

None.

(Courtesy of Gulf Coast Regional Blood Center, Houston, TX.)

BOX 12–4.   VENIPUNCTURE FOR BLOOD DONATIONS

Purpose

To provide instructions for proper performance and documentation of the venipuncture procedure.

Scope

This procedure is to be performed by a phlebotomist after proper preparation of the *venipuncture site.*

Procedure

Materials needed:
  Labeled blood bag set.
  Trip scale.
  Weight monitor.
  Donor record.
  Tourniquet.
  Tape.
  Face mask (optional).
  Hand gripper.
  Gauze.
  Hemostat.
  Gloves.
  Clock or watch with second hand.
  HOMS scale.
  Lab coat or disposable gown.

(continued)

BOX 12–4.   *(continued)*

Platform Scales/Shaker

1. Place the primary bag flat on the shaker platform.
2. Thread each side loop of the bag closest to the donor bed through the two standing metal leg supports attached to the platform and thread the slit of the bottom of the bag through the metal leg support located at the end of the metal platform.
3. Hang the satellite bags on the leg support located at the back of the platform when using an electric bag shaker.
4. Secure the labeled vacutubes through the side loops of the primary bag located on the outer edge of the platform.

Trip Scales and Weight Monitors

1. Hang the bag on a trip scale or weight monitor from the slit at the bottom of the bag. This will allow the blood to travel from the tubing up into the bag through the anticoagulant.
2. Thread the tubing through the cut-off groove on the trip scale or weight monitor and pull the tubing back and forth through the groove to ensure that it is not pinched.
3. Hang the satellite bags from the pig on the end of the weight monitor. Do not place the satellite bags on the floor or allow them to touch the floor.
4. Fold the tubing at approximately the fifth segment from the needle, and clamp the tubing with the hemostat.
5. Put on a clean pair of gloves before proceeding with the rest of the procedures. This step may be performed after step 4. Donor's arm has already been scrubbed as per Venipuncture Site Preparation Procedure.
6. Tie the tourniquet snugly around the donor's arm, and have the donor open and close his or her hand around the gripper, then make a clenched fist. Do not touch the scrubbed area.
7. Carefully remove the sterile gauze cover, and avoid touching the scrubbed area.
8. Remove the cap from the needle, retract the skin firmly below the scrubbed area, and insert the needle through the skin and into the vein in one smooth motion.
9. Release the hemostat, instruct the donor to unclench his or her fist, and watch for blood flow into the tubing.
10. If the initial venipuncture does not produce blood flow or an adequate blood flow, adjust the needle or ask for assistance. Do not probe in the donor's arm.
11. If the adjustment is unsuccessful, discontinue the phlebotomy. (See SOP #315.04.)
12. Secure the needle by taping the hub and tubing to the donor's arm.
13. Cover the venipuncture site with a dry sterile gauze.
14. Ask the donor to open and close his or her hand slowly and continuously throughout the collection.
15. If using an electric bag shaker, turn the shaker on. If using a trip scale or weight monitor, mix the blood and anticoagulant immediately after blood flow begins by gently inverting the bag several times. Mix the bag several times during the collection.
16. Release and readjust the tourniquet less tightly, if necessary, for the donor's comfort.
17. Monitor the flow of blood. If it appears to be slow or stopped, use strippers to check the flow. DO NOT USE HEMOSTATS. Excessive stripping can cause the vein to collapse and hemolyze cells.
18. Adjust the needle, if necessary, to restore blood flow. Turning the needle slightly will often be adequate.
19. If palpation of the vein after the insertion of the needle is necessary, it is recommended that the procedure be done only with a GLOVED finger above the site of insertion.
20. Monitor the donor throughout the procedure, and observe for signs of an adverse reaction.

(continued)

BOX 12–4. *(continued)*

Documentation of Phlebotomy

1. If the donor is an autologous, directed, or therapeutic donor, circle the "01-AU," "07-DE," or "14-TH," respectively, in the Donation Type box below the vital signs. If the donor is an allogeneic donor, no designation is required in this box.

2. Circle "WB" in the Procedure section of the donor record if the donor is donating whole blood. If the donor is undergoing an apheresis procedure, circle the appropriate procedure designation: PP, platelets; PL, plasma; GP, granulocytes; CO, combo; DP, double platelets.

3. Check the appropriate Left Arm or Right Arm box on line 1 of the Phlebotomy section of the donor record to indicate which arm was used for phlebotomy.

   Note: If the donor is stuck a second time, use line 2 to record the same information.

4. Record the identification number of the trip scale used in the space marked Scale on line 1 of the Phlebotomy section (line 2 in the case of a double stick).

5. Record the time, in military time, that the phlebotomy was begun on the Begin Line of the time box. Also record your initials and employee identification number on the corresponding In# Line of the Emp Box.

6. Write the time, in military time, the collection was begun on the upper right side of the primary bag base label. Do not write over the bar code on the base label.

Procedure Notes

1. If the phlebotomy is a difficult stick, needs several adjustments or strippings, has poor blood flow, or takes longer than 10 minutes, circle "01-Diff Stick" in the Venipuncture section of the donor record. Follow the procedure in SOP 315.03 "Whole blood collections that do not meet standards."

2. If the phlebotomy takes longer than 20 minutes, circle "06-NUC" in the Venipuncture section of the donor record. Follow the procedure in SOP 315.03, "Whole blood collections that do not meet standards."

3. Frequent mixture of the blood bag during phlebotomy is essential to prevent clots and provide quality blood components.

References

1. Walker RH, ed. *Technical Manual.* 12th ed. Bethesda, MD: American Association of Blood Banks; 1996.

2. Code of Federal Regulations. Current ed. 21 CFR. Washington, DC: U.S. Government Printing Office.

3. AABB Monthly Newsletter, March 1997.

Records or Reports

None.

Appendices

None.

(Courtesy of Gulf Coast Regional Blood Center, Houston, TX.)

■ THERAPEUTIC PHLEBOTOMY

Therapeutic phlebotomy is the intentional removal of blood for therapeutic reasons. It is used in the treatment of some myeloproliferative diseases, such as polycythemia, or other conditions in which there is an excessive production of blood cells. Records in the blood bank should indicate the patient's diagnosis, the physician's request for the phlebotomy, and the amount of blood to be taken. The medical director of the blood bank must decide whether the patient is to be bled in the donor room or in a private section of the blood bank. Some patients are visibly ill and weak, and their presence may have an adverse psychological effect on the healthy donors in the donor room. When a patient is obviously ill, his or her physician or the medical director of the blood bank should be present during the phlebotomy. Generally, the patient should be bled more slowly than a healthy donor, and the resting period should be extended.

The blood obtained through therapeutic bleeding may be used for homologous transfusion if the unit is deemed suitable by the director of the blood bank. If it is to be used, the recipient's physician must agree to use the blood for his or her patient, and a record of the agreement should be kept. The unit is then labeled and processed in the usual manner. The label must indicate that the blood is the result of a therapeutic bleed and must include the patient's diagnosis. If the unit is unsuitable for transfusion, the entire unit is disposed of in the usual manner for contaminated wastes.

■ AUTOLOGOUS TRANSFUSION

A practice that is frequently used is **autologous transfusion:** the patient donates his or her own blood before anticipated surgery. The reason for this type of transfusion is that the safest blood a recipient can receive is his or her own blood. The autologous transfusion prevents transfusion-transmitted infectious diseases (e.g., HIV, hepatitis) and eliminates the formation of antibodies in the transfused patient.

■ THE EMERGENCY CENTER

The atmosphere in an emergency center differs from that in any other area of the hospital. Most emergency rooms are chronically filled with people in pain whose medical problems range from relatively minor injuries or illnesses to major, traumatic injuries. In addition to those who come to the emergency center for immediate treatment of acute injuries or illnesses, some patients have no regular physician and use the local emergency center for treatment of chronic illnesses, such as coughs and colds. Family members often accompany the patients and may be highly emotional and vocal about their concern for their loved ones.

This range of patients and families with varying needs who demand attention from the limited staff can create a highly charged atmosphere. In most emergency centers, the patients are prioritized in a central reception area, often referred to as a *triage area,* as they arrive. Those who need immediate attention are seen first, and those whose conditions are more stable are seen later. Even when the patients are prioritized according to their illnesses, however, the routine can be upset if a trauma patient arrives by ambulance and requires immediate life-saving measures. Although personnel at the triage desk may attempt to maintain a stable and orderly work flow in the emergency center, medical emergencies and critically ill or injured patients are unavoidable and must be handled professionally. The emergency center is an unpredictable setting; even though guidelines are placed on the flow of patients, the unexpected can occur at any moment.

Recognizing that the emergency center setting is stressful, the health care provider has two important responsibilities. First, he or she must be completely familiar with all the equipment and well versed in all blood-collecting procedures. If called on to collect stat (immediate) blood specimens from a critically injured person about to go to surgery, the health care worker must respond quickly and must successfully obtain the correct specimen in the right volume. He or she may not have enough time to collect another specimen if the first one is unsuitable. Consequently, only experienced health care workers should accept positions in the emergency center, where skills must be well mastered and automatic. The second responsibility is to follow directions quickly and correctly. In a critical situation, the health care worker must be able to follow the orders exactly and not require extensive, time-consuming directions. Only an experienced, confident, mature health care worker is suited to the unpredictable emergency environment.

Another factor present in the emergency center, which may cause a great deal of stress in some persons, is the sight and sound of traumatically injured patients in pain. Profuse bleeding, disfigurement, moaning, and groaning are common occurrences in this setting. Health care workers should be aware of their own reactions to critically injured patients. If they find the setting too stressful, they should opt for work on the general floors of the hospital or in a clinic where the sights and sounds are more predictable and controlled. The health care worker who chooses to work in an emergency center must learn to do his or her job with single-mindedness and to ignore anything that may distract from obtaining high-quality samples with speed and accuracy.

A career in emergency medicine is not for everyone; some people can work in the stressful setting for only a limited amount of time, whereas others would work nowhere else. The excitement of being part of a team of professionals who routinely provide life-saving treatment to critically injured patients has an attraction that cannot be easily duplicated in any other area of patient care. Health care workers must choose the environment that is best suited to their temperament and where they can best deliver quality patient care.

SELF STUDY

KEY TERMS

Allen Test
Arterial Blood Gases (ABGs)
Autologous Transfusion
Bacteremia
Bleeding-Time Test
Blood Cultures
Brachial Artery
Cannula
Capillary Blood Gas Analysis
Central Venous Catheter (CVC)
Intravenous (IV) Line
Femoral Artery
Fevers of Unknown Origin (FUO)
Fistula
Glucose Tolerance Test
Heparin or Saline Lock

Implanted Port
Lactose Tolerance Test
Peripherally Inserted Central
  Catheter (PICC)
Postprandial Glucose Test
Radial Artery
Septicemia
Sodium Polyanethole Sulfonate
  (SPS)
Therapeutic Drug Monitoring
  (TDM)
Therapeutic Phlebotomy
Trace Metals
Vascular Access Devices
  (VADs)

STUDY QUESTIONS

For the following, choose the *one* best answer:

1. What is a cannula?

    a. the fusion of a vein and an artery
    b. a good source of arterial blood
    c. a tubular instrument used to gain access to venous blood
    d. an artificial shunt that provides access to arterial blood

2. Which of the following is a milk sugar that sometimes cannot be digested by healthy individuals?

    a. glucose
    b. glucagon
    c. lactose
    d. lactate

3. Which of the following is the preferred site for blood collection for ABG analysis?

    a. subclavian artery
    b. femoral artery
    c. ulnar artery
    d. radial artery

363

4. Which of the following supplies is *not* needed during an arterial puncture for an ABG determination?

   a. tourniquet
   b. heparin
   c. lidocaine
   d. syringe

5. What is the reason for performing the Allen test?

   a. to obtain the oxygen concentration of the patient
   b. to determine whether the patient's blood pressure is elevated
   c. to test for the possibility of a hematoma
   d. to determine that the ulnar and radial arteries are providing collateral circulation

6. When blood is drawn from the radial artery for an ABG determination, the needle should be inserted at an angle of no less than

   a. 20 degrees
   b. 30 degrees
   c. 45 degrees
   d. 65 degrees

7. Which of the following evacuated tubes is preferred for the collection of a blood culture specimen?

   a. yellow-topped evacuated tube
   b. green-topped evacuated tube
   c. light blue-topped evacuated tube
   d. red-topped evacuated tube

8. During a glucose tolerance test which procedure is acceptable?

   a. a standard amount of glucose drink is given to the patient, then a fasting blood collection is performed
   b. the patient should be encouraged to drink water throughout the procedure
   c. the patient is allowed to chew sugarless gum
   d. all the patient's specimens are timed from the fasting collection

9. The bleeding-time test is used for what purpose?

   a. check for vascular abnormalities
   b. diagnose diabetes mellitus
   c. determine whether the patient's blood pressure is low
   d. assess liver glycogen stores

10. Autologous transfusion is to prevent which of the following possibilities?

    a. the transfused patient will develop diabetes mellitus
    b. antibodies will form in the transfused patient
    c. antigens will form in the transfused patient
    d. polycythemia will develop in the transfused patient

References

1. National Committee for Clinical Laboratory Standards (NCCLS). *Percutaneous Collection of Arterial Blood for Laboratory Analysis.* NCCLS Document H11-A2. Villanova, PA: NCCLS; Vol 12, no 8, 1992.

2. National Committee for Clinical Laboratory Standards (NCCLS). *Blood Gas Preanalytical Considerations: Specimen Collection, Calibration, and Controls.* NCCLS Document C27-A. Villanova, PA: NCCLS; 1993.

3. Smith C. Surgicutt: a device for modified template bleeding times. *J Med Technol.* 1986;3(4).

4. International Technidyne Corporation. *Surgicutt: Package Insert of Procedure.* Edison, NJ: International Technidyne Corporation.

5. Balows A (ed). *Manual of Clinical Microbiology.* 5th ed. Washington, DC: American Society for Microbiology; 1991.

6. Koneman E, Allen S, Janda W, et al. eds. *Color Atlas & Textbook of Diagnostic Microbiology.* 5th ed. Philadelphia: Lippincott; 1997.

7. Isaacman DJ, Karasic RB. Lack of effect of changing needles on contamination of blood cultures. *Pediatr Infect Dis J.* 1990;9:274.

8. Krumholz HM, Cummings S, York M. Blood culture phlebotomy: switching needles does not prevent contamination. *Ann Intern Med.* 1990;13:290.

9. Baron EJ, Peterson LR, Finegold SM, eds. *Bailey & Scott's Diagnostic Microbiology.* St. Louis: Mosby; 1994.

10. Report of the Expert Committee on the Diagnosis and Classification of Diabetes Mellitus. *Diabetes Care.* 1997 Jul; 20(7):1183–1197.

11. Kaplan LA, Pesce AJ, eds. Therapeutic drug monitoring. In: *Clinical Chemistry: Theory, Analysis Correlation.* 3rd ed. St. Louis: Mosby; 1996.

12. Franson TR, Ritch PS, Quebbeman EJ: Aminoglycoside serum concentration sampling via central venous catheters: a potential source of clinical error. *JPEN.* 1987;11(1):77–79.

13. Guder W, Narayanan S, Wisser H, Zawta B: *Samples: From the Patient to the Laboratory.* Darmstadt: Git Verlag; 1996.

14. Quattrocchi F, Karnes H, Robinson J, et al. Effect of serum separator blood collection tubes on drug concentration. *Ther Drug Monit.* 1983;5:359–362.

15. Meranger J, Hollebone B, Blanchette G: The effects of storage times, temperature and container types on the accuracy of atomic absorption determination of Cd, Cu, Hg, Pb and Zn in whole heparinized blood. *J Anal Toxicol.* 1981;5:33–41.

16. National Committee for Clinical Laboratory Standards. *Control of Preanalytical Variation in Trace Element Determinations: Approved Guidelines.* Villanova, PA: Document C38-A. NCCLS; 1997.

17. Kennedy C, Angermuller S, King R, et al. A comparison of hemolysis rates using intravenous catheters versus venipuncture tubes for obtaining blood samples. *J Emerg Nurs.* 1996;22(6):566–569.

18. U.T.M.D. Anderson Cancer Center—Division of Laboratory Medicine/General Services/Diagnostic Center. *Drawing Blood Through Central Venous Catheters.* Houston, TX: U.T.M.D. Anderson Cancer Center, 1997.

19. Baranowski L, Lonsway RA, Hedrick C: *Intravenous Therapy: Clinical Principles and Practice.* Philadelphia: WB Saunders; 1996.

20. Vengelen-Tyler V, ed. *Technical Manual of the American Association of Blood Banks.* 12 ed. Bethesda, MD: 1996.

13

THIRTEEN

■

Elderly, Home, and Long-term Care Collections

CHAPTER OUTLINE

CHAPTER OBJECTIVES

Upon completion of Chapter 13, the learner is responsible for the following:

1. List two other terms that are synonymous with *point-of-care testing*.

2. Define five physical and/or emotional changes that are associated with the aging process.

3. Describe how a health care worker should react to physical and emotional changes associated with the elderly.

4. Identify four analytes whose levels can be determined through point-of-care testing.

5. Describe the most widely used application of point-of-care testing.

6. Given the abnormal and normal control values for glucose from a daily run, plot the control values on the appropriate quality control charts.

With new emerging technology, laboratory testing services and results delivery have expanded beyond the laboratory to the hospital bedside, the home, the nursing home, and any other direct-contact patient setting.[1] The terms used for these direct laboratory services include *decentralized laboratory testing, on-site testing, alternate-site testing, near-patient testing,* **patient-focused testing, point-of-care testing,** and *bedside testing.* With the increasing health care requirements of the growing U.S. elderly population and the innovations in point-of-care instrumentation, nurses, laboratorians, and other health care providers will increasingly perform additional on-site laboratory testing to obtain various types of laboratory test results. The demand for point-of-care testing is increasing because rapid turnaround of laboratory test results is necessary for prompt medical decision making.

The elderly or geriatric population comprises about 15 percent of the U.S. population and uses 31 percent of the nation's health care services.[2] In 25 years, the geriatric population will have reached 20 percent of the total U.S. population. Physical conditions, such as arthritis, **Parkinson's disease** (i.e., a disease causing tremors), and other debilitating diseases in the elderly will continue to increase point-of-care testing by skin puncture due to the difficulty of obtaining blood by venipuncture. In addition, this patient population will increasingly need point-of-care testing and other health care services in their homes, nursing homes, rehabilitation centers, and other long-term care facilities (where the length of stay is over 30 days).

The process of aging presents physical and emotional problems that can be challenging for health care workers. Whatever the case, elderly individuals should be treated with the utmost respect and dignity. Physical problems that are common include the following:

- Hearing loss may cause embarrassment and frustration. Repeating instructions or adjusting one's position to speak in the "good" ear may be necessary for the patient to truly understand a procedure.
- Failing eyesight is common, so the health care worker should take care to guide the elderly individual to the appropriate seat for blood collection or to the bathroom for urine collections.
- Loss of taste, smell, and feeling can accompany the aging process. Elderly people may lack an appetite, which may lead to malnourishment. They may tend to drop things or not be able to make a fist due to muscle weakness. The health care worker should make a note of these clues, particularly if the patient is homebound without a caregiver.
- Memory loss can affect the patient's ability to take medications or to remember the last time they ate. These factors may interfere with the interpretation of laboratory results.
- Epithelium and subcutaneous tissues become thinner thereby making venipuncture more difficult. The phlebotomist must hold the skin extra taut so that the vein does not "roll."
- Muscles become smaller, so the angle of penetration of a venipuncture needle may need to be more shallow.
- Increased susceptibility to accidental hypothermia (a subnormal drop in body temperature) can make the elderly patient feel cold. Thus, specimen collection may require warming of the site.

Emotional problems that are associated with aging include the possible loss of career, spouse, close friends, or relatives and can be reflected by depression or anger at life in general. Health care workers should remember to address the elderly with dignity and respect by using "Mr., Mrs., Miss," etc. Respect for privacy should also be considered.

Factors related to the physical setting can also affect a phlebotomist's work. If specimens are to be collected in homes, all procedures are similar except that extra care must be taken for the following:

- Extra supplies and equipment, including biohazard containers for disposables and a specimen transport container, should be taken into the home.
- The patient should be positively identified if possible. If not possible, then procedures of the health care organization should be developed and followed.
- The patient should be placed in a comfortable, preferably reclining position, in case of fainting.
- The phlebotomist should locate the nearest bathroom, sink, and clean towels for washing hands. It is advisable for home care workers to use hand disinfectants that are easily transportable. These are commercially available in creams and foams.
- The health care worker should carefully inspect the area after the procedure to assure that all trash and used supplies have been properly discarded.
- Specimens should be carefully labeled and placed in leakproof containers. Appropriate temperatures for transport should be checked.
- Health care workers who are working in high crime areas should take security precautions, travel with a mobile phone, and maps of the area to avoid getting lost on the way to or from the patient's home.
- Delays in returning specimens to the laboratory should be carefully documented.

■ GLUCOSE MONITORING

One of the most widely used applications of point-of-care testing is blood glucose monitoring, in which commercially available instruments, such as the one shown in Figure 13–1, are used to determine blood glucose levels. Such determinations allow the physician to choose appropriate treatment regimens for patients with **diabetes mellitus,** a chronic disease in which the pancreas cannot produce enough **insulin** or cannot use the insulin that it does produce. Insulin is a chemical that is released into the bloodstream by the pancreas when glucose levels in the blood increase after meals. Insulin causes the glucose to be absorbed from the blood into the body tissues, where it is used for energy. Because of the lack of insulin in patients with diabetes mellitus, glucose is not properly absorbed by the tissues, and the glucose levels within the blood increase.

Clinical Alert ❗

If the blood glucose levels become too elevated, the diabetic patient can enter a state of metabolic acidosis (ketoacidosis), which can result in shock and then death. Because research has shown that strict glucose control in patients with diabetes mellitus is necessary to prevent serious complications, pocket-size glucose meters are used in point-of-care testing to help these patients monitor and maintain glucose levels within the acceptable range.[3]

During the past decade, small glucose-monitoring instruments, such as those described in Table 13–1, became commonplace in the home, in the nursing home, and at the hospital bedside.

These "rapid" methods require whole blood samples collected by skin puncture from the finger, heel (for infants), or a flushed heparin line. As for any blood collection procedure, appropriate safety protocols must be followed (e.g., wearing gloves), and disposal of potentially contaminated waste must be part of the quality control and safety guidelines. These bedside procedures are handy for quick screening in a hospital or outpatient setting. *Extreme caution* must be taken, however, to provide a rigid, up-to-date, quality control and training program for personnel before they begin to implement such procedures. Variance in methodology and lack of quality control on reagents and equipment can lead to serious medical consequences for patients being tested.[4,5] Therefore, careful adherence to manufacturers' instructions, a thorough evaluation of the monitoring devices, and strict adherence to daily quality control procedures will ensure a more accurate and precise screening tool. In addition, careful recording of the results must include the date, time, and health care

Figure 13–1. HemoCue β-Glucose Analyzer.

(Courtesy of HemoCue, Inc., Mission Viejo, CA).

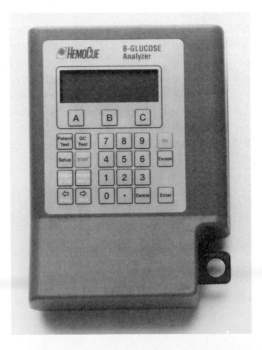

Table 13–1.   Blood Glucose Monitors

INSTRUMENT (MANUFACTURER)	FEATURES	TEST TIME
Glucometer Encore (Bayer Corp., Tarrytown, NY)	Quality control (QC) management capability Memory function includes date and time; thus, no timing Above average accuracy No wiping required Easy to operate	15–60 seconds
Accu-Chek easy (Boehringer Mannheim Corp., Indianapolis, IN)	QC and patient data management capability with AccuData GTS Memory function includes data, time, and patient identification number Above average accuracy	15–60 seconds
One Touch Profile (Life Scan Milpitas, CA)	QC data management capability Automated QC features Available for use in 19 languages Memory function includes date and time Above average accuracy Easy to use	45 seconds
β-Glucose analyzer (HemoCue, Inc., Mission Viejo, CA)	Refrigerated temperature required for test cuvettes Above average accuracy Memory capability is available Easy to operate	15–45 seconds
ExacTech (MediSense, Waltham, MA)	No wiping, blotting, or timing Credit card size and shape Blood does not enter sensor, so cleaning not required Memory function includes last reading recall and calibration code recall	30 seconds

worker identification, as well as verification that the results are from the bedside (or patient's home) rather than the clinical laboratory. In some health care facilities, bedside test results are recorded on special bedside testing forms or in a separate section of the patient's medical record.

To perform the blood glucose determinations, health care providers need to gather the appropriate supplies (Box 13–1) and must be aware of the total quality assurance procedures that are required to obtain accurate and precise results. A skin puncture is customarily performed to obtain the blood for these bedside glucose assays. The patient's finger should be cleansed with alcohol and allowed to dry. A microcollection lancet is used to puncture the finger. The first drop of blood is wiped away with a dry, sterile gauze pad, and the next drop is allowed to fall from the finger onto the reagent strip or pad. After the specified time indicated on the instrument's instruction sheet elapses, the blood drop is removed by blotting or washing, and the strip is placed in the instrument to obtain a glucose reading. The timing of the reaction is critical, and most of these instruments call the time to the attention of the operator by buzzing or by sounding an alarm.

> # BOX 13–1.   SUPPLIES AND EQUIPMENT FOR BLOOD GLUCOSE MONITORING
>
> Blood glucose testing monitor.
> Strips (or cuvettes) appropriate for the monitor.
> Calibrators and controls.
> Tissues, gauze, or cotton balls.
> 70 percent isopropyl alcohol.
> Safety blood collection lancets.
> Gloves (nonlatex if allergic to latex).
> Biohazard disposal container for lancets.
> (Timing device for visual testing.)
> Biohazard disposal trash can.

The HemoCue β-Glucose Analyzer (HemoCue, Inc., Mission Viejo, CA) (Fig. 13–1) is an instrument used for bedside glucose testing. This instrument can obtain test results from capillary, venous, or arterial whole blood. It uses a microcuvette rather than a test strip and does not require blotting. Also, it can be used to monitor blood glucose in neonates.

 Some glucose-monitoring instruments should be calibrated with glucose standards (calibrators). The glucose values must be monitored daily with **quality control material,** and whenever a battery is changed, or the meter is cleaned. This control material should be similar to the patient's specimen in order to determine if the analytic system is working properly. For example, the glucose control material should be based on the use of whole blood because this type of body fluid is used for measurements with bedside glucose-monitoring instruments.

For each day the glucose assay is performed on patients' blood specimens, control material must be analyzed. The control value obtained each day is plotted on a chart under the appropriate date, and the daily plots are joined with a straight line (Fig. 13–2). Interpretation of this chart is based on the fact that for a normal distribution, 95 percent of the values about the mean, or average ($\bar{x}$), should be within ± 2 standard deviations (SD) of the mean (average), and the fact that 99 percent of the values are within ± 3 SD of the mean. Tolerance limits are determined by pooling the data obtained during a 20-day test period and referring to the mean ± 2 SD. If a daily control value exceeds the tolerance limits, corrective action must occur according to the manufacturer's directions and be documented for future reference.

Another quality control measure that can be taken when point-of-care glucose-monitoring instruments are used is purchasing the reagent strips and controls in quantities that enable health care workers to use constant pools of the same lot number. This leads to reproducibility of the glucose results. Required preventive maintenance of each meter is critical for accurate results.

Some point-of-care glucose-testing instruments can store and download calibrators, controls, and patients' results and can, thus, provide a complete instrument log for quality

Figure 13–2. Quality control record.

QUALITY CONTROL RECORD

PRACTICE NAME

PRECISION HEALTH CARE INC.

INSTRUMENT _Glucose Monitor- Institution #55_

CONTROL LOT # _11542A_   EXPIRATION DATE _01/29/99_

Director Signature/Date:

NAME/LEVEL

TEST _Glucose *Glucose Monitor_   UNITS _mg/dl_

LOWER LIMIT _91_   MEAN _100_   UPPER LIMIT _109_

DATE	No.	VALUE	TECH	COMMENT	DATE	No.	VALUE	TECH	COMMENT
12/8/98	1	99	KBm			17			
12/9/98	2	103	KBm	prev. maintenance		18			
12/10/98	3	100	KBm			19			
12/11/98	4	100	KBm			20			
12/14/98	5	105	KBm			21			
12/15/98	6	97	KBm			22			
12/16/98	7	95	KBm			23			
12/17/98	8	96	KBm	new battery		24			
12/18/98	9	103	KBm			25			
12/19/98	10	100	KBm			26			
12/20/98	11	103	KBm			27			
12/21/98	12	97	KBm			28			
	13					29			
	14					30			
	15					31			
	16								

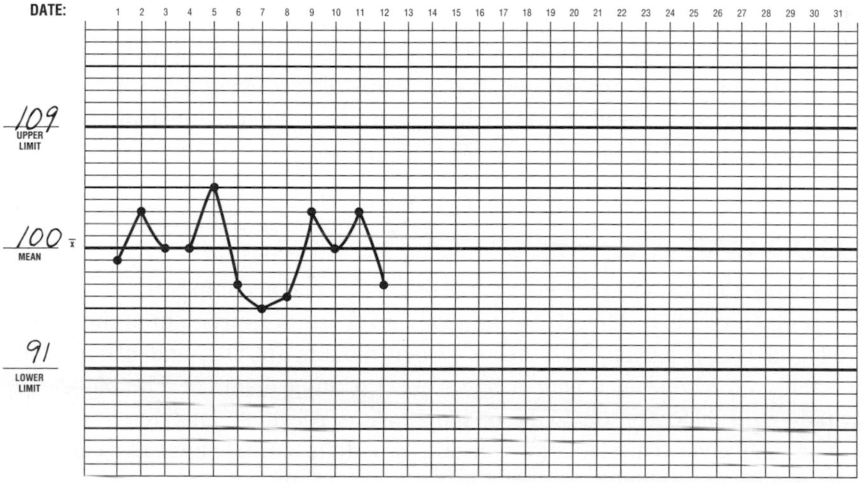

DATE: 1 2 3 4 5 6 7 8 9 10 11 12 13 14 15 16 17 18 19 20 21 22 23 24 25 26 27 28 29 30 31

_109_ UPPER LIMIT

_100_ x̄ MEAN

_91_ LOWER LIMIT

Table 13–2.   Problems to Avoid in Point-of-Care Glucose Testing

Specimen is inappropriately stored.

Contamination of the blood with alcohol. (After alcohol is used to cleanse the skin puncture site, the skin must dry *completely* before puncturing the site.)

Wrong volume of specimen is collected.

Specimen is collected at wrong time.

Instrument blotting/wiping technique is not performed according to manufacturer's directions.

Instrument is not clean.

Reagents are outdated.

Timing of the analytic procedure is incorrect.

Reagents are not stored at proper temperature, leading them to deterioration.

Patient has not dieted properly for procedure.

Patient's result/time/date/etc., are mislabeled.

Recording of result is incorrect.

Battery for instrument is weak or dead.

Calibrators and/or controls are not properly used.

Results are not sent to appropriate individuals in timely manner.

assurance interpretation. Table 13–2 provides a list that will help lead to quality results through *avoidance* of these problems.

■ BLOOD KETONE TESTING

An elevated level of metabolic acids (e.g., β-hydroxybutyric acid) occurs in a patient with uncontrolled diabetes mellitus, which can result in shock and death. A point-of-care instrument is now available that can determine the blood level of β-hydroxybutyric acid, the predominant ketone body. This reflectance meter, the Ketosite (GDS Diagnostics, Elkhart, IN), can monitor the status of **ketoacidosis.** It is a 2-minute test using a blood sample of only 25 μL. Thus, along with the glucose monitoring, this point-of-care instrument can be extremely important in diabetic monitoring for clinician use.

■ BLOOD GAS AND ELECTROLYTE ANALYSIS

Blood gas analysis for critical patient care needs can also be accomplished through patient-focused testing (Fig. 13–3). **Blood gas analysis** involves measurement of the partial pressure of oxygen (pO_2), partial pressure of carbon dioxide (pCO_2), and pH. The pO_2 and pCO_2 are analyzed whenever a patient has a heart or lung disorder. The blood pH determines whether the blood is too acidic or too alkaline. All these analytes must be closely monitored in emergency care situations, critical care units, cardiac intensive care units, and other units requiring immediate patient diagnosis and treatment.

In addition to monitoring blood gases, point-of-care testing instruments, such as those shown in Figures 13–3 and 13–4, can measure blood electrolyte levels—sodium (Na^+), potassium (K^+), chloride (Cl^-), and bicarbonate (HCO_3^-) levels. These electrolyte measurements, as well as blood gas analysis, are needed immediately in critical care situations.

Figure 13–3. i-STAT system for point-of-care testing.

(Courtesy of i-STAT Corporation, Princeton, NJ.)

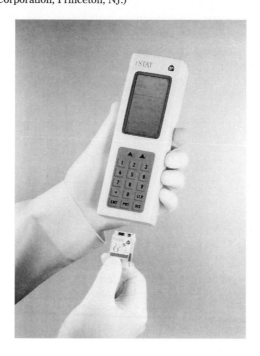

Figure 13–4. Nova Biomedical stat profile analyzer.

(Courtesy of Nova Biomedical, Waltham, MA.)

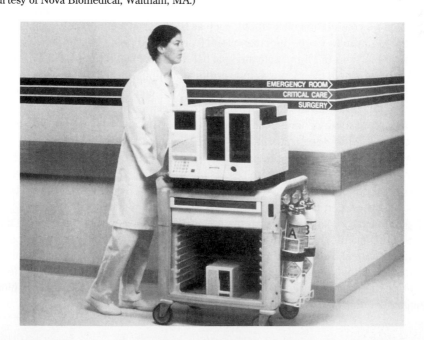

These instruments require preventive maintenance and quality control similar to the glucose-monitoring instruments; however, these instruments measure more than one analyte and, thus, have more complex operational, quality control, and maintenance needs than the glucose monitors. Consequently, as a health care professional involved in collecting blood and determining the analytes' results with these instruments, it is extremely important to be thoroughly trained in their use prior to actually testing patients' blood.

■ POINT-OF-CARE TESTING FOR ACUTE HEART DAMAGE

 Clinical Alert

 Troponin T is a protein released and detected after a myocardial infarct (heart attack). Troponin T is elevated only when heart (cardiac) damage has occurred. Boehringer Mannheim (Indianapolis, IN) has developed a point-of-care STAT test for determination of cardiac troponin T. The blood test results can be read from this rapid assay in 1 to 15 minutes, depending on the troponin T concentration in the patient's sample. If the test is positive, it indicates that the patient has had a myocardial infarction and should immediately be admitted to the hospital's coronary care unit (CCU).

■ BLOOD COAGULATION MONITORING

Similar to glucose monitoring, monitoring blood coagulation through point-of-care testing provides immediate results that can be used in controlling bleeding or clotting disorders in patients.[6] A blood coagulation instrument, such as the CoaguChek Plus Coagulation System (Boehringer Mannheim Corp., Indianapolis, IN), is a hand-held instrument that can measure prothrombin time (PT) and activated partial thromboplastin time (APTT) from an unmeasured drop of whole blood, providing results in 3 minutes (Fig. 13–5). The CoaguChek System is another near-patient testing instrument that can be used by home health care providers or other outpatient clinic providers to determine PT results on patients (Fig. 13–6). It is used to monitor long-term anticoagulation therapy in patients. The immediate test results allow rapid dose adjustments. Again, the health care provider using these instruments must be trained appropriately in the preventive maintenance and quality control parameters in order to obtain accurate results. Also, reading the manufacturer's directions is essential. For example, the CoaguChek Plus Coagulation System is calibrated to use the *first* drop of blood in skin puncture.

Other point-of-care coagulation systems are the Actalyke Activated Clotting Time Test (ACT) System (Fig. 13–7) (Array Medical, Somerville, NJ), the ProTime Microcoagulation System (International Technidyne Corp., Edison, NJ), and the Hemochron Jr. Instrument (International Technidyne Corp., Edison, NJ). These instruments are designed for use at the patient point-of-care (i.e., home, intensive care unit, physician's office) to monitor heparin anticoagulation therapy.

Figure 13–5.   CoaguChek Plus Coagulation System.

(Courtesy of Boehringer Mannheim Corp., Indianapolis, IN.)

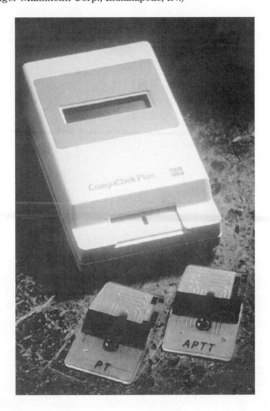

Figure 13–6. CoaguChek System.

(Courtesy of Boehringer Mannheim Corp., Indianapolis, IN.)

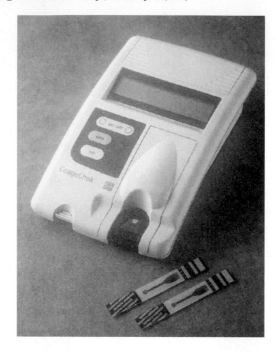

Figure 13–7. Actalyke Activated Clotting Time Test (ACT) System.

(Courtesy of Array Medical, Somerville, NJ.)

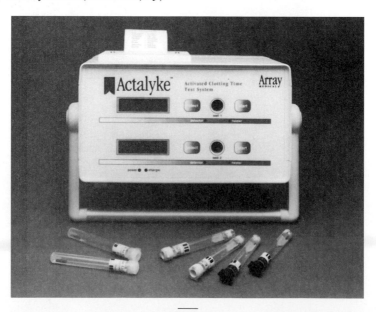

■ HEMATOCRIT, HEMOGLOBIN, AND OTHER HEMATOLOGY PARAMETERS

The hematocrit (Hct, packed cell volume [PCV], Crit) represents the volume of circulating blood that is occupied by red blood cells (RBCs). It is expressed as a percentage; thus, a hematocrit value of 38 percent indicates that 38 mL of each 100 mL of peripheral blood is composed of RBCs. Hematocrit values are obtained to aid in the diagnosis and evaluation of anemia, a less than normal number of erythrocytes, and may be used to evaluate blood volume and total RBC mass. Shown in Box 13–2 is a technical procedure for hematocrit. For

---

BOX 13–2.   THE UNIVERSITY OF TEXAS–HOUSTON HEALTH SCIENCE CENTER (UTHHSC) MEDICAL MOBILE VAN:

TECHNICAL PROCEDURE: HEMATOCRIT OR PACKED CELL VOLUME (PCV)

Principle of the Test

The hematocrit represents the volume of circulating blood that is occupied by erythrocytes and is expressed as a percentage. The method used for the determination is centrifugation with the Stat-Spin centrifuge (Norfolk Scientific, Inc., Norwood, MA) procedure. The hematocrit test helps the physician to identify patients at risk of developing anemia and manage patients who have anemia. Anemia is a less than normal number of erythrocytes in the volume of packed cells. The most common cause of anemia throughout the world is iron deficiency. A decrease in the hematocrit value results in a lack of energy, a reduced resistance to infections, and an increased risk of abnormality in pregnancy. An increased hematocrit value can result from polycythemia, hemoconcentration, and/or cardiac disease.

The reference intervals based on Texas Department of Health (TDH) values are:

40–54% (males).

38–47% (females).

44–64% (newborns).

35–49% (14–90 days).

30–40% (6 months–1 year).

31–43% (1 year–10 years).

The critical limits are based on TDH levels:

<34% or >54% (male)

<31% or >47% (female)

If levels are in critical range, rerun. If the same, Nurse Practitioner refers to rural health clinic.

Materials and Reagents Required

Heparin-coated plastic microcapillary tubes.

Gloves (non-latex if patient has latex allergy).

Microcentrifuge.

Controls.

Laboratory tissues.

(continued)

BOX 13–2. *(continued)*

Specimen Collection

The technical procedure for finger puncture should be followed for blood collection. It is extremely important to wear gloves and a protective laboratory coat during the collection and testing procedures. Plastic microcapillary tubes treated with ammonium heparin (color-coded red) should be used for the capillary blood collection. These tubes should be stored in a cool, dry place.

To perform the microcollection, hold the microcapillary tube by the end that has the color-coded band. Fill to the color-coded band. After filling, tilt the banded end downward until the blood moves halfway between the band and the end of the tube. Hold the tube in a horizontal position and push the *dry* (banded) end of the tube fully into the vertically held sealing compound. Twist and remove. Using a laboratory tissue, wipe off any blood that is forced from the other end.

Precautions

Do not squeeze, or "milk," the finger before or during the procedure; doing so can result in an abnormally low reading.

Do not collect blood in the microcapillary tube while the patient's finger is still wet with alcohol or a low reading will result. Allow the finger to air dry before collection.

Test Procedure

1. Put the microcapillary tube (sealed end toward the outer rim) in any of the 12 positions on the hematocrit microcentrifuge. This rotor need not be balanced. Screw the cover in place.

2. Holding the rotor by the black "cover knob," attach the rotor to the rotor holder. (*Important:* Always hold the hematocrit rotor by the black knob on the rotor cover when pressing it firmly in a downward motion onto the rotor holder and when removing the rotor from the centrifuge. Pressing on the outer edges of the hematocrit rotor may result in damage to the rotor.)

3. Centrifuge the hematocrit rotor.

4. After the rotor stops, remove the rotor. To read the hematocrit value, place the rotor in the middle of the illuminated magnifying reader. Follow the directions on it as follows:

   Position the reader so that the base of the red blood cell column intersects the 0 (zero) line and the 100 percent line intersects the top of the plasma. Read the height of the red blood cell column directly from the scale. Interpolate between the markings to 1 percent.

Quality Control

- On a daily basis, use the controls purchased for the microhematocrit procedure.
- To verify the adequacy of cell packing, on a daily basis select one or more tubes (preferably with a hematocrit value of more than 50 percent, if available), centrifuge, and read. Spin these tubes a second time. The difference between the initial reading and the second reading should be 1 percent or less.

Preventive Maintenance of Microcentrifuge

- The timer should be calibrated with a stopwatch every 2 weeks.
- Speed can be checked by using the cell-packing procedure described under Quality Control.

References

StatSpin Procedure.
National Committee for Clinical Laboratory Standards (NCCLS). *Physician's Office Laboratory Guidelines.* 2nd ed. Document POL1-T2. Villanova, PA: June, 1992.
Becan-McBride K, Ross D. *Essentials for the Small Laboratory and Physician's Office.* St. Louis: Mosby-Year Book; 1988.

(Courtesy of The University of Texas–Houston Health Science Center, Houston, TX.)

accurate test results, remember not to squeeze the tissue to obtain capillary blood because doing so will dilute the sample with tissue fluid.

Determining a patient's hemoglobin level is another test to aid in the diagnosis and evaluation of anemia and other blood abnormalities. The hemoglobin test has been determined by the American Medical Association (AMA) to be more accurate than the hematocrit test in diagnosis and treatment. Also, the hemoglobin procedure is a safer method to detect anemia. A point-of-care analyzer that can be used to measure hemoglobin is the HemoCue β-Hemoglobin System (HemoCue, Inc., Mission Viejo, CA) (Fig. 13–8). A patient's venous, capillary, or arterial whole blood sample placed in the microcuvette and inserted into this instrument provides the patient's hemoglobin value.

The Ichor automated cell counter (Array Medical, Somerville, NJ) is new instrumentation for hematology analysis in acute patient management (Fig. 13–9). It is the first system available for use at the point of patient care (e.g., ICU) to determine the hematology parameters that include platelet count, hemoglobin, hematocrit, WBC count, and RBC count. The results are available in about 1 minute. In blood transfusion triage, Ichor can quickly provide results to guide clinical decisions about needed blood components. Since only 12 μL of

Figure 13–8.   HemoCue β-Hemoglobin Analyzer.

(Courtesy of HemoCue, Inc., Mission Viejo, CA.)

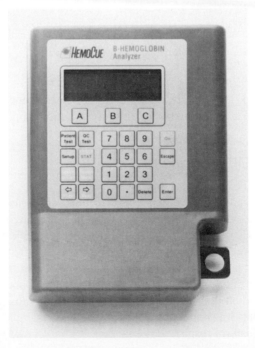

Figure 13–9.   Ichor Automated Cell Counter.

(Courtesy of Array Medical, Somerville, NJ.)

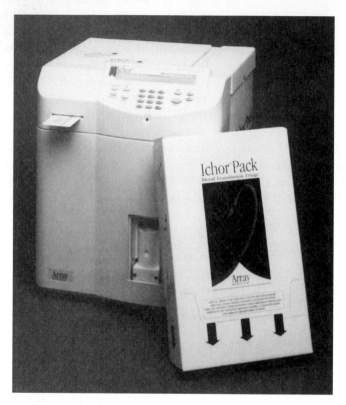

whole blood is required per analysis, the analyzer can accommodate standard, pediatric, and microsample blood collection tubes for a variety of patient populations.

■ CHOLESTEROL SCREENING

Another laboratory testing procedure that health care providers are performing through point-of-care testing is cholesterol screening. Total blood cholesterol values can be monitored with a disposable, one-step, quantitative procedure by using the AccuMeter (Chem-Trak, Inc., Sunnyvale, CA).[7] Its measurement is from finger stick whole blood or venous heparinized whole blood. This analytic system is somewhat different from other patient-focused testing systems in that it uses no instrumentation. Thus, preventive maintenance, calibration, and function checks are not necessary. After blood application, however, a visual evaluation of the colored bar height of the cholesterol reaction must occur in good lighting for accurate results. Also, it is imperative to have a sufficient sample size of 40 μL or more to obtain accurate cholesterol results.

The Accu-Chek Instant Plus (Boehringer Mannheim Corp., Indianapolis, IN) monitors both cholesterol and glucose. It uses test strips that provide cholesterol results via the monitor in 3 minutes and glucose results in 12 seconds using a finger stick drop of blood.

■ FUTURE TRENDS

More point-of-care testing procedures are evolving that will inevitably involve phlebotomists, nurses, patient care technicians, and others who are providing care at the hospital bedside, nursing home, and/or home. For each new procedure, the health care worker must make a point of learning in detail the blood collection requirements, preventive maintenance, quality control, and calibration requirements in order to provide accurate test results.

SELF STUDY

KEY TERMS

Blood Gas Analysis

Diabetes Mellitus

Insulin

Ketoacidosis

Parkinson's Disease

Patient-Focused Testing

Point-of-Care Testing

Troponin T

Quality Control Material

STUDY QUESTIONS

For the following, choose the *one* best answer:

1. Insulin is released into the bloodstream in which of these circumstances?
   a. blood cholesterol levels decrease
   b. blood glucose levels decrease
   c. blood glucose levels increase
   d. blood cholesterol levels increase

2. Diabetes mellitus is caused by the inability of the pancreas to make or to use which substance?
   a. glucose
   b. cholesterol
   c. sodium
   d. insulin

3. In which of the following organs is insulin produced?
   a. gallbladder
   b. pancreas
   c. liver
   d. kidney

4. What is the next step after the skin is punctured to obtain blood for glucose monitoring?
   a. use the first drop of blood for the glucose test
   b. use an alcohol pad to remove the first drop of blood
   c. use a dry, sterile gauze pad to remove the first drop of blood
   d. squeeze the patient's finger to make a big first drop of blood for the monitor

5. What should the blood collector do prior to using reagent strips and/or controls in point-of-care testing?
   a. check the date when the bottle was opened
   b. check the expiration date
   c. verify that they were stored at the appropriate temperature
   d. all of the above

6. How can a phlebotomist increase the blood flow from the skin puncture site for patient testing?

   a. squeeze the punctured finger
   b. massage the area
   c. puncture another site adjacent to the first puncture site
   d. none of the above

7. What do blood gas analyses measure?

   a. Na^+ and K^+
   b. pCO_2, pO_2, and pH
   c. Cl^- and HCO_3^-
   d. pCO_2, Na^+, and Cl^-

8. Which tests are measured through blood coagulation monitoring by point-of-care testing?

   a. PT and APTT
   b. PT and pCO_2
   c. pO_2 and pCO_2
   d. PT, APTT, and pH

9. Which of the following is a blood glucose monitor?

   a. One Touch Profile (Life Scan, Mountain View, CA)
   b. i-STAT (i-STAT Corporation, Princeton, NJ)
   c. AccuMeter
   d. AccuMonitor

10. Which tests can be measured by electrolyte monitoring through point-of-care testing?

   a. Na^+, K^+, PT, and APTT
   b. Pco_2, Po_2, and Na^+
   c. Na^+, K^+, Cl^-, and HCO_3^-
   d. Pco_2, Cl^-, HCO_3^-, and Po_2

References

1. Tsai WW, Nash DB, Last JV: Point-of-care testing: barriers and facilitators to implementation. *Clin Lab News.* 1994; October: 14.

2. Faulkner WR, Meites M: *Geriatric Clinical Chemistry: Reference Values.* Washington, DC: AACC Press; 1994.

3. National Committee for Clinical Laboratory Standards (NCCLS). *Blood Glucose Testing in Settings Without Laboratory Support; Proposed Guideline.* NCCLS Document AST4-P. Villanova, PA: NCCLS; 1996.

4. National Committee for Clinical Laboratory Standards (NCCLS). *Ancillary (Bedside) Blood Glucose Testing in Acute and Chronic Care Facilities (Tentative Guidelines).* NCCLS Document C30-T. Villanova, PA: NCCLS; 1994.

5. Joint Commission for Accreditation of Healthcare Organizations (JCAHO). *Accreditation Manual for Pathology and Clinical Laboratory Services.* Oakbrook Terrace, IL: JCAHO; 1993.

6. Despotis GJ, Sontoro SA, Spritznagel E, et al: Prospective evaluation and clinical utility of on-site monitoring of coagulation in patients undergoing cardiac operation. *J Thorac Cardiovasc Surg.* 1994;107(1):271–279.

7. Allen MP, DeLizza A, Ramel U, et al: A noninstrumental quantitative test system and its application for determining cholesterol concentration in whole blood. *Clin Chem.* 1990;36:1591–1597.

14

FOURTEEN

■

Urinalysis and Body Fluid Collections

CHAPTER OUTLINE

CHAPTER OBJECTIVES

Upon completion of Chapter 14, the learner is responsible for the following:

1. Identify the types of body fluid specimens, other than blood, that are analyzed in the clinical laboratory, and the correct procedures for collecting and/or transporting these specimens to the laboratory.

2. Identify the various types of specimens collected for microbiological, throat, and nasopharyngeal cultures and the protocol that health care workers must follow when transporting these specimens.

3. List the types of patient specimens that are needed for gastric and sweat chloride analyses.

4. List three types of urine specimen collections and differentiate the uses of the urine specimens obtained from these collections.

In addition to collecting and transporting blood specimens, health care workers usually are involved in the collection and/or transportation of urine and other body fluid specimens. The health care worker should be careful when transporting body fluids because they are difficult to obtain and because the quality of the clinical laboratory test result is only as good as the specimen that is collected and transported to the testing site as quickly as possible under appropriate environmental conditions. Also, because such specimens may be biohazardous, the health care worker must adhere to universal standard precautions (see Chapter 4, Infection Control, and Chapter 5, Safety and First Aid) during collection and transportation of these specimens. Just as for blood collections, the laboratory request slip must accompany the specimen, which must be properly labeled with the patient's name, the patient's identification number, the date, the time of collection, the type of specimen, and the attending physician's name.

■ URINE COLLECTION

Routine urinalysis (UA) is one of the most frequently requested laboratory procedures because it can provide a useful indication of body health. It can be performed on a "first morning" or "random" urine specimen. Various diseases and disorders, such as those listed in Table 14–1, can be detected through a routine UA. Some of the more common types of urine specimen collections and their uses are provided in Table 14–2.

The routine UA includes a physical, chemical, and sometimes microscopic analysis of the urine sample. The physical properties include the following: color, transparency v. cloudiness, odor, and concentration as detected through a specific gravity measurement. The chemical analysis for abnormal constituents is determined by using plastic strips impregnated with color-reacting substances that test for the presence of glucose, protein, blood (red blood cells [RBCs] and hemoglobin), white blood cells (WBCs), bacteria, bilirubin,

Table 14–1.   Abnormal Urine Test Results and Associated Conditions

ABNORMAL URINE TEST RESULT	ASSOCIATED CONDITION
Presence of protein urine (proteinuria)	Kidney disease Prolonged exercise Chemical poisoning
Presence of hemoglobin in urine (indicates blood destruction)	Kidney disease Malaria Severe burns Chemical poisoning
Presence of bilirubin in urine	Liver disease Obstructive jaundice
Presence of glucose in urine (glycosuria)	Diabetes mellitus
Presence of leukocytes in urine (white blood cells)	Infection of the kidney Infection of the urinary bladder Infection of the urethra
Presence of ketone bodies in urine (ketosis)	Diabetes mellitus Starvation

Table 14–2. Types of Urine Specimen Collections and Their Uses

SPECIMEN TYPE	REASON FOR COLLECTION	USE
Random	This type of specimen is most convenient to obtain.	Routine urinalysis (UA) Quantitative and qualitative
First urine of the morning	This urine excretion is the most concentrated.	Protein, nitrite, microscopic analysis Routine urinalysis (UA)
Fasting	Metabolic abnormalities are suspected.	Glucose level determinations for diabetes mellitus testing
Clean-catch midstream	The specimen is free of contamination.	Culture for bacteria and/or microscopic analysis
Timed (e.g., 2 hour, 4 hour, 24 hour)	The excretion rate of the analyte can be determined.	Creatinine clearance test, urobilinogen determinations, hormone studies
Tolerance test	Timed blood and urine specimens are obtained to detect metabolic abnormalities.	Glucose tolerance test (GTT) and other tolerance tests

and other constituents. The plastic strip, which has a separate reagent pad for each chemical test, is dipped into the urine briefly. The color of each reagent pad is compared to a color chart usually shown on the outer label of the reagent strip container. The results are reported according to the reagent label specifications (e.g., trace, $1+$, $2+$, and so on for a positive result, or negative when no reaction occurs). The strip is discarded after it is used one time. The urine may also be viewed microscopically for the presence of blood cells, bacteria and other pathogenic microorganisms, crystals, and casts.

Other tests that can be performed on urine specimens are the pregnancy, myoglobin, and porphyrin tests. Urine is also the specimen of choice for drug abuse testing. Other laboratory procedures associated with the urinary system include the **creatinine clearance test** to determine the ability of the kidneys to remove creatinine from the blood and the **blood urea nitrogen (BUN) test** to measure the amount of urea in the blood.

PREGNANCY TEST

Human chorionic gonadotropin (HCG) is the first detectable analyte produced in pregnancy. Thus, its determination in the urine or serum is the basis of pregnancy tests. HCG is a hormone produced by the placental cells beginning approximately 10 days after conception (implantation of the ovum).

The urinary excretion of HCG peaks during the first trimester of pregnancy at approximately 10 weeks. Several types of assays are used to determine urinary HCG levels. An example of a frequently used enzyme immunoassay for HCG is the Hybritech Icon II HCG urine assay (Hybritech, Inc., San Diego, CA). The procedure for this assay follows:

1. Obtain a **random urine sample** from the patient. If possible, use the first urine specimen of the morning because it has the highest concentration of HCG.
2. Drop five drops of patient's urine onto the center of the Icon II HCG membrane, allowing each drop to absorb into the membrane before adding the next.

3. Drop three drops of the antibody–enzyme conjugate reagent (bottle A) in rapid sequence onto the Icon II membrane so that the reagent covers the entire surface.
4. Wait 1 minute.
5. Dispense wash solution (buffer in kit) by directing flow toward the inner wall of the test cylinder. Fill the cylinder to the fill line and wait for drainage of the wash solution before proceeding.
6. Dispense three drops of the substrate reagent (bottle B) in rapid sequence onto the membrane so that the reagent covers the entire surface of the membrane.
7. Wait 2 minutes.
8. Stop the reaction by filling the cylinder to the fill line with wash solution.
9. With the indicator mark facing the user, observe the color development at the test zone and the positive reference zone. Formation of a circular blue dot in the test area confirms the presence of HCG. A built-in negative control indicates when a test result is invalid because of interfering substances.

Pregnancy tests are performed not only because of inquiry regarding pregnancy, but also for other medical reasons. Some of these reasons include the following:

- Certain surgical and diagnostic procedures (e.g., x-rays, colon surgery) are postponed or reconsidered if the patient is pregnant.
- Genetic counseling and/or plans to investigate, through cytogenetic and genetic studies, the possibility of any familial defects in the infant that may occur if the pregnancy test is positive.
- The HCG level is elevated in the urine of persons having various types of neoplasms and tumors (e.g., lung carcinoma).

SINGLE-SPECIMEN COLLECTION

The preferred urine specimen for most analyses is the first voided urine of the morning, when urine is the most concentrated. The urine collection containers must be clean and dry prior to the collection process. For routine UA procedures, appropriate containers include plastic disposable cups or bags (for infants) with a capacity of 50 mL. The containers must be properly labeled, free of interfering chemicals, able to be tightly capped, and leakproof. The specimen should be transported to the UA section promptly for analysis within 2 hours after the patient voids. If transportation or analysis cannot occur within this time period, the urine should be refrigerated.

Another type of single-specimen urine test is the urine **culture and sensitivity (C&S).** This specimen requires a **clean-catch midstream** urine collection. The patient is instructed to void approximately one half of the urine into the toilet, a portion is collected in a readily available sterile container (Fig. 14–1), and the rest is allowed to pass into the toilet.[1]

If asked, "What is a *clean-catch urine specimen?*," the procedure should be described, stating that this type of specimen is used to detect the presence or absence of infecting organisms. The specimen must be free of contaminating matter that may be present on the external genital areas. Thus, the steps in Box 14–1 should be explained to a female patient who is to obtain a clean-catch midstream urine specimen.

Figure 14–1.   Midstream urine collection catch kits.

(Courtesy of Evergreen Scientific, Los Angeles, CA.)

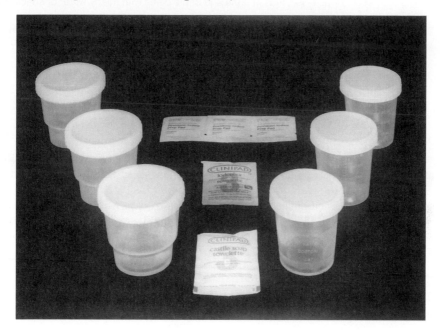

For a male patient, the procedure in Box 14–2 should be adhered to for obtaining a clean-catch midstream urine specimen.[2]

The urine specimen must be transported to the microbiology section promptly. If it cannot be taken to the area for microbiological culturing within 1 hour of collection, the specimen should be refrigerated to prevent an overgrowth of contaminate bacteria. Figure 14–2 provides examples of various types of urine collection containers for culture or urinalysis.

BOX 14–1.   CLEAN-CATCH MIDSTREAM URINE COLLECTION INSTRUCTIONS FOR WOMEN

1. After washing her hands, the woman should separate the skin folds around the urinary opening and clean this area with mild antiseptic soap and water or special towelettes.

2. Holding the skin folds apart with one hand and after urinating into the toilet, the patient should urinate into a sterile container. The container should not touch the genital area. It must be covered with the lid provided after urination. It is extremely important not to touch the inside or lip of the container with the hands or other parts of the body.

3. The health care worker or sometimes the patient will label the container with her name and the time of collection and deliver it to the requested location.

4. Health care personnel should refrigerate the urine specimen immediately.

BOX 14–2.   CLEAN-CATCH MIDSTREAM URINE COLLECTION INSTRUCTIONS FOR MEN

1. The man should wash his hands and the end of his penis with soapy water or special tow-elettes and then let dry.
2. After allowing some urine to pass into the toilet, the patient should collect the urine in the sterile container. The container should not touch the penis. Steps 3 and 4 are the same as those for a woman.

TIMED COLLECTIONS

For some laboratory assays, such as the creatinine clearance test, urobilinogen determinations, and hormone studies, 24-hour (or other timed period) urine specimens must be obtained. Incorrect collection and improper preservation of this type of specimen are two frequent errors affecting timed collections. Thus, the health care worker should be aware of the protocol for collecting a 24-hour urine specimen so that he or she can assist other health care professionals and the patient in preventing collection errors. The steps in Box 14–3 should be followed for a 24-hour urine collection.[3]

Figure 14–2.   Urine collection containers.

(Courtesy of Bio-Medical Products Corp., Mendham, NJ.)

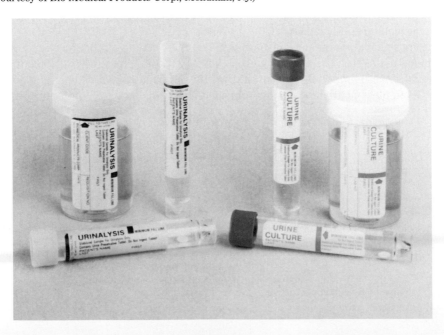

BOX 14–3.   INSTRUCTIONS FOR A 24-HOUR URINE COLLECTION

1. The patient should be given a chemically clean, wide-mouthed, 3- to 4-L container with a tight-fitting lid. The laboratory personnel should add any required preservatives to the container prior to giving it to the patient. Patients should not be allowed to submit urine specimens in their own jars because the jars might not be chemically clean and would not contain the required preservatives. The preservative and any associated precautions should be written on the collection container label. The label should be placed on the container, not on the lid. Other information on the label should include the following:

   - Patient's name.
   - Patient's identification number.
   - Starting collection date and time.
   - Ending collection date and time.
   - Name of the requested laboratory test.

   Other information that may be required by the facility includes

   - Physician's name.
   - Patient's location (e.g., hospital room, outpatient).

2. The patient should be instructed verbally that the collection of the 24-hour urine specimen begins with emptying the bladder and discarding the first urine passed. This first step in the collection process should start between 6 and 8 AM, and the exact time should be written on the container label.

3. Except for the first urine discarded, all urine should be collected during the next 24-hour period. The patient should be reminded to urinate at the end of the collection period and to include this urine in the 24-hour collection. The patient should be told to urinate before having a bowel movement because fecal material in the urine specimen will make the specimen unacceptable for collection.

4. Because urine is an ideal culture medium for microorganisms that decompose chemical constituents, the patient should be instructed to refrigerate the entire specimen after adding each collection during the 24-hour period, except for urate testing.

5. Some preservatives for 24-hour urine collection are corrosive if accidentally spilled or if the patient comes in contact with them during collection. Thus, the patient should be warned of any preservatives in the container.

6. The patient should be informed not to add anything except urine to the container and not to discard any urine during the collection period.

7. A normal intake of fluids during the collection period is desirable unless otherwise indicated by the physician.

8. Some laboratory assays require special dietary restrictions; these instructions should be given to the patient.

9. If possible, medications should be discontinued for 48 to 72 hours preceding the urine collection as a precaution against interference in the laboratory assays.

10. The 24-hour urine specimen should be transported to the clinical laboratory as soon as possible. The specimen should be placed in an insulated bag or a portable cooler to maintain the cool temperature.

11. Following the verbal instructions for the 24-hour urine collection, the patient should be provided with written instructions (non–English speaking patients should receive instructions in their native language) as a reminder.

TOLERANCE TESTS

The glucose tolerance test (GTT) (see Chapter 12 for detailed steps) requires individual urine specimens collected serially at times that correlate with the timing of the blood specimens (i.e., fasting, 30 minutes, 60 minutes). The diagnosis and treatment regimen depend on the interpretation of the timed specimens. Thus, specimens must be collected according to the schedule established for the patient. Each specimen must be labeled appropriately, including the time of collection and the specimen type (i.e., fasting, 30-minute collection). This protocol also applies to other tolerance tests.

■ CEREBROSPINAL FLUID

Cerebrospinal fluid (CSF) is obtained by a physician through a spinal tap or lumbar puncture. The fluid is usually collected in three sterile containers numbered in the order in which they were collected. The first tube is usually contaminated with blood. Thus, the second and third tubes are usually used for analysis. Tests commonly performed on CSF include total protein level, glucose level, cell count, microbiological, chloride level, and cryptococcal antigen determinations. CSF must be transported at room temperature immediately to the clinical laboratory for stat analysis. Transportation can occur to a reference laboratory if the CSF is maintained in an ice slurry,[4] however, it should not be frozen.

■ FECAL SPECIMENS

Stool (fecal) specimens are commonly collected in order to detect parasites (e.g., **ova and parasites [O&P]**), enteric disease organisms (e.g., *Salmonella, Shigella, Staphylococcus aureus*), and viruses. The specimen is collected in a wide-mouthed plastic or waxed cardboard container with a tight fitting lid. If the patient is to collect the stool specimen at home, he or she should be given a collecting container and instructed to avoid urinating in the container because urine can kill the microorganisms in the collected stool specimen. For children, the container can be placed under the toilet seat so that the child can sit on the toilet. The patient should be instructed to wash the outside of the specimen container after collection and to wash his or her hands thoroughly. The specimen container must be properly sealed to prevent leakage and contamination because fecal material from patients with infectious intestinal diseases is extremely hazardous. The specimen must be transported to the laboratory immediately and maintained at body temperature (37°C) for detection of parasitic infections.

In addition to the collection of stool specimens for microorganism detection, feces are collected to detect invisible (occult) quantities of blood that do not alter the appearance of the stool. Laboratory determination of **occult blood** assists in the confirmation of the presence of blood in black stools and can be helpful in detecting gastrointestinal (GI) tract lesions and colorectal cancer. Feces for occult blood tests are often collected by the patient using special test cards, such as Hematest (Bayer Corp., Tarrytown, NY). The cards can be mailed or brought to the health care facility after collection. Manufacturers have also developed occult blood tests that can be performed at home without collecting a stool specimen. A chemically impregnated pad is dropped into the toilet by the patient after he or she has a bowel movement. The patient watches for a color change that he or she reports to the physician via a special test result card supplied with each patient kit. The health care workers involved in specimen collection and transportation should be aware of the procedural steps for these occult blood tests to instruct the patient for proper collections.[5]

■ SEMINAL FLUID

Semen is examined in the clinical laboratory to (1) determine the effectiveness of vasectomy, (2) investigate the possibility of sexual criminal charges, and (3) assess fertility. Before collection of a semen specimen, the patient should be given clear instructions for proper specimen collection. Semen must be collected in containers that are clean and free of trace detergents. Condoms can be used but must be washed free of spermicidal substances prior to use. Specimens must not be exposed to extremes of temperature or light prior to being submitted to the clinical laboratory and should be transported within 2 hours of collection.

■ AMNIOTIC FLUID

Fluid that bathes the fetus within the amniotic sac is called **amniotic fluid.** It may be collected by a physician when the pregnant patient is at approximately 16 weeks' gestation so that fetal abnormalities can be detected through chromosomal analysis and chemical tests, such as the alpha-fetoprotein (AFP) assay. Occasionally, amniotic fluid is obtained in the last trimester of pregnancy to determine the lung maturity of the fetus. When transporting amniotic fluid to the laboratory, the specimen must be protected from light and transported immediately.

■ OTHER BODY FLUIDS

In addition to the fluids just discussed, other types of body fluids that sometimes must be transported to the laboratory include **synovial fluid,** which is extracted aseptically from joint cavities, and fluid aspirated from body cavities (e.g., **pleural fluid** obtained from the lung cavity, **pericardial fluid** from the heart cavity, **peritoneal fluid** from the abdominal cavity).

Upon receiving any type of body fluid for transportation, it is important to verify that the container is properly labeled with the patient's name, the patient's identification number, the date, the time of collection, and the type of body fluid collected.[5]

■ CULTURE SPECIMENS

Other specimens that the health care worker may be requested to transport to the clinical laboratory include **sputum** (fluid from the lungs containing pus), throat and sinus drainage cultures, wound cultures, ear or eye cultures, and skin cultures. The health care worker should be extremely careful while transporting each type of specimen because the specimens can easily become contaminated and may be biohazardous. For safety, the health care worker needs to wear gloves when handling and transporting these specimens in their containers.

■ OTHER NONBLOOD PROCEDURES

THROAT AND NASOPHARYNGEAL CULTURE COLLECTIONS

Nasopharyngeal cultures are often performed to detect carrier states of *Neisseria meningitidis, Corynebacterium diphtheriae, Streptococcus pyogenes, Haemophilus influenzae,* and *Staphylococcus aureus.* For infants and children, from whom significant sputum cultures are difficult to obtain, nasopharyngeal cultures may be used to diagnose whooping cough, croup, and pneumonia. Throat cultures are most commonly obtained to determine the presence of streptococcal infections. Because coughing may force organisms from the lower respiratory tract into the nasopharynx, it may be best to perform a throat culture on a child or an infant and stimulate coughing in order to obtain a more significant nasopharyngeal culture. Health care workers should be thoroughly taught the correct procedures before they are allowed to acquire specimens from patients.

When a throat culture is ordered, the patient should be instructed to open the mouth wide, as if to yawn. A light source should be directed into the mouth and throat so that areas of inflammation, ulceration, exudation, or capsule formation can be readily seen. A tongue blade or spoon is used to depress the tongue and to prevent contamination with organisms from the oral cavity. A sterile cotton swab should be used to brush both tonsillar areas, the posterior pharynx, and all other areas of possible infection.[6]

The swab can then be placed in a special transport medium or the fluid on the swab can be inoculated directly onto agar in a Petri dish by rolling the swab across a small area of the medium. The specimen can then be transported to the laboratory, where it may be spread out, or "streaked," for distribution of the microorganisms. A Gram-stained smear is often useful to provide preliminary indications of infection and should be made with the swab by rolling it across a sterile slide before placing it in a transport medium or inoculating plate agar. The slide, the swab, and any inoculating media should be taken to the laboratory and processed as soon as possible after collection. The culture should be placed under optimal growth conditions for suspected pathogens (i.e., the culture should be incubated). Timely processing of the specimen helps prevent overgrowth of normal flora, which can inhibit or mask any pathogenic organisms present.

Nasopharyngeal specimens should be obtained with a Dacron- or cotton-tipped flexible wire that can be easily sterilized prior to use. Commercially packaged sterilized swabs are also available. The swab is passed gently through the nose and into the nasopharynx, where it is rotated. Then, the swab is carefully removed and placed in a transport medium or the fluid on the swab is inoculated onto a medium for isolation. Again, the timely processing of all specimens is crucial for best results.

SKIN TESTS

On occasion, a nurse or other health care worker may be asked to perform a **skin test.** The health care worker should check the policies of the health care facility prior to performing the procedure. Skin tests are simple and relatively inexpensive. They determine whether a patient has ever had contact with a particular antigen and has produced antibodies to that antigen. A wide range of disease states stimulate antibody responses in individuals. Tests range from detection of ragweed and milk allergies in hypersensitive individuals, to detection of tuberculosis (TB) and fungal infections in persons who have had contact with these organisms.

The TB skin test can be administered using an automatic device or by pulling 0.1 mL of diluted antigen into a tuberculin syringe. All air bubbles should be expelled by holding the syringe vertically and tapping the sides of the barrel. The volar surface of the patient's forearm should be cleaned with alcohol and prepared in the same manner as for a venipuncture (see Chapter 8). The area should be devoid of scars, skin eruptions, and excessive hair. Holding the syringe at a slight angle (approximately 20 degrees), the needle should be slipped just under the skin. The plunger should be pulled back to ensure that a blood vessel has not been entered. The fluid may be slowly expelled into the site. The needle should be promptly removed, and only slight pressure applied, with gauze, over the site. Care should be taken that the fluid does not leak onto the gauze or run out of the injection site. The patient should hold the arm in an extended position until the site has time to close and retain the fluid. A bandage should not be used over the site because it may absorb some of the fluid and distort the results of the skin test by causing skin irritation from the adhesive.

The patient should report any reaction, no matter how slight, to the physician. Also, a return visit for proper interpretation of the skin reaction should be scheduled with the physician. At some health care agencies, the patient is asked to note the exact size of the reaction site or to compare their reaction with pictures on a prelabeled card that can be mailed back to the institution. When this is the case, patients should be fully informed about how to read positive and negative reactions.

GASTRIC ANALYSIS AND HOLLANDER TEST

Gastric analysis and the **Hollander test** both involve gastric (stomach) fluid to determine gastric function in terms of stomach acid production. The gastric analysis measures gastric acid secretion in response to stimulation from histamine or pentagastrin, whereas the Hollander test uses insulin to stimulate gastric secretions. Both tests involve passing a tube through the patient's nose and into the stomach. Both tests also require intravenous (IV) administration of the stimulant. The health care worker may be asked to assist and collect specimens as required. The responsibility for properly intubating the patient (using fluoroscopic examination) and administering the stimulant intravenously usually rest with the physician or the nurse. The health care worker can be present to assist in patient care and to draw any required blood specimens, but under *no* circumstances should be expected to carry out the procedure unless properly trained. Improper placement of the tube poses a high risk to the patient and could result in a punctured lung if the tube enters the bronchial system instead of the esophagus. The health care worker can and should be responsible for proper labeling of gastric and blood samples when he or she is present and assisting during the procedure.

SWEAT CHLORIDE BY IONTOPHORESIS

The **sweat chloride test** is used in the diagnosis of cystic fibrosis.[7,8] Cystic fibrosis is a disorder of the exocrine glands, generally thought to be enzymatic in nature, that causes changes in mucus-producing glands in the body. Primarily affected are the lungs, upper respiratory tract, liver, and pancreas. Patients with cystic fibrosis produce chloride in their sweat at two to five times the level produced by healthy individuals.

For the laboratory evaluation, pilocarpine hydrochloric acid (HCl) is iontophoresed into the skin of the patient to stimulate sweat production. The sweat is absorbed onto preweighed gauze pads, then the weight of the sweat is determined. The pad is then diluted with deionized water, and the chloride is generally read by titration with a chloridometer.

When a health care provider receives an order to perform a sweat chloride test on a patient, he or she should properly prepare for the procedure under the supervision of a medical technologist. Four cups and lids should be preweighed with two 2-in. square gauze pads in each cup. Only two cups are normally used, but the other two can be used as backups, if needed.

Choosing a site with the largest surface area (in children and infants, the leg is best suited), the health care worker should wipe the surface of the skin with a gauze pad soaked in deionized water. Next, the area is wiped dry. Another 2-in. square, eight-ply gauze pad is soaked in 0.07 moles/liter sodium bicarbonate and placed on the cleaned area. The negative electrode is placed on the gauze and taped securely to the skin. The electrode should not come into direct contact with the skin at any time when the current is on.

Another gauze square is soaked in 0.33 percent pilocarpine HCl and placed on the skin next to the sodium bicarbonate square but not touching it. The positive electrode should be placed on this piece of gauze and taped securely in place. Again, care should be taken that the electrode does not come into direct contact with the skin at any time during the procedure. Before the current is turned on, the area between and around the secured gauze squares should be wiped dry.

Next, the current is turned on and very slowly increased to 1 mA. The current must be incremented slowly because a sudden increase may electrically shock the patient. After 10 minutes, the current is decreased to zero. The switch is turned off and the electrodes and gauze squares are removed and discarded. Reagent-grade water is used to wipe off the pilocarpine HCl area, which is then wiped dry.

A 2 × 2-in. square of thin waxed film, such as Parafilm, should be cut out and handled with clean forceps. Using the forceps, the film can be placed against the cleaned area and taped securely onto the skin on adjacent sides. Still using the forceps, two gauze pads from a preweighed cup are removed and placed between the Parafilm and the skin. The remaining side can be taped securely. Tape may also be applied across the top of the Parafilm to prevent it from tearing. A timer should be started for 1 hour. During that period, the procedure should be repeated on the other arm or leg.

After 1 hour, the tape should be carefully removed, and the gauze sponges removed with forceps and returned to the original cup. The lid must be placed tightly on the cup and the cup weighed again. After weighing, 200 μL of deionized water should be added to the cup. The lid should be replaced and wrapped securely with Parafilm. The gauze sponges should equilibrate 2 to 3 hours or overnight. The cups and a record of the weights measured during the procedure should be taken to the laboratory, where a clinical laboratory scientist will determine the chloride and calculate the results.

SELF STUDY

KEY TERMS

Amniotic Fluid
Blood Urea Nitrogen (BUN)
Cerebrospinal Fluid (CSF)
Clean-Catch Midstream
Creatinine Clearance Test
Culture and Sensitivity (C&S)
Gastric Analysis
Hollander Test
Occult Blood

Ova and Parasites (O&P)
Pericardial Fluid
Peritoneal Fluid
Pleural Fluid
Random Urine Sample
Skin Test
Sputum
Sweat Chloride Test
Synovial Fluid

STUDY QUESTIONS

For the following, choose the *one* best answer:

1. What type of urine specimen is needed to detect an infection?

   a. random
   b. clean catch
   c. routine
   d. 24 hour

2. Which of the following types of specimens is most frequently collected for analysis?

   a. amniotic fluid
   b. urine
   c. CSF
   d. pericardial fluid

3. Which of the following body fluids is extracted from joint cavities?

   a. pleural fluid
   b. peritoneal fluid
   c. synovial fluid
   d. pericardial fluid

4. The O&P analysis is requested on what type of specimen?

   a. CSF
   b. amniotic fluid
   c. fecal
   d. synovial fluid

5. Fetal abnormalities are detected through analysis of which fluid?

   a. pleural
   b. peritoneal
   c. amniotic
   d. CSF

6. The occult blood analysis is frequently requested on what type of specimen?

   a. CSF
   b. fecal
   c. throat culture
   d. seminal fluid

7. Ketosis is frequently detected with which of the following conditions?

   a. liver disease
                 c. chemical poisoning

   b. diabetes mellitus
            d. infection

8. Which of the following body fluids is obtained from the abdominal cavity?

   a. synovial fluid
            c. peritoneal fluid

   b. pericardial fluid
          d. CSF

9. Which of the following can be used in children and infants to diagnose whooping cough?

   a. CSF culture
            c. amniotic fluid culture

   b. nasopharyngeal culture
      d. pericardial fluid culture

10. What is the specimen of choice for drug abuse testing?

   a. CSF
                c. synovial fluid

   b. urine
              d. gastric fluid

References

1. Garza D. Urine collection and preservation. In: Ross DL, Neely AE, eds. *Textbook of Urinalysis and Body Fluids.* New York: Appleton-Century-Crofts; 1983, p 61.

2. Free AH, Free HM. *Urinalysis in Clinical Laboratory Practice.* Cleveland: CRC Press; 1975.

3. National Committee for Clinical Laboratory Standards (NCCLS). *Routine Urinalysis and Collection, Transportation, and Preservation of Urine Specimens.* NCCLS Document GP16-T. Villanova, PA: NCCLS; December 1992.

4. Guder WG, Narayanan S, Wisser H, Zawta B. *Samples: From the Patient to the Laboratory.* Darmstadt, Germany: Git Verlag Pub.; 1996.

5. Jacobs ES, Horvat R, Demott W et al., eds. *Laboratory Test Handbook.* 4th ed. Cleveland: Lexi-Comp Inc.; 1996.

6. Becan-McBride K, Ross D. *Essentials for the Small Laboratory and Physician's Office.* Chicago: Mosby-Year Book; 1988.

7. National Committee for Clinical Laboratory Standards (NCCLS). *Sweat Testing: Sample Collection and Quantitative Analysis.* NCCLS Document C34-A. Wayne, PA: NCCLS; 1994.

8. *Clinical Practice Guidelines for Cystic Fibrosis.* Bethesda, MD: Cystic Fibrosis Foundation; 1997.

FIFTEEN

Specimen Collection for Forensic Toxicology, Workplace Testing, Sports Medicine, and Related Areas

CHAPTER OUTLINE

CHAPTER OBJECTIVES

Upon completion of Chapter 15, the learner is responsible for the following:

1. Define *toxicology* and *forensic toxicology*.

2. Give five examples of specimens that can be used for forensic analysis.

3. Describe the role of the health care worker or "collector" in federal drug testing programs.

4. List security measures and minimum site requirements for urine collection for federal drug testing programs.

5. Describe the function of a chain-of-custody, and the Custody and Control Form.

6. List the basic steps in specimen collection for urine drug tests and blood alcohol levels.

■ OVERVIEW AND PREVALENCE OF DRUG USE

The use of alcohol, tobacco, and **illicit drugs** (illegal drugs including opiates, cocaine, amphetamines, etc.) has been declining in recent years; however, a significant percentage of the U.S. population uses at least one of these substances. Alcohol is the most commonly used substance. In a 1992 survey, approximately 48 percent had consumed alcohol in the past month and approximately 11 percent acknowledged using illicit drugs in the past 12 months. Persons between the ages of 18 to 25 years are the most likely to use illicit drugs, and approximately 30 percent of high school seniors are classified as heavy users of alcohol (having five or more drinks in the previous 2 weeks). Teenagers use alcohol and tobacco more than any other drugs. They are sometimes referred to as **"gateway drugs"** because adolescents with substance abuse problems tend to begin with alcohol and cigarettes, progress to marijuana, and then move on to using other drugs or combinations of drugs.[1]

The leading cause of death among people between 15 to 24 years of age is violence, including accidents, homicides, and suicides. Often these deaths are attributed to the use of drugs and alcohol.[1]

Among pregnant women approximately 25 percent use nicotine, 5 to 8 percent are at risk for alcohol-related prenatal problems, and the prevalence of illicit drug use is undefined. Treatment of heroin addiction during pregnancy, however, is particularly important for the health of the mother and the baby. Heroin produces wide swings in blood levels, can lead to premature labor, spontaneous abortion, and other severe adverse effects. If an addicted mother is treated by methadone maintenance, pregnancy tends to increase methadone metabolism so some patients require two doses per day to maintain stable blood levels. Infants born to mothers on methadone therapy are dependent on opioids but are not addicted and are more easily treated.[1]

The development of modern screening techniques, clinical laboratory automation, molecular advances, and computer technology have increased the variety of laboratory testing options available for diagnosis and treatment of drugs of abuse and analysis of specimens in remote locations or from crime scenes. The following sections will provide basic guidelines and resources for further information.

■ FORENSIC TOXICOLOGY SPECIMENS

Toxicology is the scientific study of poisons (including drugs), how they are detected, their actions in the human body, and the treatment of the conditions they produce. **Forensic specimens** are those involved in civil or criminal legal cases. Forensic toxicology usually involves testing specimens for drugs of abuse in legal cases.

In toxicologic analysis, very small amounts of analytes are usually found in the blood, urine, or other specimens obtained for analysis. Thus, the type of specimen (e.g., venous blood, arterial blood, urine, hair), materials, and equipment used for collecting specimens for toxicologic analysis can greatly affect analytic results. The type of glass or plastic composing the collection tube, cover, or both may contain materials that will contaminate

BOX 15–1.   FORENSIC SPECIMENS

Specimens that may be used in forensic analyses[4–7]:
- Arterial blood
- Bones
- Capillary blood
- Clothing
- Dried blood stains
- Hair
- Nails
- Saliva
- Skin
- Sperm
- Sweat
- Teeth
- Urine
- Venous blood

and/or react with or absorb the analytes. Even oils or bacteria from dirty fingers that handle specimens may cause contamination. Thus, for toxicologic specimens, the health care worker must strictly adhere to the facility's laboratory guidelines for collection of these types of specimens. Extensive training, experience, and supervision are required for collecting specimens for forensic analyses. Box 15–1 includes types of specimens that may be used for forensic toxicology studies or other medical applications of a criminal investigation.

■ CHAIN-OF-CUSTODY

The chain-of-custody is a process for maintaining control and accountability of each specimen from the point of collection to final disposition of the specimen. The process documents the identity of each individual that handles the specimen and each time a specimen is transferred in the chain. A **chain-of-custody** form is also required that indicates specific identification of the patient or subject, the individual who obtained and processed the specimen, the date, the location, and the signature of the subject documenting that the specimen in the container is the one that was obtained from the person identified on the label. The specimen must be placed in a specimen transfer bag that is permanently sealed until it is opened for analysis. The seal ensures a "tamper-evident" transfer of contents until it reaches its destination for analysis.[2] Even after the specimen reaches its destination, each individual who handles every aliquot should sign and complete the chain-of-custody forms.

■ FEDERAL WORKPLACE DRUG TESTING

Workplace drug testing programs initially began in the mid-1980s when Mandatory Guidelines were published by the **Department of Health and Human Services (HHS)**. This initiative established scientific and technical guidelines for federal drug testing programs,

BOX 15–2.   FORENSIC SPECIMENS

Initial tests (using immunoassays):

- Marijuana metabolites.
- Cocaine metabolites.
- Opiate metabolites.
- Phencyclidine.
- Amphetamines.

Confirmatory tests (using gas chromatography/mass spectrometry techniques):

- Marijuana metabolite: delta-9-tetrahydrocannabinol-9-carboxylic acid.
- Cocaine metabolite: benzoylecgonine.
- Opiates: morphine and codeine.
- Phencyclidine.
- Amphetamines: amphetamine and methamphetamine.

as well as standards for certification of laboratories engaged in urine drug testing for federal agencies, such as the **Department of Transportation (DOT).** The standards relate to the testing of specimens, quality assurance and quality control, the chain-of-custody form called the **Custody and Control Form (CCF),** personnel, and results reporting. They require that each certified laboratory be inspected at least twice a year to document performance. Box 15–2 indicates the classes of drugs that the DOT requires in initial testing and confirmatory testing, and Box 15–3 indicates the format of the CCF. The Substance Abuse and Mental Health Services Administration (SAMHSA) has published a useful handbook for urine collection procedures in federal workplace drug testing programs.[3] It provides guidance to health care workers responsible for collecting urine specimens for these programs.

> The collector is the key to the success of a drug testing program and is the one individual with whom all donors will have direct, face-to-face contact. If the collector does not ensure the integrity of the specimen and adhere to the collection process, the specimen may not be considered a valid piece of evidence. If a specimen is reported positive for a drug or metabolite, the entire collection process must be able to withstand the closest scrutiny and all challenges to its integrity.[3]

■ SPORTS MEDICINE AND PRIVATE INDUSTRIES

Workplace drug testing programs have moved beyond the federal arena to sports associations, such as the National Basketball Association (NBA) and the National Football League (NFL), and major companies and industrial complexes that require drug screening for their employees. Usually, the screening is done without prior notice to the employee, therefore, the procedures for specimen collection, processing, analysis, and reporting are very strict and well defined. Companies that enforce workplace drug testing programs typically use

BOX 15–3. USE OF THE OMB-APPROVED CUSTODY AND CONTROL FORM (CCF) TO DOCUMENT THE COLLECTION OF A URINE SPECIMEN

The CCF is usually obtained from the laboratory performing the testing. The CCF consists of seven copies with the color of each copy noted in parentheses:

1. Original—must accompany specimen to laboratory (white).
2. Second original—must accompany specimen to laboratory (white).
3. Split specimen—must accompany split specimen to laboratory (white). *This is discarded for single specimen collections.*
4. Medical review officer copy (pink).
5. Donor copy (green).
6. Collector copy (yellow).
7. Employer copy (blue).

Information (steps) required on the CCF.

1. Name, address, and identification number of the employer, specific name and address of the Medical Review Officer (MRO), donor's social security number or other employee identification number, reason for the test, and tests to be performed (e.g., random, pre-employment). (See below for special considerations for identification.)
2. Record temperature measurement of the specimen as "acceptable" or "unacceptable."
3. Record the actual temperature.
4. The donor provides a daytime phone number, evening phone number, date of birth, printed name, signature, and date of collection.
5. The health care worker provides the name and address of the collection facility, collector's business phone number, printed name and signature of the collector, date of collection, time of collection, and an indication of whether the collection was a single or split specimen collection.
6. This step is used to document the transfer and handling of the specimen at the collection site. On the first line, the collector records the date and prints and signs his or her name in the column labeled "Specimen received by." The collector should complete the first line immediately after receiving the specimen from the donor. A slight delay may be necessary while the temperature is being taken (within 4 minutes).

Special Considerations for Identification of Donor.

1. The donor must be positively identified by a photo identification, an authorized agency/employer representative, or any other identification specifically allowed under the agency's drug testing plan.
2. The following are *not* acceptable: identification by a co-worker or another donor or a single, nonphoto identification card. If the donor has no photo identification, the collector must document in the "Remarks" section of the CCF that none was available. If the donor can provide two items of identification bearing his or her signature (e.g., social security card, credit card, union or other membership cards, pay vouchers, voter registration card), the collector must confirm signature identification and may proceed with the collection process. If the signature identification is unconfirmed the collection may be discontinued. The collector must include ample information in the "Remarks" to help make a determination regarding the validity of the specimen collection process.

HHS-certified reference laboratories to test their specimens. Many, however, have not required using the HHS-collection procedures. Additionally, some employers may request
that the certified laboratory test for several drugs or drug classes other than those required
by HHS. They may also use different testing levels for initial or confirmatory tests. These
differences are very important in determining whether an employer has adopted the federal
Mandatory Guidelines or not.

■ SPECIMEN COLLECTION SITES

According to federal guidelines, collection sites can be permanent or temporary facilities located at remote sites or in the workplace. The minimum site requirements are:

1. The site must allow the donor to have privacy while providing the urine specimen.
2. A source of water or moist towelettes must be available for washing hands.
3. There must be a work area for the collector.
4. The collector must be able to restrict access to the site during the collection.

Security measures should include:

1. Access should be restricted to authorized personnel only.
2. Only collection supplies/materials should be taken into the collection site.
3. Unobserved entrances/exits should be prohibited.
4. Secure handling/storage should be provided.
5. Access to water supply should be controlled by using tape to prevent opening/turn-
   ing faucet handles, or closing the shut off valve for the water supply.
6. Bluing or other color-appropriate agents must be added to any tank or toilet bowl
   that is accessible to the donor.[3]

■ SPECIMEN COLLECTION PROCEDURES

COLLECTING URINE FOR DRUG TESTING

When a site has been selected, the health care worker should assure that the appropriate
supplies are available. These are noted in Box 15–4.

The actual collection steps for a typical urine collection procedure for drug testing (noted
in Box 15–5) under the HHS Mandatory Guidelines are extensive and highly regulated. Facilities that perform these tests and health care workers responsible for collecting the specimens must be adequately trained.[3]

Without appropriate documentation and meticulous attention to the details of the procedure, a specimen can be rejected for testing or results can be invalidated. This results in
enormous losses, both financial and emotional, to the donor being tested, the agency or employer, and/or to the collector who may lose his or her job. Box 15–6 indicates documentation errors that may result in specimen rejection.

 If the specimen collector omits information, HHS recommends that laboratories retain
specimens for a minimum of 5 days to allow the collector to provide a **Memorandum for
Record (MFR),** a document that provides the appropriate correction, if possible. The laboratory should contact the collector immediately after a specimen is received to determine

BOX 15–4.   URINE COLLECTION SUPPLIES FOR DRUG TESTING[3]

The following supplies should be available to conduct proper collections:

1. Clean, single-use, wrapped or sealed specimen bottles with appropriate caps/lids.

2. Clean, single-use, wrapped or sealed collection containers for each donor to urinate into. These have wider bottle necks so they are easier to use.

3. Temperature strips that can be attached to the exterior surface of collection containers or specimen bottles to measure the temperature within 4 minutes after the donor gives the specimen bottle/container to the collector.

4. Temperature measuring devices that can be used to measure a donor's body temperature if the temperature of the specimen is outside of the mandatory range (32 to 38°C or 90 to 100°F).

5. Approved Chain-of-Custody Forms. The Office of Management and Budget (OMB) has approved Custody and Control Forms (CCFs), but they *cannot* be used by private sector companies for their workplace testing programs.

6. Tamper-evident labels/seals for the specimen bottles that have the same preprinted specimen ID number that appears on the CCF. Appropriate labels/seals are provided with each CCF.

7. Separate supply of tamper-evident seals in case the one provided does not properly adhere to the specimen container.

8. Leak-proof plastic bags in which sealed specimen containers are placed prior to shipment to the laboratory.

9. Absorbent material that is placed inside the leak-proof plastic bag in case the specimen container breaks or leaks during shipment.

10. Shipping containers/mailers that can be labeled for transporting specimens to the laboratory and that can be securely sealed to eliminate the possibility of undetected tampering.

11. Bluing or other coloring agent to add to the toilet bowl or tank to discourage adulteration/dilution of the specimen.

12. The health care worker should have appropriate identification. He or she is required to provide identification if requested by the donor. There is no requirement for the collector to have a picture ID or to provide his or her driver's license with an address. Also, the collector is not required to provide any certification or other documentation to the donor proving the collector's training in the collection process. It may benefit the health care worker to have his or her agency representative's name and telephone number to call should the donor request it.

13. Storage box, area, or place where specimens can be stored before shipment to the laboratory. It may be necessary to temporarily use a refrigerator or cabinet that can be secured. The health care worker should be within sight of the temporary storage area to ensure that no one has access to the specimens.

14. Single-use disposable gloves for use while handling specimens.

whether the collector can provide a means that would recover an error or omission in their documentation. If the collector indicates that the information can be recovered, the laboratory may test the specimen, but it may not report the results until the correction MFR is received.[3] Box 15–7 provides a sample MFR.

COLLECTING SPECIMENS FOR ALCOHOL LEVELS

Many states have provisions under which drivers suspected of being intoxicated by the arresting police officer must voluntarily give implied consent to the performance of certain laboratory assays to determine the level of blood alcohol. In some states, this statute applies

(text continues on p. 411)

BOX 15–5.   A TYPICAL URINE COLLECTION PROCEDURE FOR DRUG TESTING (FEDERAL MANDATORY GUIDELINES)[3]

The following procedure describes a typical urine collection for drug testing. Changes in the sequence of steps, errors, or omissions in some steps may result in a specimen being unacceptable for testing at the laboratory or the results being declared invalid.

1. After the collection site has been prepared and the donor identified, the collector (health care worker) should ensure that the CCF has appropriate information. The collector should request that the donor read the instructions on the CCF to ensure that he or she knows what to expect.

2. The donor should be asked to remove unnecessary clothing, such as coat, jacket, sweater, or hat, and to leave any briefcase, purse, or other personal belongings with the outer garments. The donor may retain his or her wallet.

3. The donor must *not* be asked to empty his or her pockets or to remove other articles of clothing, *nor* to remove all clothing to wear a hospital gown. If the collector, during the course of the procedure, notices unusual behavior that may indicate the donor is trying to tamper with the specimen (as evidenced by a bulging or overstuffed pocket), the collector may request that the donor empty the pockets, display the items, and explain the need for such items during the collection. This procedure may be done only when individual suspicion exists.

4. The collector should instruct the donor to wash and dry hands, preferably under observation. The donor should not be allowed any further access to water or other materials that could be used to tamper or dilute the specimen.

5. The collector gives the donor or allows the donor to choose the collection container or bottle to be used from the available supply. If the container or specimen bottle is wrapped/sealed, the collector must observe unwrapping or breaking the seal. It is recommended that the collection containers and bottles be wrapped or sealed separately.

6. For a **single-specimen collection,** only one container should be taken into the rest room. If the container is part of a prepackaged set of two, the collector should note in the "remarks" that only a single specimen was collected.

For a **split-specimen collection,** if the container and two specimen bottles are wrapped together, *only one* collection container should be taken into the rest room. The donor should not be allowed to split the specimen.

7. The donor takes the collection container into the restroom, toilet stall, or partitioned area to provide the specimen in private. The collector instructs the donor not to flush the toilet or to use any source of water. The collector should remind the donor to leave the restroom or toilet stall as quickly as possible after the donor has voided because it is required that the temperature of the specimen be determined within a few minutes. The donor is always permitted to provide a specimen in private unless a direct observed collection has been authorized.

8. The donor gives the specimen to the collector immediately upon leaving the restroom. Both collector and donor should maintain visual contact of the specimen until the label/seal is placed over the specimen bottle lid.

9. The collector performs the following checks:

   a. Checks the volume to ensure there is at least 30 mL of urine. If it is a split-sample collection, a minimum of 45 mL is required. If the volume is less than required, the collector may request a second specimen. (The donor should be given a reasonable amount of time and liquid to drink.)

   b. Reads the specimen temperature within 4 minutes of receiving the specimen and marks the section on the CCF along with recording the actual temperature. If the collector must transfer the specimen to a bottle, the temperature should be taken before the transfer. If the temperature is outside the acceptable range, a second specimen may be collected under direct observation, and both specimens are sent to the laboratory. A separate CCF for each specimen and appropriate comments should be provided. The collector should *never collect and add or combine urine* from two separate voids. Further detailed

(continued)

BOX 15–5.   (*continued*)

procedures are available in the Mandatory Guidelines for extenuating circumstances involving volume, temperature, and direct observations.

c. Inspects the specimen for unusual color, odor, or other signs of adulteration or tampering. If it is apparent that the donor has tampered with the specimen (e.g., blue dye in the specimen), the collector will collect another specimen under direct observation, and both specimens will be sent to the laboratory for testing.

10. If a collection container is used and the collector must transfer the specimen to a bottle, the lid should be placed on the bottle and the "A" seal should be affixed on it. If a split specimen is needed, the first bottle should contain 30 mL of urine and be sealed with the "A" seal, while the second bottle should contain at least 15 mL of urine and be sealed with the "B" seal. The donor should be present to observe the sealing of the specimens.

11. The collector documents the date and he or she initials the CCF labels/seals. The donor must also initial the seal. If the seal is damaged or will not adhere, a second seal should be placed perpendicular to the CCF seal to avoid obscuring information on the original seal. The second seal should also be dated and initialed by the collector and donor. Remarks should be made on the CCF form as to why a second seal was used.

Since the specimen is now sealed with tamper-evident tape, it no longer has to be in the direct observation of the donor and he or she may be allowed to wash hands.

12. The donor must then read and sign the certification statement of the CCF, provide their date of birth, printed name, and day and evening contact phone numbers. If the donor refuses to sign the form, the collector must document it.

13. The collector completes the remaining sections of the CCF.

14. The collector signs the CCF, indicating he or she has received the specimen from the donor, and prints his or her name and the date. The donor does not sign anywhere in the chain of custody block.

15. The donor may list any prescription and/or over-the-counter medications they may have taken recently on the back of their copy. The collector gives the appropriate copy to the donor who may then leave the site.

16. If the collector is going to ship the specimen immediately, he or she should complete the next line of the chain of custody by signing and printing his or her name in the "Specimen released by" section and completing the "Specimen received by" section with the name of the courier or shipping service and the date. The section "Purpose of change" should be completed by an indication such as, "shipment to lab."

17. The collector places the specimen bottle and appropriate copies of the CCF inside a leak-proof plastic bag that serves as a secondary barrier to prevent any leakage from damaging the shipping container or documents. If the collection involved a split sample, there would be an additional specimen bottle (B) and another copy of the CCF inside the leak proof plastic bag. Some bags have an outside pouch for the copies of the CCF. Bags should use the appropriate seal(s) to prevent access to the specimen and copies of the CCF. The US Postal Service and other carriers require the use of a secondary barrier that is leak-proof (such as a plastic bag containing absorbent material) when shipping potentially hazardous biologic materials.

A collector may place numerous specimens into a single-shipping container, as long as each CCF is completed with the specific carrier and in a leak-proof bag, and visual contact of each plastic bag is maintained until all are sealed in the single-shipping container.

18. The sealed leak-proof plastic bag(s) are placed in the shipping container and sealed. The shipping container should be designed to minimize damage during handling and be securely sealed to indicate any tampering during transit to the laboratory. Couriers and Postal Service employees are not required to make chain-of-custody entries on the CCF.

19. The collector sends the appropriate copy of the CCF to the Medical Review Officer and to the employer. One copy of the CCF is for the collector to retain.

20. Following the procedure, the site should be checked to ensure that the donor did not leave anything that could have been used by him or her or by the next donor to dilute or tamper with the specimen. At this point, the collector should flush the toilet and add bluing to the toilet in preparation for the next collection.

BOX 15–6.   DOCUMENTATION ERRORS ASSOCIATED WITH URINE DRUG TESTING

The following errors and omissions on the part of the collector may result in a specimen being rejected[3]:

1. The preprinted number on the custody form does not match the specimen ID number on the seal of the specimen bottle.
2. There is no specimen ID number on the seal.
3. There is an insufficient quantity of urine.
4. The seal is missing, broken, or shows evidence of tampering.
5. The specimen has been obviously tampered with (e.g., color, foreign objects, unusual odor).
6. The collector signed the certification statement but forgot to sign the line on the chain-of-custody.
7. The donor's social security number or ID number is omitted on the CCF, and the collector did not state that the "donor refused to provide information" in the "Remarks."
8. The donor's certification statement is not signed and there is no indication that the "donor refused to sign."

BOX 15–7.   SAMPLE MEMORANDUM FOR RECORD[3]

A *Memorandum For Record* is a statement prepared by an individual that provides or corrects information on any documents associated with a drug test.

(*Use appropriate letterhead*)
Memorandum For Record

Date: _____

From: _____ (*Collector's printed name*) _____

To: _____ (*Drug Testing Laboratory Name and Address*) _____

Subject: Memorandum to recover missing information

Re: Specimen ID Number
            Donor SSN or other ID Number

On (*date of collection*) I served as the collector for the above specimen. While completing the custody and control form, I inadvertently forgot to (*insert appropriate phrase that describes the issue*). I have reviewed the collection procedure and am certain that I followed all other parts of the collection procedure (*may list other parts of the procedure here*) as required.

To ensure that this omission will not happen again, I am planning to review the entire custody and control form before I separate the copies and seal the specimen bottles and the form in the leak-proof plastic bag.

_____
(*Collector's signature*)

cc: Medical Review Officer

only to the testing of urine and breath samples. Therefore, it is advisable to determine the medically acceptable manner for obtaining blood specimens from patients in each state. If blood alcohol specimens are collected by venipuncture, all procedures are similar to routine collections except that the health care worker performing the phlebotomy *must use a non-alcoholic disinfectant* to cleanse the site. If an alcohol wipe is used to cleanse the site it may interfere with test results. Correct identifications, precautions, and labeling procedures apply to these situations as well. The National Committee for Clinical Laboratory Standards (NCCLS) recently published *Blood Alcohol Testing in the Clinical Laboratory: Approved Guideline,* that provides technical and administrative guidance on laboratory procedures associated with blood alcohol testing, including specimen collection, analytic methods, quality assurance, and result reporting.[9]

■ TAMPERING WITH SPECIMENS

Sometimes the health care worker may suspect that the individual from whom a urine specimen has been collected has tampered with or substituted another specimen. Reasons for this may include that there is blue dye in the specimen, he or she may hear something unusual or smell something while the donor is providing the specimen, or actually see other evidence of tampering after the procedure. The health care worker must always seek approval to conduct another collection procedure under "direct observation." Federal guidelines are very strict about the circumstances for this measure, however, there are situations when it is required.[3]

SELF STUDY

KEY TERMS

Chain-of-Custody
Custody and Control Form (CCF)
Department of Health and Human
    Services (HHS)
Department of Transportation
    (DOT)
Forensic Specimens

Gateway Drugs
Illicit Drugs
Memorandum for Record
    (MFR)
Single-Specimen Collection
Split-Specimen Collection
Toxicology

STUDY QUESTIONS

The following questions may have *one* or *more* answers.

1. Persons in which of the following age categories are most likely to use illicit drugs?

   a. 12–17 years old
   b. 18–25
   c. 25–40
   d. 41–70

2. Specimens that can be used in forensic analysis include which of the following?

   a. hair
   b. urine
   c. blood
   d. nails

3. "Gateway drugs" include which of the following?

   a. alcohol
   b. tobacco
   c. heroin
   d. cocaine

4. Forensic specimens are those involved in which of the following?

   a. routine testing for diabetes
   b. legal cases/criminal
      investigations
   c. urine screening for
      pre-employment physicals
   d. Pap smears

5. What is the purpose of a chain-of-custody process?

   a. maintain control of the donor
      who gives the specimen
   b. maintain control and
      accountability of a specimen
      from point of collection to
      final results
   c. specimen identification
   d. provide privacy to the donor

6. Appropriate seal(s) on the specimen containers used in the chain-of-custody assures which of the following?

   a. tamper-evident
   b. privacy
   c. aliquot identification
   d. confidentiality

7. Which of the following agencies/organizations are likely to conduct drug testing programs?

   a. NFL
   b. DOT
   c. NBA
   d. international chemical company

8. Minimum requirements for a urine collection site for drug testing includes which of the following?

   a. privacy for the specimen donor
   b. water source for washing hands
   c. work area for the collector
   d. access to site must be restricted during the collection

9. Skin preparation for blood alcohol levels must be cleansed with which of the following?

   a. 70 percent ethyl alcohol
   b. iodine
   c. 70 percent isopropyl alcohol
   d. nonalcoholic disinfectants

10. Which of the following is not acceptable for positive identification of a urine donor for drug testing?

   a. a co-worker
   b. nonphoto identification card
   c. social security card
   d. driver's license

REFERENCES

1. National Institute on Drug Abuse (NIDA). *Diagnosis and Treatment of Drug Abuse in Family Practice—Epidemiology.* Web page: http//165.112.78.61/Diagnosis-Treatment/Diagnosis3html, December, 1997.

2. Bittikofer J. Toxicology. In: Bishop M, Duben-Englekirk J, Fody E, eds. *Clinical Chemistry: Principles, Procedures, Correlations.* Philadelphia; JB Lippincott; 1992.

3. Substance Abuse and Mental Health Services Administration (SAMHSA). *Urine Specimen Collection Handbook for Federal Workplace Drug Testing Programs.* US Department of Health and Human Services, DHHS Publication No. (SMA)96-3114, 1996.

4. Swan N. Sweat testing may prove useful in drug-use surveillance. *NIDA Notes.* September/October, 1995.

5. Cone EJ, Hillsgrove MJ, Jenkins AJ, et al. Sweat testing for heroin, cocaine, and metabolites. *J Analyt Toxic.* 1994;18:298–305.

6. Federal Bureau of Investigation (FBI). *DNA Evidence Extraction Procedures.* FBI DNA Testing. Website: www.fbi.gov, October, 1997.

7. Tracqui A, Kintz P, Ludes B, et al. The detection of opiate drugs in nontraditional specimens (clothing): a report of 10 cases. *J Forens Sciences.* March, 1995;40(2):263–265.

8. US Department of Transportation. Part 40: *Procedures for Transportation Workplace Drug Testing Programs*. US Government Printing Office. 49CFR40, October 1, 1997.

9. National Committee for Clinical laboratory Standards (NCCLS). *Blood Alcohol Testing in the Clinical Laboratory: Approved Guideline*. T-DM6-A. (NCCLS, 940 West Valley Road. Ste. 1400, Wayne, PA 19087-1898, (610) 688–1100) 1997.

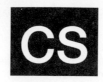

PHLEBOTOMY CASE STUDY

■

Home Care Collections

Mr. Albert A. Thomson, a 55-year-old white man, was released from Nicholson Community Hospital on March 25. He had been in the hospital for 14 days as a result of undergoing cardiac bypass surgery and experiencing some complications. On March 29, Ms. Terry Alright, a home health care phlebotomist from Nicholson Community Hospital saw that her schedule included a visit to Mr. Thomson for blood collection for the following laboratory test:

- Chemistry screen
- Protime
- CBC
- APTT
- Calcium, ionized

When she arrived at Mr. Thomson's home and began her preparations for blood collection, she noticed that Mr. Thomson had hematomas in both antecubital fossa areas of the left and right arms. Thus, she checked the right hand and found a vein that looked suitable for collecting blood with a safety winged infusion set with small blood collection vacuum tubes. She prepared the site for blood collection, and using a 23-gauge safety winged infusion needle, she inserted the needle into the vein and first collected blood in a red-speckled-topped vacuum tube, followed by a purple-topped tube, two light blue–topped tubes, and then a green-topped tube. As she collected each tube, she mixed the blood and additive in the blood collection tube. After completing the blood collection, she labeled the tubes, discarded the biohazardous blood collection items in her biohazardous disposal container, and left Mr. Thomson's home with the collected blood and her blood collection items.

She traveled next to Ms. Jennifer Smith's home to collect blood from Ms. Smith for a digoxin assay and a plasma potassium level determination. Ms. Smith, an 85-year-old African American woman, was homebound because of arthritis and a cardiac arrhythmia problem. Collecting blood from the median cubital vein in Ms. Smith's left arm, the phlebotomist used a syringe because of the fragility of the vein. After collecting 5 mL of blood in the syringe, Ms. Alright placed 2 mL of blood in a small red-speckled-topped blood collection tube and 3 mL of blood in a small purple-topped blood collection tube. She labeled the tubes, discarded the biohazard blood collection items, and left Ms. Smith's house to travel to the hospital laboratory and drop off the blood specimens.

QUESTIONS

1. For each of the following laboratory tests, what color should the top of the blood collection tube be?

Laboratory Assay	Color of Blood Collection Tube Top
Calcium, ionized	
APTT	
CBC count	
Protime	
Chemistry screen	
Digoxin	
Plasma potassium	

2. Did the home health care phlebotomist use the proper order of draw for Mr. Thomson's laboratory tests? If not, what was the proper order of draw?

3. Did the phlebotomist use the proper order to fill tubes for Ms. Smith's laboratory tests? If not, what was the proper order of draw?

Bedside Glucose Testing

A 59-year-old Hispanic woman having non–insulin diabetes mellitus tested her glucose level at home on March 14, 1998, and obtained a glucose reading of 320 mg/dL using a test strip. Because she was having symptoms of sweating, feeling bad, and feeling lightheaded, the woman went to her physician the next day. Her physician immediately hospitalized her for treatment of uncontrolled diabetes. During the hospitalization, the following glucose meter v. clinical laboratory comparisons were performed:

DATE	GLUCOSE METER RESULTS (mg/dL)	LABORATORY TEST RESULTS (mg/dL)
3/15/98	151	198
3/16/98	192	238
3/17/98 (AM)	96	267
3/17/98 (PM)	120	246

From product performance specifications, hospital personnel determined that the comparisons for March 15 and March 16 were within the acceptable product performance variation range. The last two comparisons, however, fell outside the acceptable range. The patient indicated that she followed the preventive maintenance schedule described in the documentation packaged with the glucose meter. The calibration was checked weekly, and the last calibrator reading, which was performed on March 17, was in range. A control run on March 16 resulted in a reading of 129 mg/dL, with confidence limits of 90 to 120 mg/dL.

QUESTIONS

1. What is the problem in this case study?
2. What troubleshooting technique(s) should have been implemented to resolve this problem?

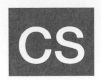

PHLEBOTOMY CASE STUDY

■

Newborn Nursery Collections

Two health care workers oversee blood collections in the newborn nursery on Saturday and Sunday of each week. On Sunday morning, the clinical laboratory scientist (CLS) overseeing the clinical chemistry section noticed that the bilirubin value for Baby McPherson was as follows:

DAY	TIME	BILIRUBIN VALUE (mg/dL)
Friday		15
Saturday	8:15 PM	12
Sunday	7:10 AM	2

Knowing that the ultraviolet light on newborn Baby McPherson could not make the bilirubin value decrease that dramatically from Saturday to Sunday, the CLS called in the health care worker who had collected the Sunday morning blood sample to ask him questions regarding the collection.

QUESTIONS

1. What type of microcollection container should have been used to collect the bilirubin sample?

2. Does taking the blood immediately to the laboratory for testing make any difference?

3. Give two reasons why the Sunday bilirubin value for Baby McPherson was so different from the values of the previous 2 days.

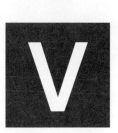

QUALITY MANAGEMENT AND LEGAL ISSUES

T HE FINAL PORTION OF THIS TEXTBOOK covers professional issues, such as assessment of the quality of services that are provided in phlebotomy practice, professional and ethical communication and management practices, and the sensitive issues of legal risk and regulatory matters.

Chapter 16, Quality, Competency, and Performance Assessment, describes the role of quality-monitoring activities in improving the practice of phlebotomy and related procedures. Specific examples are provided that demonstrate how quality-improvement tools (e.g., flowcharts, Pareto charts, cause-and-effect diagrams) can enhance services to customers, who include patients, families, physicians, nurses, and other health care professionals.

Chapter 17, Legal and Regulatory Issues, describes general legal principles, such as statutory, administrative, and judicial law, and provides definitions of legal terminology. Also covered are the following legal issues, that are particularly important to health care professionals who practice phlebotomy: confidentiality, human immunodeficiency virus (HIV) exposure, informed consent, implied consent, and legal claims. In addition, legal cases that are related to phlebotomy and laboratory practices are cited, and issues of how to manage legal risk, malpractice insurance, and protective equipment are highlighted.

16

SIXTEEN

■

Quality, Competency, and Performance Assessment

CHAPTER OUTLINE

CHAPTER OBJECTIVES

Upon completion of Chapter 16, the learner is responsible for the following:

1. Describe the importance of quality improvement and total quality management.

2. Describe the "5 Ds" in terms of negative patient outcomes.

3. Identify steps in monitoring and evaluating a specimen collection process.

4. Distinguish between quality control and quality improvement.

5. Give examples of improved patient outcomes for phlebotomy services.

Most of the credit for initiating the quality revolution in the United States goes to **Dr. W. Edwards Deming,** an American statistician who spent time in Japan and helped develop modern Japanese management theories. His work focused on minimizing variation in the manufacturing processes, such as those in the automotive industry. This is similar to a laboratory's goal of minimizing the variations in laboratory testing. Other noted quality innovators are Drs. Joseph Juran, Avedis Donabedian, Philip Crosby, and Donald M. Berwick. Dr. Donabedian, a physician, pinpointed key aspects (structure, process, outcomes) of health care functions that needed to be monitored for quality improvement. The contribution of this framework has shaped the way health care providers view quality assessments.

The Joint Commission on the Accreditation of Healthcare Organizations (JCAHO) has been instrumental in bringing quality-improvement methodologies to health care. This commission based its guidelines on Juran's model of **total quality management (TQM)** and Deming's principles of **continuous quality improvement (CQI).**[1,2] One widely used strategy for quality assessment of health care performance is the **JCAHO 10-step process** (Box 16–1). It provides a systematic process for improving health care processes and outcomes. Another commonly used strategy for quality improvement is the plan–do–check–act (PDCA) approach (Box 16–2). Both are examples of how health care organizations can use a common method to assess the quality of their services systematically.

BOX 16–1.   JCHAO 10-STEP PROCESS FOR QUALITY ASSESSMENT

1. *Assign responsibility*. The director or chairperson is responsible for monitoring and evaluating service quality. A written plan should describe responsibilities, the laboratory setting, the populations served, and the quality assessment activities.

2. *Delineate the scope of care.* All major sections of the laboratory must be covered.

3. *Identify key aspects of care.* These include high-volume procedures, high-risk procedures, problematic procedures, high-cost procedures and specific patient outcomes.

4. *Construct indicators.* Indicators should specify which activities, events, or patient outcomes will be monitored.

5. *Define thresholds of evaluation.* Thresholds specify the lower limits of acceptable quality. Exceeding them should stimulate further evaluation and problem resolution.

6. *Collect and organize data.* Two basic types of monitors should be used: scanning monitors (to provide important statistics about the laboratory's operations) and focused monitors (to collect data periodically so that the causes, nature, or scope of a problem can be determined).

7. *Evaluate data.* This includes comparing performance to standards, analyzing patterns and trends, evaluating statistical significance and clinical relevance, and analyzing causes.

8. *Develop a corrective action plan.* The plan should detail who or what is to change and what specific actions will be taken and when; it should focus on improving the system or behavior.

9. *Assess actions and document improvement.* The corrective actions must be monitored until the problem is resolved.

10. *Communicate relevant information.* Complete reports (including objectives, findings, conclusions, corrective actions, and follow-up results) must be forwarded to the appropriate officials in a timely manner.

(From Martin BG, ed. *The CLMA Guide to Managing a Clinical Laboratory.* Malvern, PA: Clinical Laboratory Management Association; 1991, with permission.)

> **BOX 16–2.**   PLAN–DO–CHECK–ACT (PDCA) CYCLE
>
> **Plan** a change.
> **Do** the improvement, data collection, and analysis.
> **Check** the results to see the effect of the change.
> **Act** on what was learned by either rejecting the change, adjusting the change, or adopting the change as a standard part of the process.

Many terms are used to convey the idea of improving the quality of services. These include *total quality management, continuous quality improvement, quality assurance,* and *integrated quality assurance,* to name a few. The current JCAHO standards include wider accountability for performance improvement. The JCAHO describes a framework of performance as follows:

> Performance is what is done and how well it is done to provide health care. The level of performance in health care is
>
> —the degree to which what is done is efficacious and appropriate for the individual patient; and
> —the degree to which it is available in a timely manner to patients who need it, effective, continuous with other care and care providers, safe, efficient, and caring and respectful of the patient.
>
> These characteristics of what is done and how it is done are called "dimensions of performance."[1]

Box 16–3 defines the JCAHO dimensions of performance. Key elements of the theorists' various approaches are briefly summarized in Table 16–1.

> **BOX 16–3.**   DEFINITIONS OF DIMENSIONS OF PERFORMANCE
>
> **I. Doing the Right Thing**
>
> The *efficacy* of the procedure or treatment in relation to the patient's condition
>   The degree to which the care of the patient has been shown to accomplish the desired or projected outcome(s)
> The *appropriateness* of a specific test, procedure, or service to meet the patient's needs
>   The degree to which the care provided is relevant to the patient's clinical needs, given the current state of knowledge
>
> **II. Doing the Right Thing Well**
>
> The *availability* of a needed test, procedure, treatment, or service to the patient who needs it
>   The degree to which appropriate care is available to meet the patient's needs
> The *timeliness* with which a needed test, procedure, treatment, or service is provided to the patient
>   The degree to which the care is provided to the patient at the most beneficial or necessary time
> The *effectiveness* with which tests, procedures, treatments, and services are provided
>   The degree to which the care is provided in the correct manner, given the current state of knowledge, to achieve the desired or projected outcome(s) for the patient
> The *continuity* of the services provided to the patient with respect to other services, practitioners, and providers, and over time

(continued)

> ## BOX 16–3. *(continued)*
>
> The degree to which the care for the patient is coordinated among practitioners, among organizations, and over time
>
> The *safety* of the patient (and others) to whom the services are provided
>
> The degree to which the risk of an intervention and the risk in the care environment are reduced for the patient and others, including the health care worker
>
> The *efficiency* with which services are provided
>
> The relationship between the outcomes (results of care) and the resources used to deliver patient care
>
> The *respect and caring* with which services are provided
>
> The degree to which the patient or a designee is involved in his or her own care decisions and to which those providing services do so with sensitivity and respect for the patient's needs, expectations, and individual differences
>
> (From Joint Commission on the Accreditation of Healthcare Organizations (JCAHO). *1995 Comprehensive Accreditation Manual for Hospitals.* Oakbrook Terrace, IL: JCAHO; 1995, with permission.)

■ TOTAL QUALITY MANAGEMENT

TQM is a process aimed at continuous quality improvement, not just meeting a minimum standard. The focus is on improving the entire process of health care so that patient outcomes are positive. It includes, but is not limited to, reducing repeat procedures, outliers, variations, or errors in all types of health care settings. And, perhaps most important, it focuses on meeting the needs of persons who are being served, or **customer satisfaction.** Customers include patients and other health care workers, such as technologists, nurses, students, pathologists, and all physicians who use or are a part of the specimen collection

Table 16-1. Summary of Theoretical Approaches to Quality Improvement

THEORIST	APPROACH
Deming	Do not tolerate poor service.
	Constantly improve production and service.
	Institute training for all workers.
	Institute effective leadership.
	Drive out fear. Create a climate of trust and innovation.
	Break down barriers between departments.
	Eliminate slogans.
	Remove barriers to pride in job performance.
	Take action.
Juran	Promote customer satisfaction.
Donabedian	Structure.
	Process.
	Outcomes.
Crosby	Zero defects.
	Strive to be error free.
Berwick	*Kaisen,* the Japanese term for "continuous search for opportunities for all processes to get better."
	Shift away from a regulatory model or seeking out the "bad apples," and move to seeking opportunities for improvement through mistakes.
	Learn from the mistakes.

> ## BOX 16–4.   THE CUSTOMERS
>
> Internal inpatients
> Outpatients
> Patients' families and friends
> Patients' support groups
> Blood donors
> Clinical laboratory scientists
> Clinical laboratory technicians
> Secretaries and clerks
> Pathologists
> Nurses
> Administrators
> Human resources personnel
> Attending physicians
> Students
> Research staff
> Research granters
> Anyone who provides financial support (e.g., insurance companies, tax-payers, foundations)

and laboratory services. Examples of customers might include a patient care aide or clerk responsible for charting a result, a patient who needs blood drawn for surgery the next morning, an anesthesiologist waiting for a stat blood gas analysis result, and a pathologist who needs to review an abnormal blood smear (Box 16–4). Even the JCAHO current accreditation guidelines recognize the need for "customer input through patient feedback."[1]

TQM is an umbrella concept that encompasses quality and performance assessment of

> ## BOX 16–5.   CHARACTERISTICS OF HOSPITALS WITH TOTAL QUALITY MANAGEMENT
>
> The six major characteristics of hospitals with successful TQM are as follows:
> 1. The organized TQM approach permeates the hospital horizontally and vertically through the organizational chart.
> 2. The objective of TQM is continuous improvement in performance and outcomes instead of meeting fixed, predetermined standards.
> 3. Work groups, teams, or quality circles include multidisciplinary individuals, preferably experts from the major groups that contribute to the process being studied. Improvements are made across departments and units.
> 4. The groups or teams are accountable to customers (patients and other members of the health care team).
> 5. The professional standards improve with time.
> 6. There is a commitment to customer satisfaction.
>
> When these six characteristics are adopted, the success of a hospital, team, service, private practice, clinic, or entire laboratory can then be measured by the rate of improvement, not just by compliance with preexisting standards.

structures, processes, outcomes, prevention, and customer satisfaction. Traditionally, clinical laboratory services have focused primarily on **quality control (QC),** or monitoring the testing process, and secondarily on quality assurance, or outcomes assessment. Box 16–5 describes TQM traits of successful hospitals. Box 16–6 defines traditional laboratory QC and CQI.[2,3]

STRUCTURE

In a TQM framework, **structure** is defined as physical or organizational properties of the settings where care is provided. Assessments of structural components include the following:

- *Physical structure.* Facilities where services are provided, adequacy of supplies, safety measures, and availability and condition of equipment, such as computers, sterilizers, refrigerators, thermometers, centrifuges, autoclaves, and glucose-monitoring devices.
- *Personnel structure.* Numbers of personnel and support staff for each service, ratios of staff to patients, qualifications of staff, and availability of the medical director or supervisors.
- *Management–administrative structure.* Updated, available procedure manuals; multidisciplinary composition of committees; adequacy of systems for record keeping; and open lines of communication throughout the organization.

Structural components in quality assessment may reveal potential problems that other assessments (process and outcome) cannot. For example, the use of outdated blood collection tubes may cause faulty laboratory test results, even though the blood collection, testing, and reporting (processes) are perfect and the treatment plan for the patient (outcome) is appropriate.

BOX 16–6.   CONTINUOUS QUALITY IMPROVEMENT AND QUALITY CONTROL—SIMILARITIES AND DIFFERENCES

Continuous Quality Improvement (CQI)

CQI is a theoretical framework and management commitment to improve health care structures, processes, outcomes, and customer satisfaction. It is ongoing and involves all levels of the administrative structure of an organization.

Quality Control (QC)

QC monitors a process. It adjusts the analytic process to meet specific standards. It includes activities, such as developing technical policies and procedures, ensuring that supplies are functional and not outdated, calibrating and maintaining equipment, and performing function checks. QC involves running QC samples in parallel with patient samples and participating in proficiency-testing programs.

PROCESS

Process is defined as what is done to the patient or client. Process assessments are common throughout the specimen collection and clinical testing arenas and include procedures and skill assessment. This is where traditional QC measures are applicable. In addition to the normal laboratory data collection routines, however, other methods are effective for monitoring processes. These include evaluation of patient records for complications, correct technical skills, and correct documentation procedures; direct observation of practices; videotaping of health care interactions and practices; patient interviews; and questionnaires.

OUTCOMES

Outcomes are what is accomplished for the patient. The ultimate goal of CQI is to improve patient outcomes. Most outcomes assessments rely on information in the patient's medical record. Chart reviews usually evaluate the health status after services are provided. Timing is usually an important component of these measures. Outcomes assessments are typically the most difficult to measure and often relate to recovery rates, cure rates, nosocomial infection rates, return to normal functions, and so on. Poor patient outcomes have been described as the "5 Ds"[4]:

- Death
- Disease
- Disability
- Discomfort
- Dissatisfaction

Unfortunately, health care workers can have negative effects in each of these categories. For example, misidentification of a patient can result in an erroneous cross-match and blood transfusion, which could be fatal to a patient (death). Inappropriate cleansing techniques or hand washing could result in transmitting nosocomial infections (disease). Poor venipuncture techniques, such as improper needle insertion or excessive probing, could result in nerve damage (disability) or severe pain (discomfort). And lengthy waiting times, rude behavior, or messy work sites can contribute to an overall feeling of patient dissatisfaction. Even though these examples are extreme, they do exist in reality and need to be improved.

Quality improvement efforts for phlebotomy services often involve evaluating the following: the health care worker's technique, complications such as hematomas, recollection rates resulting from contamination, and multiple sticks on the same patient. All these issues have the potential to result in a negative outcome for the patient. Thus, continuous improvement in minimizing these problems would be most beneficial to the patient and the health care worker.

SATISFACTION

The study of satisfaction among patients and health care workers is usually accomplished by using questionnaires, mail outs, and telephone or personal interviews. Although the information gathered by using these techniques may be subjective, knowing *why* customers are dissatisfied and *which* customers are unhappy is extremely valuable. This information can be used to improve targeted services or aspects of a service. Health care workers must remember that positive patient outcomes usually result in positively satisfied customers.

■ TOOLS AND TRENDS FOR PERFORMANCE ASSESSMENT

In a laboratory, check sheets, run charts, and statistical tests can be used to review both the analytic and nonanalytic parts of the laboratory. In an analytic sense, clinical laboratory scientists and technicians use data collection to ensure test sensitivity, specificity, precision, and accuracy. In a nonanalytic sense, data can be used to assess the timeliness of responses to requests, turnaround time for reporting test results, and effective communication. Tools for implementing CQI include the following[3]:

- **Flowcharts.** Useful for breaking a process into its components so that people can understand how it works (Fig. 16–1).
- **Pareto charts.** Bar charts that show the frequency of problematic events; the Pareto principle suggests that "80 percent of the trouble comes from 20 percent of the problems" (Fig. 16–2).
- **Cause-and-effect (Ishikawa) diagrams.** Diagrams that identify interactions between equipment, methods, people, supplies, and reagents (Fig. 16–3).

Figure 16–1.   Flowchart.

(Adapted from Martin BG, ed. *The CLMA Guide to Managing a Clinical Laboratory.* Malvern, PA: Clinical Laboratory Management Association; 1991.)

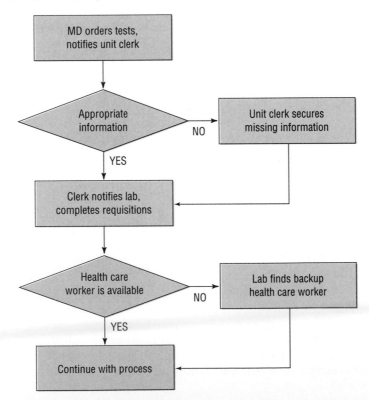

Figure 16–2.   Pareto chart.

(From Martin BG, ed. *The CLMA Guide to Managing a Clinical Laboratory.* Malvern, PA: Clinical Laboratory Management Association; 1991, with permission.)

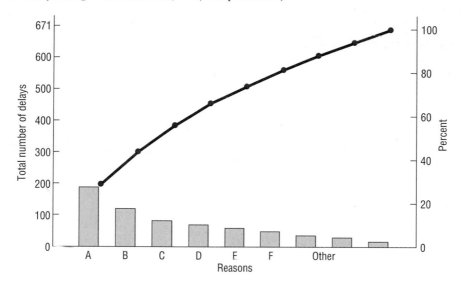

Figure 16–3.   Ishikawa diagram, ER, emergency room.

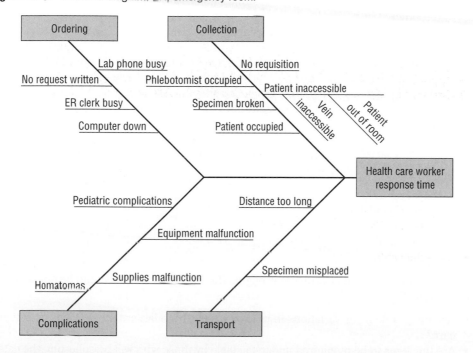

- **Line graphs, histograms, scatter diagrams.** Pictorial images representing performance trends.
- **Brainstorming.** Method used to stimulate creative solutions in a group.

Westgard and associates[4] suggest a **"5 Q" framework** for clinical laboratories that focuses on the following:

- Quality planning (QP).
- Quality laboratory practices (QLP).
- Quality control (QC) of processes.
- Monitoring performance, quality assessment.
- Quality improvement (QI) when problems occur.

This is a self-perpetuating, cyclic process that should become a way of life for all employees in the laboratory. Each health care institution has different characteristics, however, and the laboratory's quality-management program will vary based on philosophy, mission, and tools selected for use.

There are many varied strategies for assessing performance of laboratories, most of which are highly effective. The role of the individual health care worker, through his or her technical competence, however, is equally important and should also be a routine part of quality and performance assessments. Basic competencies were covered in Chapter 1, but, in addition, each health facility may have its own additional required competencies.

■ CQI FOR SPECIMEN COLLECTION SERVICES

CQI studies for specimen collection services can be very revealing for laboratory employees, supervisors, and managers. A study by Howanitz and colleagues[5] indicated that 98.6 percent of patients in a study group from numerous hospitals were satisfied with many aspects of the phlebotomy services that they received. In this group, 97.3 percent of the patients had blood collected on the first phlebotomy attempt, and 16.1 percent of the punctures resulted in ecchymosis. In 25 percent of the cases, the time required for the phlebotomy procedure was 5 minutes or less. Each of these factors, in addition to numerous others, was analyzed, and areas for targeted improvement were identified. One of the general areas cited for suggested improvement was reduction of discomfort or pain caused by the puncture. Examples of CQI assessments that should be considered in specimen collection services are listed in Box 16–7.

Monitors or indicators for quality assessment should fit specific criteria in order to be useful and valid. The **RUMBA model** is an easy check for determining the feasibility of monitoring a particular procedure or process.

- R—Relevant
- U—Understandable
- M—Measurable
- B—Behavioral
- A—Achievable

Before a study of a particular problem is begun, the RUMBA criteria should be applied. The following questions should be asked:

- Are the problems or variations in practices relevant to laboratory services or patient care?

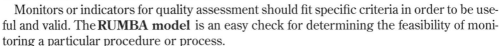

- Are the items to be monitored understandable by those who will be collecting the data?

BOX 16–7. CONTINUOUS QUALITY IMPROVEMENT ASSESSMENTS FOR SPECIMEN COLLECTION SERVICES

- Health care worker response time (for inpatients).
- Patient waiting time (for outpatients).
- Time required for completion of the phlebotomy procedure.
- Percentage of successful blood collections taken on the first attempt.
- Number of phlebotomy attempts beyond the first attempt.
- Number of phlebotomy attempts per patient by the medical service.
- Number and size of hematomas.
- Number of patients who faint.
- Amount of time spent and number of telephone calls needed to acquire appropriate identification.
- Number of redraws requested because of inadequate specimens.
- Contribution of health care worker to turnaround times of designated laboratory tests.
- Number of incomplete forms, documents, logs, and so forth.
- Number of therapeutic drug monitoring tests that have incorrect documentation or timing.
- Number of specimens received in incorrect tubes.

- Can measurable objective data be collected?
- Are there behavioral aspects that can be changed if necessary?
- Is the project realistic and achievable?

An important factor that can sometimes become a stumbling block for quality assessment is the data collection process. Most of the data can be collected from information already available in the patient care unit of the hospital or the laboratory, or by adding a brief tally or list to forms already in existence (Box 16–7). In addition, there are many other accessible sources of information (refer to Box 16–8), although the use of some of these sources may require special permission.

BOX 16–8. SOURCES OF INFORMATION FOR QUALITY ASSESSMENT

Medical records	Committee reports
Incident reports	Staff meetings
Accident reports	Marketing agents
Written complaints	Pathologists
Patient questionnaires	Attending physicians
Customer focus groups	Direct observation
Quality circles	Laboratory employees

■ COLLECTION PROCEDURES TO ENSURE QUALITY

Health care workers can consider the clinical laboratory testing process in several phases. The primary goal of specimen collection is to obtain an accurate sample for analysis. Many variables exist, however, before the specimen is actually analyzed. Box 16–9 depicts preanalytic, analytic, and postanalytic phases in specimen collection, processing, and testing. For purposes of this text, the quality assessment efforts focus on the preanalytic phases. Analytic and postanalytic phases involve rigorous quality control procedures and other types of quality assessment procedures, including proficiency testing using specimens from outside approved sources, and periodic inspections from authorized agencies. Table 16–2 indicates examples of preanalytic processes that are subject to quality reviews and monitoring. Each health care worker should be trained.

Each health care facility should target specific issues for quality assessment based on recognized concerns, incident reports, and/or recurring problems. A monthly review of the laboratory's collection procedures and policies is recommended to reduce collection errors. The clinical laboratory should provide the nursing staff with a floor book that describes laboratory services, preparation of the patient, and special handling of patients' specimens. In addition, the phlebotomist should have access to a pocket-sized collection booklet that contains the same information as that found in the floor book, along with other useful information for specimen handling, transporting, and processing.

BOX 16–9.   PREANALYTIC, ANALYTIC, AND POSTANALYTIC PHASES IN SPECIMEN COLLECTION, PROCESSING, TESTING, AND REPORTING

Preanalytical Phase Outside the Laboratory

Patient identification and information
Isolation techniques
Correct venipuncture or skin puncture
Appropriate use of supplies and equipment
Appropriate transportation and handling

Preanalytical Phase Inside the Laboratory

Sample treatment
Specimen registration and distribution
Centrifugation
Identification of aliquots
Appropriate storage

Analytical Phase

Testing the specimen

Postanalytical Phase

Reporting the results
Appropriate follow-up or repeat testing

Table 16-2.   Examples of Preanalytic Variables and Processes That Are Subject to Quality Control and Monitoring

PREANALYTIC VARIABLES AND PROCESSES	SUPPLIES AND MATERIALS

Patient preparation
  Identification
  Dietary information (fasting)
  Posture
  Previous complications (syncope)
  Providing information to patient
  Warming the site of collection
	Blood collection tubes
	Urine containers
	Expiration dates on all supplies
	Warming devices

Preparation of specimen
  Entering requests
  Appropriate labeling
	Request forms
	Sample identification

Specimen procurement
  Timing
  Cleansing the site
  Vein selection
  Needle positioning
  Order of draw for multiple tubes
	Needles
	Collection tubes
	Disinfectants

Transporting specimen
  Appropriate timing
  Transporting on ice
  Protection from light sensitivity
  Avoidance of leakage or breakage
	Transport containers
	Pneumatic tube systems
	Cooling systems

Processing the specimen
  Readiness for testing
  Aliquot preparation
  Centrifugation
	Identification and tracking software
	Centrifuge
	Pipettes

Storing the specimen
  Timing
  Site and temperature
  Preparation after storage
	Refrigerators
	Freezers
	Containers

ANTICOAGULANTS AND PRESERVATIVES: QUALITY ASSURANCE

As discussed in Chapters 7 and 8, the health care worker uses various anticoagulants and preservatives in the collection of blood specimens. These tubes containing anticoagulants must be inverted promptly after blood is drawn to ensure mixture of the anticoagulant and the blood and, thus, to provide quality assurance of a perfectly collected specimen. As reviewed in Chapter 8, when several evacuated tubes of blood are collected from a patient, tubes containing anticoagulants should be filled in the appropriate order so that proper inversion can occur and carryover of anticoagulants to clotted tubes will not occur.

For quality assurance, the anticoagulants and preservatives should meet the requirements established by the National Committee for Clinical Laboratory Standards (NCCLS). The manufacturer of the anticoagulants and preservatives must provide the shelf-life or expiration date of these additives on the packages so that the user will know how long these additives are effective. When restocking the supply of collection tubes, health care personnel should place the tubes with a shelf-life (expiration date) nearest the current date at the front of the shelf so that these tubes are used first. Manufacturers of collection tubes must test and verify draw and fill accuracy until the stated expiration date. The health care worker should be cognizant of expiration dates on any item used in specimen collection. Quality assurance accreditation standards require the health care institution to establish QC procedures for proper inspection of new lot numbers of evacuated blood collection tubes. In addition, quality can be obtained in specimen collection only with fresh specimens. If the blood specimen is not to be tested immediately, the health care worker must make certain that it is stored properly until the test is run.

REQUIREMENTS FOR A QUALITY SPECIMEN

The clinical competency of health care workers is ultimately linked to the quality of the specimen delivered.

 Clinical Alert

The requirements for a quality specimen include the following:

1. Using universal precautions, the patient is prepared properly and medication interference is avoided, if possible.
2. Collecting specimens from the correct patients and proper labeling are done. Because the policy of most clinical laboratories is to discard specimens that are unlabeled or labeled incorrectly, the health care worker must abide by the written laboratory policy describing acceptable identification of specimens. The potential errors in after-the-fact reidentification of a specimen by floor personnel can be extremely detrimental to the patient in question and must be avoided. (See Chapter 8 for identification and labeling procedures.)
3. The correct anticoagulants and preservatives must be used with the sufficient amount collected (see Chapters 7 and 8).
4. Specimens should not be hemolyzed.
5. Fasting specimens should be collected in a timely fashion and should actually be fasting samples.
6. Timed specimens should be correctly timed and documented.
7. Specimens without anticoagulants should be allowed to stand a minimum of 30 minutes so that clot formation can occur completely. (Gel separator tubes will shorten the time of clot formation, depending on the manufacturer's tubes.)
8. Specimens should be transported to the clinical laboratory in a timely fashion to maintain freshness (within 45 minutes). If the laboratory does not have designated delivery times for specimens, the health care worker may suggest to his or her laboratory supervisor that such a system would ensure fresh specimens and, thus, high-quality laboratory test results. A list of the specimens that are delivered after the designated time limits should be maintained in a logbook. Such a list can usually help personnel detect the source of the problem so that quality assessments can be evaluated. The list reveals the number of specimens that were delivered after the allowable limits and how late they were. The supervisor of specimen control usually decides whether the late specimen should be discarded and a new one collected.

NUMBER OF BLOOD COLLECTION ATTEMPTS

Another way to provide quality services to patients is by monitoring and reducing the number of unsuccessful collection attempts. If the health care worker has had consecutively unsuccessful phlebotomy attempts on different patients, the supervisor and the health care worker will know that the problem in blood collection must be identified and solved to prevent future unsuccessful attempts. Most clinical laboratories have a written procedure on the inability to draw specimens that describes the steps that should be taken by the health care worker when (1) collection attempts are unsuccessful (usually no more than two sticks), (2) the patient is unavailable, or (3) the patient refuses to have blood drawn.

QC AND PREVENTIVE MAINTENANCE

The health care worker should be aware that QC checks and preventive maintenance of certain instruments and equipment most often occur in the specimen control section of larger clinical laboratories or by trained laboratory personnel in smaller facilities. Instruments that must be monitored and maintained for quality by blood collection personnel may include:

- Thermometers
- Sphygmomanometers
- Centrifuges

In addition to undergoing preventive maintenance procedures, the centrifuge that is used to spin down the blood must be checked for accurate speed. The speed of the centrifuge can be checked with a tachometer, which indicates the speed in revolutions per minute (RPM). The relative centrifugal force, or g value, is then determined from a nomogram available in laboratories. The g value, gives the efficiency of the instrument by determining the true force exerted by the centrifuge. A g force of approximately 1000 for 10 minutes is usually efficient for good separation of cells or clotted blood from plasma or serum. The health care worker, however, must be sure to follow the manufacturer's directions when using gel separator devices to separate blood specimens. These collection tubes usually require a specified force higher than 1000 g for complete separation. The NCCLS publishes a manual entitled *Procedures for the Handling and Processing of Blood Specimens,* which provides more information on centrifugation of blood specimens.

SELF STUDY

KEY TERMS

Assessments
Cause-and-Effect (Ishikawa) Diagrams
Continuous Quality Improvement
  (CQI)
Customer Satisfaction
Dr. W. Edwards Deming
"5 Q" Framework
Flowcharts
Histograms

JCAHO 10-Step Process
Outcomes
Pareto Charts
Process
Quality Control (QC)
RUMBA Model
Structure
Total Quality Management
  (TQM)

STUDY QUESTIONS

The following questions may have *one* or *more* answers:

1. Of the following, which are examples of customers for phlebotomy services?

    a. outpatients
    b. patient's family members
    c. attending physicians
    d. nursing staff

2. Examples of unfavorable patient outcomes include which of the following?

    a. excessive probing for a vein
    b. multiple sticks on the same
       patient
    c. nosocomial infections
    d. hematomas

3. Which of the following are examples of structural components of quality that should
   be periodically checked?

    a. expiration dates
    b. condition of supplies
    c. adequacy of supplies
    d. nosocomial infections

4. Which of the following are examples of process components of quality that should
   be checked?

    a. documentation procedures
    b. hematomas
    c. multiple sticks
    d. use of incorrect anticoagulants

5. Why is rapid delivery of specimens important?

    a. because cells should not remain in contact with sera for excessive periods
    b. so that the health care worker can hurry to the next patient
    c. to reduce turnaround time for results
    d. because laboratory test results are most accurate when fresh specimens are used

References

1. Joint Commission on Accreditation of Healthcare Organizations (JCAHO). *1995 Comprehensive Accreditation Manual for Hospitals.* Oakbrook Terrace, IL: JCAHO; 1995.

2. Simpson KN, Kaluzny AD, McLaughlin CP. Total quality and the management of laboratories. *Clin Lab Manage Rev.* November/December, 1991; 448–462.

3. Graham NO. *Quality in Health Care: Theory, Applications, and Evolution.* Gaithersburg, MD: Aspen Publishers; 1995.

4. Westgard JO, Barry PL, Tomar RH. Implementing TQM in health care laboratories. *Clin Lab Manage Rev.* 1991;5(5):354.

5. Howanitz PJ, Cembrowski GS, Bachner P. Laboratory phlebotomy—CAP Q-probe study of patient satisfaction and complications in 23,783 patients. *Arch Pathol Lab Med.* 1991; 115:867–872.

6. Martin BG, ed. *The CLMA Guide to Managing a Clinical Laboratory.* Malvern, PA: Clinical Laboratory Management Association; 1991.

17

SEVENTEEN

∎

Legal and Regulatory Issues

CHAPTER OUTLINE

CHAPTER OBJECTIVES

Upon completion of Chapter 17, the learner is responsible for the following:

1. Define major legal terms and explain how they relate to the health care setting.
2. Define risk and describe the major elements in a risk management program.
3. Describe the basic functions of the medical record.
4. Define *informed consent.*
5. Describe how to avoid litigation as it relates to specimen collection in a health care environment.
6. Describe CLIA '88 in perspective to blood collection and transportation responsibilities.

■ GENERAL LEGAL PRINCIPLES

The laws governing medicine and medical ethics complement and overlap one another. For many years, even centuries, the decision of the physician or health care professional was unquestioned. This has changed. Health care consumers and patients have become more aware, more critical, and much more willing to sue anyone that their lawyer believes has been at fault, including health care workers who are collecting blood specimens.

The legal system in the United States falls under legislative, regulatory, and judicial procedures at the federal, state, and local levels.

STATUTORY LAW

Statutes are written laws enacted by state legislatures and the US Congress. Legislative activities performed by local government lead to written laws referred to as *ordinances.* Statutes and ordinances are **statutory laws** that are binding but in certain instances may require the courts (judicial law) to interpret how the statutory law applies to a given set of facts. For example, a statute may state that no sexual harassment will be allowed in the workplace. A court then may be called on to decide whether certain actions by a person are considered sexual harassment and, therefore, violate the law.

ADMINISTRATIVE LAW

Once enacted, statutes and ordinances must be implemented; this is **administrative law.** This process is performed by the executive branch, which has numerous departments and agencies. Administrative agencies (e.g., Health Care Financing Administration) write regulations that enforce the laws created through the legislative body. One department under the executive branch that has a major effect on administrative laws regarding health care workers is the US Department of Health and Human Services (HHS). The HHS is the main source of regulations affecting the health care industry.

JUDICIAL LAW

The function of the judicial branch of local, state, and federal governments is to resolve disputes in accordance with law. Most of the nation's **judicial law** actions occur at the state level. State and federal systems have trial courts, which are the first level. The second level within the court system includes intermediate courts (appeals courts), which review the decisions of the trial courts. The highest level within the judicial system is the supreme court of each state and of the federal system; these courts will hear only specific cases. Most of the written legal decisions occur from the appeals and supreme courts. More than 90 percent of all lawsuits are settled out of court, however, and many that are tried are settled before a final verdict is rendered.[1] Usually, phlebotomy cases are tried in state courts. If federal laws or regulations pertain to the case, however, the federal court system is used.

LEGAL TERMINOLOGY

If a health care worker understands basic legal concepts, this understanding can help to define how personnel involved in the specimen collection process can be liable for activities that may occur in this field of health care. Such understanding can also reduce the conflicts between law and the health care workers. Liability for the lack of a proper standard of health care may be imposed on any health care worker, including health care institutions, physicians, nurses, laboratorians, patient care technicians, and phlebotomists. The number of substantial awards against health care workers as a result of improper care has grown in recent years as patients have become more sensitive to treatment complications.

Lawyers have become advisers to health care professionals and institutions in matters ranging from termination of treatment to approval of experimental protocols. Some lawyers specialize in hospital law or food and drug law; personal injury lawyers handle malpractice claims, and others are especially knowledgeable about Medicaid and workers' compensation benefits. No one lawyer can master all these areas. William J. Curran defined *health law* as a "specialty area of law and law practice related to the medical and other health fields—such as dentistry, nursing, hospital administration, and environmental law."[2]

To grasp the legal implication of health care, the health care provider must have some knowledge of basic legal terminology. The avoidance of legal conflicts through education and planning is called **preventive law.** Thus, there is a need to understand basic legal definitions and, it is hoped, to develop a preventive law approach in the procedures and techniques of blood collection. A few major definitions with health care examples can be found in Box 17–1.

Negligence

In the past decade, the number of legal cases in which the laboratory has been directly or indirectly involved has increased noticeably. Negligence is "a violation of a duty to exercise reasonable skill and care in performing a task."[3] Four factors, or key points, must be considered in alleged negligence cases.[3]

1. *Duty*—relates to what duties or responsibilities the hospital or health care worker had toward the patient; it also includes all the individuals who had a duty toward the patient to use the appropriate standard of care.
2. *Breach of duty*—relates to whether the duty was breached and if it was avoidable. The plaintiff must be able to show what actually happened and that the defendant acted unreasonably.
3. *Proximate causation*—relates to whether the breach of duty actually contributed to

BOX 17–1. LEGAL TERMINOLOGY

- **Assault.** The unjustifiable attempt to touch another person or the threat to do so in such circumstances as to cause the other to believe that it will be carried out, or to cause fear. An assault may be permissible if proper consent has been given (e.g., consent to obtain a blood specimen).

- **Battery.** The intentional touching of another person without consent; also, the unlawful beating of another or carrying out of threatened physical harm. Because battery always includes an assault, the two are commonly combined in the phrase *assault and battery*. The receiver of the battery does not have to be aware that a battery has been committed (e.g., a patient who is unconscious and has surgery performed on him or her without his or her approval, either expressed or implied). The law provides a remedy to the individual when consent to a touching has not been obtained or if the act goes beyond the consent given. Thus, the injured person may initiate a lawsuit against the wrongdoer for the damages suffered. Liability of hospitals, physicians, and other health care workers for acts of battery is most common in situations involving lack of or improper consent to medical procedures, such as blood collecting. For example, a small boy who refused to have his blood drawn was locked in the blood collection room by the health care worker and was forced to have his blood drawn by the health care worker. The patient's parents sued and won. As another example, a patient is feeling stressed because of pain and not knowing what medical procedures will be occurring. If a health care professional displays behavior in a threatening manner, this can lead to legal intervention. The health care worker must obviously avoid directing threatening language to a patient (e.g., "If you don't let me collect your blood, your illness will probably become critical"). If the patient feels threatened by these words, he or she can "claim intentional infliction of emotional distress." The stress of collecting blood from numerous patients in a short period can lead some health care workers to think about threatening difficult patients, but, of course, this could be detrimental to all involved.

- **Breach of duty.** An infraction, violation, or failure to perform.

- **Civil law.** Not a criminal action; the plaintiff sues for monetary damages.

- **Criminal actions.** Legal recourse for acts or offenses against the public welfare; these actions can lead to imprisonment of the offender.

- **Defendant.** The health care worker or institution against whom the action or lawsuit is filed.

- **False imprisonment.** The unjustifiable detention of a person without a legal warrant.

- **Felony.** Varies by state but generally is defined as public offenses, if the defendant is convicted, he or she will spend time in jail.

- **Invasion of privacy.** Physical intrusion upon a person; the publishing of confidential information, although true, but of such an objectionable or personal nature as to be offensive.

- **Liable.** Under legal obligation, as far as damages are concerned.

- **Litigation process.** The process of legal action to determine a decision in court. Many malpractice cases are negotiated and settled out of court.

- **Malice.** Knowing that a statement is false or making a statement with reckless disregard of the truth.

- **Malpractice.** Improper or unskillful care of a patient by a member of the health care team, or any professional misconduct, unreasonable lack of skill, or infidelity in professional or judiciary duties. Malpractice may be described as *professional negligence*.

- **Misdemeanor.** The general term for all sorts of criminal offenses not serious enough to be classified as felonies.

- **Misrepresentation.** Use of misleading information or omission of important facts.

- **Negligence.** Failure to act or to perform duties according to the standards of the profession.

- **Plaintiff.** The claimant who brings a lawsuit or an action.

(continued)

BOX 17–1 *(continued)*

- **Respondeat superior.** The concept whereby actions of one individual may be imputed to another person having control. This suggests that a technician's negligent act can be imputed to a laboratory corporation. Under this concept, supervisors and directors may be held liable for the negligent actions of their employees. This concept is also referred to as **vicarious liability.**

- **Tort.** A legal wrong in which the person who commits it is liable for damages in civil action. The tort system is a substructure of the judicial system. It is basically concerned with resolving two-party disputes over whether some harm to one party, or his or her property, was caused by the actions or inactions of another party. A tort is a harm or an injury that is civil, not criminal, in nature and does not constitute a breach of contract. Civil law does not deal with crimes. Torts and other civil wrongs must be proved by a *preponderance of the evidence. Preponderance* is taken to mean a majority; 51 percent or more implies that the defendant more likely than not committed the act.

- **Whistle-blowing.** Public disclosure of perceived wrongdoing by an employee(s) of the same organization. This usually occurs when a dedicated employee has observed something at work that may cause serious harm to one or more patients or that may be illegal. In most of these cases, the employee has reported the occurrence(s) to supervisors with no remedy to the situation. Whistle-blowers may report to governmental agencies, accreditation agencies, etc. Employees who speak out may fear reprisals that could include dismissal, blacklisting, threats of violence, and/or harassment. Numerous laws are in place, however, to protect employees who report legitimate wrongdoing.

or caused injury; also concerns all the parties involved in contributing to the alleged injury. There must be a direct line from the conduct to the injury.

4. *Damages*—relates to whether the plaintiff was actually injured and when these injuries were discovered. Once negligence and causation are established, plaintiffs must be able to show that they were actually damaged by the negligent act.

Many circumstances could be considered negligence if health care workers are not extremely careful. For example, there have been legal cases in which confusion of patient samples led to a patient's death.[4]

Patient Confidentiality

Negligence cases can also arise out of violation of the right to privacy or of **patient confidentiality.** "No one except the patient may release patient results without a clinical need to know." Patient or employee laboratory test results must be considered *strictly* confidential. Negligence can be claimed if employees' or patients' drug abuse test results are released to anyone other than the attending physician or other authorized individuals. This is particularly true regarding employee or athlete drug or alcohol abuse screening and human immunodeficiency virus (HIV) testing. Confidential materials include communications between the physician and the patient, the patient's verbal statements, and nonverbal communications, such as laboratory test results.

■ CONFIDENTIALITY AND HIV EXPOSURE

An increasing concern for health care workers collecting blood from patients who are homebound is the health care worker's rights in relation to accidental exposure to blood or body fluids, whether by a needlestick or some other means. In some states, laws allow health care workers to know the identity of a patient who has acquired immunodeficiency syndrome (AIDS) or who is HIV positive. Many states, however, do not provide for the easy acquisition of this sensitive patient information. A home health care worker who routinely collects blood specimens from homebound patients should obtain information on the state's law regarding confidentiality and HIV status.[5] It can be obtained from the health care worker's employer, from legal counsel, or from a national or state health professional organization.

It is important to use the proper blood collection techniques with safety precautions and required infection control procedures for homebound patients. If exposure to the blood occurs through a needlestick, a lancet, or another means, the home health care worker needs to be certain of obtaining the patient's HIV status to ensure that the proper immediate and long-term self-protective procedural steps can be taken. Even if the report from the HIV test is negative for the health care worker, continued negative status is not guaranteed. Just because a patient's status is HIV positive, however, the health care worker exposed to the blood may not become HIV positive.

If employed by a health care facility, the health care worker should follow the guidelines established by the facility. If he or she is self-employed, it is important to monitor his or her own HIV status. Also, counseling should be sought to obtain emotional support during this stressful time.

 Clinical Alert

If employed by a health care facility, the exposed health care worker must immediately file an incident report concerning the accidental exposure. If the health care worker is self-employed and working for various agencies, he or she must report the incident to these agencies. Employers are responsible for postexposure follow-up testing. The health care institutions and agencies must report accidental exposure incidents to the **Centers for Disease Control and Prevention (CDC).** The CDC maintains national surveillance of health care workers' accidental exposures. These statistics assist in developing better safeguards (e.g., new blood collection equipment) against accidental exposure.

■ MALPRACTICE

Malpractice, or professional negligence, is defined as improper or unskillful care of a patient by a member of the health care team, or any professional misconduct or unreasonable lack of skill.

The relationship between doctor and patient is, in the legal sense, a contractual one. The basic elements involved are common with those of other contracts. The elements of contracts are as follows:

- **Offer.** The physician offers to provide a service, either by opening an office or being on a hospital staff or both. Thus, he or she has made him- or herself available to patients who seek care.

- **Acceptance.** The patient visits the physician for treatment of a disease or a disorder and may agree to accept medical care.
- **Consideration.** The patient accepts treatment and pays for the care provided by the physician.

By completing these steps, the physician and the patient engage in a contract that implies obligations on both their parts. The physician is obligated to provide medical care to the patient if he or she follows directions and pays for the service. There is even a question about the length of grace period in terms of payment. Also, the patient generally must refuse treatment before the physician is legally freed from his or her obligation. By agreeing to provide service, the physician is required to provide a standard of care.

If the physician is the medical director overseeing clinical laboratory testing, in most cases he or she is responsible under the law for the standard of care and the performance of all aspects of laboratory testing. Therefore, a breach of standard on the part of the health care worker collecting blood for laboratory assays could place both the physician and the health care worker at risk.

■ STANDARD OF CARE

If a patient has suffered injury due to blood collection for laboratory testing, the patient must show that the health care worker who collected the blood failed to meet the prevailing **standard of care.** All health care workers must conform to a specific standard of care to protect patients. In legal cases, the standard of care is determined by what a reasonably prudent person would do under similar circumstances. It is a measuring stick representing the conduct of the average health care worker in the community. The community has been expanded to be a national community as a result of national laboratory standards and requirements. Examples of setting the standard of care include statutes, licensing requirements, rules and regulations of regulatory or professional organizations (e.g., American Hospital Association, Joint Commission for Accreditation of Healthcare Organizations [JCAHO], Health Care Financing Administration, etc.), internal health care facility rules and regulations, and professional publications.

■ INFORMED CONSENT

Informed consent is voluntary permission by a patient to allow touching, examination, and/or treatment by health care providers. It allows patients to determine what will be performed on or to their bodies. Without informed consent, intentional touching can be considered a criminal offense. This type of consent can be obtained through word or action. Thus, the consent may be given orally, expressed by nonverbal behavior, or expressed in writing.

> The following is an example of nonverbal consent. The physician orders laboratory tests for diagnosis and the patient comes to the laboratory with a rolled-up sleeve and outstretched arm. The patient is giving consent for the health care worker to take the blood samples. Integral to consent is the patient's belief that the person to whom consent is given has the knowledge, skills, and technical ability to perform such tasks. Consequently, the patient can expect the blood collector to know the

proper venipuncture, arterial puncture, and/or skin puncture technique. For the blood collection, the health care worker should briefly explain to the patient the procedure used to collect the blood specimen. It is important for the health care worker collecting the blood to stress that the physician ordered the test.

 Clinical Alert

Health care workers are becoming more cognizant of the informed consent principle because this is the largest area of litigation. Minors *must* have the consent of their parents or legal guardians for medical care, including blood collections. With the increased amount of immigration to this country, language can be a barrier to informed consent. An interpreter may be necessary so that information for consent may be given in the native tongue.

Most states have enacted legislation requiring that informed consent be obtained before most HIV testing is performed. The statutes indicate the type of information that must be given for the patient to be considered informed. These laws usually require that the patient be counseled on the following: (1) an explanation of the test, including its purpose; (2) potential uses of the HIV test; and (3) testing limitations and the meaning of its results.

■ IMPLIED CONSENT

Implied consent exists when immediate action is required to save a patient's life or to prevent permanent impairment of the patient's health. In other words, an emergency removes the need for consent. Implied consent differs legally from one state to another. Health care providers need to know the legal boundaries of implied consent because they may become involved in an emergency situation (e.g., giving cardiopulmonary resuscitation).

■ STATUTE OF LIMITATIONS

The **statute of limitations** is a law that defines how soon after an injury (e.g., malpractice) a plaintiff must file the lawsuit or be forever barred from doing so. The purpose of this law is to prevent the threat of a lawsuit from hanging over a possible defendant's (e.g., health care worker's) head forever and to force legal action before memories and records are not available and witnesses die. The statute of limitations for professional negligence in most states is 2 years. A complete and accurate medical record with laboratory testing results is the best defense in these cases because the attending physician and health care workers for the patient may have little recollection of the events in question.

■ LEGAL CLAIMS AND DEFENSE

In a malpractice lawsuit, the first pleading filed in a negligence action is the complaint. It is the first statement of a case by the plaintiff(s) against the defendant(s) and states a cause of action, notifying the defendant(s) as to the basis for suit.

Several steps follow, and if the case is not dismissed before trial, the parties to a lawsuit have the right to **discovery**—to examine the witnesses before the trial. Examination before trial is a method used to enable the plaintiff(s) and defendant(s) to learn more regarding the nature and substance of each other's case. This discovery process consists of oral testimony under oath and includes cross-examination by the lawyers. The **deposition** is the testimony of a witness that has been recorded in a written legal format. Either party in the lawsuit—plaintiff or defendant—may obtain a court order permitting examination and copying of laboratory reports, incident reports from personnel files, medical records, phlebotomy and laboratory policies and procedures, training manuals, and so forth, and other facts and information that may help in the discovery.

In addition to the deposition, the parties may undergo cross-examination at the time of the trial. They will provide testimony that will be recorded and filed with the court regarding the cause for the case.

If a health care worker receives a summons to provide a deposition before a trial and/or testimony during a trial for a lawsuit, some helpful guidelines include the following:

- Answer only the questions asked.
- Be organized in your recollection of the facts regarding the incident.
- Do not be antagonistic in answering the questions.
- Explain the laboratory and/or blood collection procedures and policies in simple terminology for the jury.
- Do not overdramatize the facts that you are presenting.
- Dress neatly and be groomed appropriately.
- Be polite, sincere, and courteous.
- Be sure to ask for clarification of questions that you did not clearly hear and questions that you did not understand.
- If you are not sure of an answer, indicate that you do not know the answer or that you are not sure.
- Above all, be truthful.

EXPERT WITNESS

Expert testimony, as well as scientific or medical data, is sometimes used to assist in establishing the standard of care required in any given situation. An **expert witness** may be used to assist a plaintiff in proving the wrongful act of a defendant or to assist a defendant in refuting such evidence. At the time of testifying, each expert's training, experience, and special qualifications will be explained during the deposition and later to the jury during the trial.

EVIDENCE

Evidence during the trial is used to prove or disprove the lawsuit. Evidence must be competent, relevant, and material. It may include such items as vacuum tube holders and tubes, needles, safety apparatuses such as biohazardous waste containers, infection control logs and reports, JCAHO standards, board certification standards for health care workers, and laboratory policies and procedures.

> ## BOX 17–2. TIPS FOR AVOIDING MALPRACTICE LITIGATION
>
> - Provide the patient with proper blood collection techniques comparable to national standards (e.g., National Committee for Clinical Laboratory Standards [NCCLS] guidelines, JCAHO regulations).
> - Obtain consent for collection of specimens.
> - Regularly participate in continuing education programs.
> - Properly handle all confidential communications (e.g., HIV testing) without violation.
> - Maintain all required blood collection equipment on trays and/or in collection areas for proper collection, including safety apparatuses, such as gloves and disposal containers.
> - Be a good listener and let the patient identify his or her anxieties.
> - Report incidents immediately and document them.

ADVICE TO AVOID LAWSUITS

Justice is expensive in the United States. Lawyers' fees typically range from $100 to $500 per hour, and associated costs can lead to thousands of dollars in legal fees. Also, legal proceedings are time consuming, expensive, and, most of all, emotionally devastating to both the plaintiff(s) and the defendant(s). Thus, to avoid a malpractice lawsuit, the health care provider should heed the advice in Box 17–2.

If the health care worker is involved in home health care collections, he or she needs to have the right types and amounts of insurance coverage to address liability exposures with respect to handling and transporting patients' specimens and wastes across the city.[6]

RESPONDEAT SUPERIOR

Respondeat superior (Latin term meaning "let the master answer") is the concept whereby the actions of one individual may be imputed to another person having control. It is a legal doctrine that holds employers responsible for acts of their employees within the scope of the employment relationship. Liability predicated on respondeat superior may be imposed on an employer only if a master–servant relationship exists between the employer and the employee and the wrongful act of the employee occurs within the scope of employment. Because the law holds negligent persons responsible for their negligent acts, employees are not released from liability when the health care institution is held liable through the application of respondeat superior. Not only may the injured party sue the employee directly, but the employer, if sued, may also seek indemnification from the employee. Indemnification is compensation for the financial loss suffered by the employee's act.

■ MEDICAL RECORDS

Medical records are vital. A health care worker cannot be expected to remember a patient from whom blood was drawn 3 to 4 years ago. The medical records must be neat, legible, and accurate. They are extremely important if a medical malpractice case goes to court. Medical records have four basic purposes:

1. Allow for continuity of the patient's care plan.
2. Provide documentation of the patient's illness and treatment.

3. Document communication between the physician and the health care team.
4. Provide a legal document that can be used by patients and hospital or health care workers to protect their legal interests.

Medical records are also used for nonmedical reasons that are not directly tied to medical services, such as billing, utilization review, quality improvement, and so on.

Health care workers and their supervisors have a legal duty to keep records, documentation, and laboratory test results confidential. This duty may be waived only if a patient has given express permission for the information to be released, if the patient has sued the institution or its health care personnel, or if the health care worker is specifically obligated to release patient information (e.g., to the CDC). But even in these situations, the confidentiality of patient records and reports cannot be breached while they are communicated or in transit.

■ LEGAL CASES RELATED TO CLINICAL LABORATORY ACTIVITIES

Most phlebotomy cases are settled after a lawsuit is filed but before the court renders a judgment. It is important to remember that many cases are not cited in the literature because often health care institutions or health care workers negotiate, arbitrate, and settle out of court. The following sections discuss cases that are of interest to health care workers involved in blood collection.

SCHMERBER V. STATE OF CALIFORNIA

Nurses, technologists, and health care workers are concerned about drawing a blood sample from an unconscious patient or lacking the patient's consent when requested by police. The US Supreme Court ruled in *Schmerber v. State of California* that tests performed on a blood sample drawn by a hospital physician from a person arrested by the police were admissible in a court action. This may vary by state.

LAZERNICK V. GENERAL HOSPITAL OF MONROE COUNTY (PA 1977)

A patient who was pregnant for the first time had her blood typed in January 1971. The report sent to her physician indicated that her blood type was A-positive. The patient gave birth to her second child on June 1977. The child was brain damaged and paralyzed on the right side of the body as a result of hemolytic blood disease. The laboratory records in 1971 and 1977 showed that the mother's blood type was O-negative. In a malpractice suit, the parents charged that the physician's and his employees' negligence caused the child's injuries. The physician, who was chief of the laboratory when the blood test was performed, was found liable, as was the health care worker.

WALTON V. PROVIDENCE HOSPITAL

A patient was admitted to Providence Hospital for treatment of pneumonia. On the second day, the patient complained of coldness and numbness in his right hand. On the fourth day, a vascular surgeon examined the hand and ordered 4000 U of heparin in hopes of restoring blood flow. The hand had to be amputated. In court, the expert witness testified that a blood pressure cuff had been left on for an extended period. The patient was awarded $40,000.

HELMANN V. SACRED HEART HOSPITAL

Failure to follow proper isolation techniques, such as proper hand washing and prevention of cross-contamination, is a major area of concern for hospitals. The patient in *Helmann v. Sacred Heart Hospital* (62 Wash. 2d 136, 381 P. 2d 605 [1963]) had multiple fractures in the area of the left hip socket. After surgery on his hip, he was returned to a semiprivate room. His roommate complained of a boil under the right arm. Eight days later, a culture was taken of the roommate's wound drainage. Three days later, the laboratory identified the wound infection as *Staphylococcus aureus*. The infected roommate was immediately placed in isolation for the wound. For the preceding 11 days, however, the hospital attendants administered care to both patients without washing their hands between patient care.

The patient with the hip injury developed a *S. aureus* infection at the site of his hip incision. The infection penetrated into the hip socket, destroying tissue and leading to additional surgery and a hip fused in a nearly immovable position. Negligence on the part of the hospital personnel was identified as the cause of the injury as a result of deviation from the accepted standard of care.

STEPP V. REVIEW BOARD OF THE INDIANA EMPLOYMENT SECURITY DIVISION

Another type of legal case involved a laboratory technician in *Stepp v. Review Board of the Indiana Employment Security Division* (521 N.E. 2d 350 [Ind. Ct. App. 1988]). She was found to have been properly dismissed from her position in the laboratory because of her refusal to perform laboratory tests on patients' specimens with AIDS warnings attached.

PAROS V. HOEMAKO HOSPITAL

The chief x-ray technician in *Paros v. Hoemako Hospital* (681 P. 2d 918 [Ariz. Ct. App. 1984]) was found to have been properly dismissed because of a chronic hostile and argumentative attitude inconsistent with managerial supervisory responsibilities. The ruling was appealed, and the appeals court upheld the lower court's decision.

CASES RESULTING FROM IMPROPER TECHNIQUE AND NEGLIGENCE

Health care workers who collect blood by venipuncture must be thoroughly trained and skilled in proper technique, safety, and the use of collection equipment. Problems that can arise include:

- Wristband or identification error
- Hematoma
- Abscess at the puncture site
- Patient falls
- Fainting

- Nerve damage
- Emotional distress

In one case settled out of court, a health care worker had not received proper blood collection training. She performed a venipuncture by inserting the needle approximately 2 inches above the antecubital fold. The needle went through the vein, through muscle, and into the nerve, severely injuring the patient's arm, which remained permanently damaged even after three surgeries to repair the damage from the resultant hematoma and nerve injury.

Another case involved a medical technologist under pressure to collect specimens from ambulatory patients as quickly as possible. One of the patients stated prior to blood collection that she had fainted during the blood collection at a previous time. The phlebotomist, however, took no precautions to avoid syncope, collected the patient's blood, and allowed the patient to leave immediately. The patient fainted at the elevator and suffered permanent loss of smell and had a permanent "ringing sound" in her ears.

In another case, a health care worker collecting and performing bedside glucose results misread the glucometer and caused the deaths of three patients with diabetes. The errors might have been avoided with better training, supervision, and quality monitoring.

DiMARCO V. LYNCH HOMES–CHESTER COUNTY, INC.

In *DiMarco v. Lynch Homes–Chester County, Inc.* (Pennsylvania Superior Court, April 14, 1989, 559 A. 2d 530 [PA Super 1989]), a blood collector suffered a needle puncture wound when a nursing home patient from whom she was collecting blood kicked her. The blood collector received follow-up treatment from her physician, who advised her that she may contract hepatitis up to 6 weeks after the incident. Thus, she was told, she should avoid sexual relations during this time to prevent the possibility of infecting her boyfriend. After 8 weeks, the blood collector resumed her relationship with her boyfriend. After this length of time, however, the blood collector contracted hepatitis and her boyfriend also was diagnosed with the disease. The boyfriend sued the physician and the nursing home. Through the appeals process within the state, the boyfriend won the case. The Pennsylvania Superior Court concluded that someone who renders services to another should recognize the need to protect the third party (the boyfriend) and is liable to the third party who is injured.

BOOKER V. DUKE MEDICAL CENTER

A similar case was *Booker v. Duke Medical Center* (2565.E. 2d 189 [N.C. 1979]), in which compensation was awarded to the wife of a laboratory technician who died after being exposed to viral hepatitis. The court ruled that the technician's employment exposed him to a greater risk of contracting the disease than members of the public or employees in general.

VERONICA PREGO V. THE CITY OF NEW YORK

In *Veronica Prego v. The City of New York* (Kings County Hospital, New York City Health and Hospital Corporation, Kings County, New York Supreme Court, Index No. 14974/88), in January 1983 a health care worker at Kings County Hospital pricked her finger on a needle used to collect blood from a patient dying of AIDS. The plaintiff tested positive for AIDS in March 1985. The health care worker stated that the hospital failed to dispose of used necdles properly, claiming that needle boxes should have been provided in each room. The health care worker won the lawsuit and more than $1 million in damages.

■ HIV-RELATED ISSUES

If a health care worker becomes infected with HIV during employment at a health care facility, coverage by workers' compensation benefits are usually available. The health care worker must, however, demonstrate a causal connection between his or her HIV infection and his or her employment. This causal connection includes having a documented incident report at the health care facility involving a needlestick injury, a puncture wound, or other exposure to HIV-contaminated blood or body fluids. In addition, the health care worker's lifestyle will be investigated to determine whether the exposure occurred elsewhere. Pre-employment health evaluations may prove useful later should the health care worker allege contraction of infection during the time of employment. Employers are legally responsible for monitoring postexposure follow-up.

If a health care worker resigns because of contracting AIDS, unemployment benefits may be available if the worker can show that he or she believed in good faith that continued employment would jeopardize his or her health.

In a letter to the *New England Journal of Medicine,*[7] a resident physician who acquired HIV from a patient stated the following: "Workers' compensation works well to cover medical expenses and income lost because of occupational injuries that result in temporary or minor disabilities such as muscle tears or bone fractures. But these are not the accidents that a physician (health care provider) is likely to suffer at work. The main threats today are catastrophic, and workers' compensation is grossly inadequate for catastrophic illness."

■ LEGAL CASE PROTECTION

 Clinical Alert

If an incident occurs (e.g., a patient develops a hematoma), the blood collector *must* write an incident report and give it to the supervisor. The incident report can be helpful in a lawsuit to identify the real cause, the time, and other details of the incident. It may be of great assistance to the health care worker who is the defendant in the case in recalling the reason for the patient's (plaintiff's) alleged suffering and truth. The health care worker, however, must not misrepresent or tamper with evidence in a lawsuit by writing an incident report after being sued by a patient for malpractice.

In one case in which a health care worker was sued for damaging a patient's median nerve as a result of probing with a needle to find the vein, the health care worker "after the alleged fact" wrote an incident report for the incident that occurred prior to the filed suit. Eventually, through court proceedings, it was discovered that the health care worker had not actually filed an incident report at the time of the patient's needlestick injury. The falsification of documentation with malice immensely affected the plaintiff's award for damages.

■ LAWS ON MEDICAL DEVICES AND PROTECTIVE EQUIPMENT

Blood collection involves the use of many types of equipment and supplies. Blood collectors and patients have been injured as a result of malfunctioning equipment. In 1990, the federal government issued the Safe Medical Devices Act, which states that any malfunctioning devices (e.g., in vitro diagnostics, reagent kits, clinical analyzers, blood collection equipment) must be immediately reported to the federal government with a description of the malfunctioning incident (e.g., breakage of needle in arm). After an investigation of the incident, a nationwide alert is generally provided to health care institutions regarding the failure(s) of the health care device. This law was enacted to protect health care workers and patients from injuries due to health care devices.

To avoid the possibility of malfunctioning equipment, the **Food and Drug Administration (FDA)** evaluates the safety, clinical efficacy, and medical efficacy of the equipment and supplies used in blood collection. Another federal agency, the **Environmental Protection Agency (EPA)** monitors and enforces environmental requirements for the safe disposal of chemical and biological hazards.

Another federal rule affecting health care workers who collect blood is the Occupational Safety and Health Administration (OSHA) rule for personal protective equipment (PPE) that became effective on July 5, 1994. The rule describes the following:

- PPE must be of a safe design and construction for the work to be performed.
- PPE must be provided, used, and maintained in a sanitary and workable condition.
- PPE must be selected for employees based on an assessment of the hazards of the work environment (e.g., safety shields over needle apparatus).
- Employees must be trained in the proper use of PPE.

■ MALPRACTICE INSURANCE

Because hospitals are places where seriously ill patients are admitted and treated with highly sophisticated medical technology, the likelihood for problems is greater there than in other health care settings. Often, the health care staff in the hospital or clinical laboratory are part of a blanket malpractice insurance policy. If, however, the health care worker is employed by a pathologist who has a contract with an institution or owns a clinic, the staff may be protected by the pathologist's malpractice insurance policy.

Malpractice insurance rates for pathologists are generally the lowest premiums charged among physicians because of their low risk level. Laboratory personnel in administrative or technical positions in laboratories have rarely been named in malpractice suits. Part of the reason for so few cases is that under the legal concept of respondeat superior, responsibility for wrongful acts of the employee (agent–servant) rests on the employer (principal–master). Also, another reason for not being named in a suit is the *deep pocket concept.* The health care worker, with less money or no insurance, in the past has not been a target for suit. The advances in technology and increased complexity of health care have, however, increased legal exposure for allied health and nursing professionals. The health care worker that routinely deals with the public in patient–health care worker relationships is indeed liable. Therefore, each individual should examine the possibility of malpractice suits and the need for malpractice insurance from a personal standpoint.[8]

If the health care worker decides to purchase malpractice insurance, the following factors should be carefully considered[9]:

1. Does the employer carry liability insurance?
2. Is adequate dollar value coverage provided? In recent lawsuits, total damages of $1 million or more have been awarded against physicians.
3. What are the coverage limitations? How much does one have to lose if sued?
4. What are the procedures that must be followed for the policy to provide coverage? Some policies state that divulging the amount of coverage or the fact of coverage voids the policy.
5. The health care worker should not assume that the lawyers representing the hospital, laboratory, or clinic will have his or her best interests at heart. The attorney's first obligation is to serve those who have hired him or her. There have been cases in which the hospital was cleared of all charges but the health care professional was held liable for damages. For the health care worker, if an adult patient seems alert and does not object to the blood specimen collection, consent is implied. Proceeding without consent may give rise to assault and battery charges, as well as civil suits.
6. Is a job change expected soon?
7. Are specimen collecting services provided off site or in patient's homes?

With the purchase of malpractice professional liability insurance, the attorney's fee and court costs are usually covered. Some professional organizations offer professional liability insurance at a reasonable or reduced rate. With the advent of organ transplantations, renal dialysis, hyperbaric care, home care, and bedside testing, the avenues of liability are widened. A genuine concern for others and careful attention to technique are good investments of the health care worker's time. A record of continuing education courses, seminars, workshops, and academic credits should be a part of each health care worker's personal file.

■ MANAGEMENT OF RISK

CONCEPTS OF RISK

Risk can be described as "exposure to the chance of injury or loss."[10] Health care workers face many risks daily. It is important for health care workers, supervisors, and managers to reflect on their personal risk and that of their employers. Active steps should be taken to understand risk factors and to minimize areas of risk for the benefit of patients and the protection of employees and employers. Risk can be managed by using carefully planned objectives that can be categorized as preloss (to reduce or prevent losses) and postloss (how the facility can recover from a loss). **Risk management programs** reduce preventable injuries and accidents and minimize financial loss. The goals and objectives of the institution or department can guide the risk management program. A generic model of **risk management** might involve the following levels:

- *Risk identification and analysis*—analysis and measurement of identified risks.
- *Risk treatment*—use of tools (e.g., safety manuals, policies and procedures, public relations tactics) to prevent harm or losses.
- *Education*—of patients, employees, and visitors.

- *Risk transfer or postponement*—shifting risk to other parties (e.g., liability insurance, contract services, and employees).
- *Risk evaluation*—assessment of what should be done.

One way to identify risk is to review *incident* or *occurrence* reports that involve laboratory or phlebotomy services. Employees must be continually encouraged to use these tools because without an effective reporting system, proper investigations and risk assessments cannot be made. An incident or occurrence does not have to result in injury. The older term *accident report* is rarely used anymore because it implies that an error occurred, which may not always be the case. Trends of events that deviate from normal, but fortunately do not harm any patients, are most revealing and controllable.

Risk treatment has two elements: loss or risk control, and risk financing.[10] Loss or risk control means that the department should attempt to reduce the frequency of errors or events that can potentially cause financial loss. Similar to quality-improvement programs, the aim would be to reduce adverse outcomes, such as excessive venipunctures on the same patient, reducing the number of hematomas, and so on. *Risk financing* refers to how to pay for losses once they occur (liability insurance or other means). If a patient faints during venipuncture and injures him- or herself, care should be taken to assist and provide free services for the person to recover. Documentation should clearly indicate the details of the incident and each step of the follow-up.

Education and communication are also vital to the risk management process. If employees do not know about new procedures, they cannot be expected to follow them.

Risk transfer through the use of liability insurance is also an important part of the risk management process. Contracting for services has also traditionally shifted some of the liability to other parties. Federal and state laws are changing, however, to include contract personnel and contract services (e.g., reference laboratories, diagnostic radiology services) under the *respondeat superior* concept. This trend suggests that health care facilities might be held liable for services performed by those with whom they have contracts.

Evaluation of all the elements of risk management just discussed may show a need for changes in procedures, employee counseling, or educational programs. Table 17–1 indicates some common sense tips for minimizing risk in a phlebotomy setting.[10–13]

CLINICAL LABORATORY IMPROVEMENT AMENDMENTS (CLIA)

In October 1988, the US Congress passed Public Law 100-578, **Clinical Laboratory Improvement Amendments (CLIA).** This public law is administered by the **Health Care Financing Administration (HCFA).** CLIA '88 regulations became effective on September 1, 1992, as a means to ensure the quality and accuracy of laboratory testing by creating a uniform set of provisions governing all laboratories that examine human specimens either for the diagnosis, prevention, or treatment of disease or for the impairment of, or the assessment of the health of human beings.[12] CLIA '88 essentially applies to every clinical laboratory testing facility in the United States and requires that the facility be certified by the federal government. The certification requires an inspection by federal and/or state agencies to determine whether the laboratory testing facility uses methods to test patients' specimens that lead to accurate, reliable, and quality test results. Only laboratories or clinics that perform "waived" laboratory tests (e.g., simple tests such as dipstick urinalysis) are not required to undergo an inspection. If the laboratory test is not categorized as waived by the CLIA '88 federal regulations, it falls into the category of "moderately complex" or "highly

Table 17–1. Lawsuit Prevention Tips for Minimizing Risks

COMMON ISSUES IN LAWSUITS AGAINST HEALTH CARE PROVIDERS	PREVENTION TIPS FOR PHLEBOTOMISTS, NURSES, AND OTHERS INVOLVED IN BLOOD COLLECTION
Documentation	Always document the time, date, and blood collector's initials on the blood collection containers.
Reporting of incidents	Document the information legibly and spell correctly. If an adverse incident occurs to the patient and/or the blood collector before, during, or after blood collection, report the incident to your immediate supervisor and complete the appropriate documentation in a legible manner.
Failure to follow health care facility's procedure	Be knowledgeable of the health care facility's and clinical laboratory's policies and procedures. If you must deviate from a policy or a procedure, discuss the incident with your immediate supervisor and decide on the appropriate action.
Failure to ensure patient's safety	Monitor the patient in an appropriate, timely manner during and after blood collection. Return bed rails to the raised position if the bed rails were raised prior to blood collection. Lock the patient in the blood collection chair for the duration of blood collection procedure. If an outpatient says that he or she faints during blood collection, place the patient in a supine position to collect blood, and monitor the patient for at least 20 minutes after collection before allowing him or her to stand up and leave the facility. Remove all supplies and equipment after the procedure.
Improper treatment and performance of treatment	Use proper technique and equipment (e.g., gloves) when performing procedures. Follow the health care facility's and clinical laboratory's procedures when perfoming treatments. Update your collection skills and techniques through continuing education classes.
Failure to monitor and to report	Report any significant changes in a patient's condition (e.g., patient continues to bleed from puncture site after blood collection).
Equipment use	Learn how to use blood collection equipment as designed. Use biohazardous waste containers as indicated in procedures. If involved in off-site blood collections, carry biohazardous waste containers. If involved in off-site collections, have correct types and amounts of insurance coverages to address liability exposures with respect to transporting biohazardous specimens.

Patients with HIV	Be conscious of actions that could result in a lawsuit:
	  Discrimination in treatment
	  Nosocomial transmission of the virus
	  Breach of confidentiality
	Follow health care facility's procedures for blood collection and disposal of biohazardous waste.

complex," depending on the difficulty of conducting the test and the risk of harm to the patient if the test is not performed correctly. For the moderately complex or highly complex testing, the inspection considers all procedural steps in laboratory testing—preanalytic, analytic, and postanalytic.

Thus, the blood collection procedures area is a major part of CLIA inspections. The HCFA states that a laboratory with moderately complex or highly complex testing must have available and follow written policies and procedures for the following:

- Protocols for the preparation of patients
- Specimen collection
- Specimen labeling
- Specimen preservation
- Conditions for specimen transportation

SELF STUDY

KEY TERMS

Administrative Law
Assault
Battery
Breach of Duty
Centers for Disease Control and
    Prevention (CDC)
Civil Law
Clinical Laboratory Improvement
    Amendments (CLIA)
Criminal Actions
Defendant
Deposition
Discovery
Environmental Protection
    Agency (EPA)
Evidence
Expert Witness
False Imprisonment
Felony
Food and Drug Administration (FDA)
Health Care Financing
    Administration (HCFA)
Implied Consent

Informed Consent
Invasion of Privacy
Judicial Law
Liable
Litigation Process
Malice
Malpractice
Medical Records
Misdemeanor
Misrepresentation
Negligence
Patient Confidentiality
Plaintiff
Preventive Law
Respondeat Superior
Risk Management
Standard of Care
Statute of Limitations
Statutory Laws
Tort
Vicarious Liability
Whistle-blowing

STUDY QUESTIONS

For the following, choose the *one* best answer:

1. What is the legal term for improper or unskillful care of a patient by a member of the health care team, or any professional misconduct, unreasonable lack of skill, or infidelity in professional or judiciary duties?

    a. a misdemeanor
    b. malpractice
    c. litigation
    d. liability

2. What are the factors, or key points, that must be considered in alleged negligence cases?

   1. duty
   2. breach of duty
   3. proximate causation
   4. damages

   Select one choice:
   a. 1, 2, and 3 are correct
   b. 1 and 3 are correct
   c. 2 and 4 are correct
   d. only 4 is correct
   e. all are correct

3. One agency affecting regulations on blood collection is HCFA. It stands for which of the following?
   a. Home Care Financing Administration
   b. Health Care Financing Administration
   c. Health Care Financial Agency
   d. Health Care Funding Agency

4. Which of the following legal branches writes regulations that enforce the laws?
   a. administrative branch
   b. judicial branch
   c. U.S. Supreme Court
   d. executive branch

5. The avoidance of legal conflicts in blood collection through education and planning is considered which type of law?
   a. administrative law
   b. executive law
   c. preventive law
   d. preparatory law

6. A child who refused to have his blood drawn was locked in a room by a phlebotomist and was forced to have his blood collected. This is an example of which legal concept?
   a. invasion of privacy
   b. informed consent
   c. a misdemeanor
   d. assault and battery

7. The standard of care currently used in malpractice legal cases involving health care providers is based on the conduct of the average health care provider in which area?
   a. state
   b. city
   c. national community
   d. local community

8. Which legal concept refers to the voluntary permission by a patient to allow touching, examination, and/or treatment by health care providers?
   a. implied consent
   b. assault and battery
   c. battery
   d. informed consent

9. Which of the following evaluates the safety, clinical efficacy, and medical efficacy of the equipment and supplies used in blood collection?
   a. EPA
   b. OSHA
   c. CDC
   d. FDA

10. When should incident reports involving accidental HIV-exposures be reported?
    a. at the end of the work shift
    b. immediately
    c. after 24 hours
    d. after seeing the employee health physician

References

1. Richards EP, Rathburn KC. *Law and the Physician.* Boston: Little, Brown and Company; 1993.

2. Curran WJ, Hall MA, Kaye DH. *Health Care Law, Forensic Science, and Public Policy.* Boston: Little, Brown and Company; 1990.

3. Rakich JS, Longest BB, Darr K. *Managing Health Services Organizations.* Baltimore: Health Professions Press; 1992.

4. *Parker v. Port Huron Hospital,* 105, N.W. 2d 854 (1981).

5. Brent NJ. Confidentiality and HIV status: the nurse's right to know. *Home Healthcare Nurse.* 1990;8(3):6–8.

6. Rozovsky F, Rozovsky L. *Home Health Care Law: Liability and Risk Management.* Boston: Little, Brown and Company; 1996, pp. 1–13.

7. Aoun H. When a house officer gets AIDS. *N Engl J Med.* 1989;321(10):695.

8. Pozgar GD. *Legal Aspects of Health Care Administration.* Gaithersburg, MD: Aspen Publishers; 1993.

9. Markus K. Your legal risk in giving advice or care. *Healthweek.* Oct 6, 1997; 5.

10. Troyer GT, Salman SL. *Handbook of Health Care Risk Management.* Rockville, MD: Aspen Publishers; 1986.

11. Bunting RF. Risk management and prevention in the clinical laboratory. *Clin Lab Sci 5.* 1992;(Jan/Feb):1, 35–37.

12. Department of Health and Human Services (DIIHS), Health Care Financing Administration (HCFA), Public Health Service: 42 CFR 405 *et seq,* 57 FR 7002–7186, Feb 28, 1992.

13. Fiesta J. *20 Legal Pitfalls for Nurses to Avoid.* Albany, NY: Delmar Publishers; 1994.

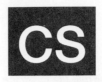

PHLEBOTOMY CASE STUDY

■

Communication

Ms. Nancy Garcia, a 78-year-old Hispanic woman, was admitted to River Bend Hospital as a result of complications from diabetes mellitus. When the health care worker arrived at her hospital room to collect blood for laboratory tests, he introduced himself and asked her name. She did not respond and looked perplexed.

QUESTIONS:

1. What should the health care worker do next?
2. What could a health care facility provide to assist in this situation?
3. Has the patient implied her consent to the venipuncture?

APPENDIX

■

Units of Measurement and Symbols

α	alpha
Å	angstrom
amp	ampere (unit of electric current)
c	centi- (10^{-2})
°C	degrees Centigrade or Celsius (unit of temperature; convert to Fahrenheit by multiplying by 1.8 and adding 32)
cc	cubic centimeter (same as mL, $^{1}/_{1000}$ L)
cd	candela (unit of luminous intensity)
cm	centimeter
cu mm	cubic millimeter
d	deci- (10^{-1})
dL	deciliter ($^{1}/_{10}$ of a liter)
°F	degrees Fahrenheit (unit of temperature; convert to Centigrade by subtracting 32 and multiplying by 0.555)
g or gm	gram ($^{1}/_{1000}$ of a kilogram, unit of mass)
G%	grams in 100 mL
h	hecto- (10^{2})
hpf	high-power field on microscope
IU	international unit
k	kilo- (10^{3})
°K	degrees Kelvin (thermodynamic temperature; convert to Centigrade by subtracting 273.15)
kg	kilogram (1000 g, or 2.2 lb)
L	liter (1000 mL or 1000 cc, unit of volume)
lpf	low-power field on microscope
μ	micro- (10^{-6})
μci	microcurie ($^{1}/_{1000}$ mCi)

μg or mcg	microgram ($^{1}/_{1000}$ mg)
μm	micron
m	meter (unit of length)
m	milli- (10^{-3})
mCi	millicurie
mEq or meq	milliequivalent
mg or mgm	milligram ($^{1}/_{1000}$ g)
mg%	milligrams in 100 mL (same as dL)
min	minutes
mIU	milli-international unit ($^{1}/_{1000}$ IU)
mL	milliliter ($^{1}/_{1000}$ L, same as cc)
mm	millimeter ($^{1}/_{10}$ cm)
mm^3	cubic millimeter
mm Hg	millimeters of mercury
mmole	millimole
mol, M	mole (unit of substance)
mOsm	milliosmol
N	normality
n	nano- (10^{-9})
ng	nanogram ($^{1}/_{1000}$ mg)
p	pico- (10^{-12})
pg	picogram ($^{1}/_{1000}$ ng)
QNS	quantity not sufficient
sec or s	second (unit of time)
SI	international system
sp g	specific gravity
U	international enzyme unit
WNL	within normal limits
WNR	within normal range
wt	weight
w/v	weight/volume
$\cong$	approximately
$\leq$	less than or equal to
$\geq$	greater than or equal to
+ or (+)	positive
− or (−)	negative
Σ	summation

2

APPENDIX

■

Metric Conversion Chart

LENGTH OR DISTANCE

1 inch (in.) = 2.54 centimeters (cm)
1 foot (ft) = 30.48 centimeters (cm)
39.37 inches (in.) = 1 meter (m)
1 mile (mi) = 1.61 kilometers (km)

MASS OR WEIGHT

1 ounce (oz) = 28.35 grams (g)
1 pound (lb) = 453.6 grams (g)
2.205 pounds (lb) = 1 kilogram (kg)

VOLUME

1 fluid ounce (fl oz) = 29.57 milliliters (mL)
1.057 quarts (qt) = 1 liter (liter or L)
1 gallon (gal = 3.78 liters (liter or L)

3

APPENDIX

■

Formulas and Calculations

Area	square meter (sq m or m^2)
Blood volume	Total blood volume = weight (kg) × average blood volume (defined by age)
Clearance	liter/second (L/s)
Concentration and conversions	
Mass	kilogram/liter (kg/L)
Substrate	mole/liter (mol/L)

% w/v to M or vice versa:

$$M = \frac{\% \, w/v \times 10}{molecular \; wt \; (mol \; wt)}$$

% w/v to N or vice versa:

$$N = \frac{\% \, w/v \times 10}{eq \; wt}$$

mg/dL to mEq/L or vice versa:

$$mEq/L = \frac{mg/dL \times 10}{eq \; wt}$$

M to N:

$$N = M \times valence$$

N to M:

$$M = \frac{N}{valence}$$

Density	kilogram/liter (kg/L)
Dilutions	Final concentration =
	Original concentration × dilution 1 × dilution 2, etc.
Electrical potential	volt (V) = kg m²/s³A
Energy	joule (J) = kg m²/s²
Force	Newton (N) = kg m²/s²
Frequency	hertz (Hz) = 1 cycle/s
Hematology math	Mean corpuscular volume (MCV) = average volume of red blood cells (RBCs); expressed in cubic microns (μm³) or femtoliters (fL)

$$\mathrm{MCV} = \frac{\mathrm{Hct} \times 10}{\mathrm{RBC\ count\ (in\ millions)}}$$

Hct = hematocrit value

Mean corpuscular hemoglobin (MCH) = Average weight of hemoglobin in RBC; expressed in picograms (pg)

$$\mathrm{MCH} = \frac{\mathrm{hgb\ (g)} \times 10}{\mathrm{RBC\ count\ (in\ millions)}}$$

hgb = hemoglobin value

Mean corpuscular hemoglobin concentration = Hemoglobin concentration of average RBC

$$\mathrm{MCHC} = \frac{\mathrm{hgb\ (g)}}{\mathrm{Hct}} \times 100\%$$

RBC distribution width (RDW) = numerical expression of variation of RBC size, dispersion of RBC volumes about the mean

$$\mathrm{RDW} = \frac{\mathrm{SD\ (standard\ deviation)\ of\ RBC\ size}}{\mathrm{MCV}}$$

Military Time	Military time uses a 24-hour time clock and eliminates the need for AM or PM designations. Time is expressed by up to four numbers; the first set is in hours (0 to 24) and the second set is minutes (0 to 59). Each day begins at midnight, 0000 and ends at 2359.

The first 12 hours are equivalent in military time (3:00 AM is equivalent to 0300 in military time), but conversion of afternoon and evening times on a 12-hour clock to military time requires adding 12 hours (2:00 PM is 1400 in military time).

Military time is usually stated in terms of hundreds (e.g., 1500 is stated as "fifteen hundred hours"; 0300 is stated as "zero three hundred").

Pressure	$Pascal (Pa) = (kg/m)s^2$
Quality control math:	

   Variance (s^2)

$$s^2 = \frac{(x - \bar{x})^2}{n - 1}$$

   Standard deviation (s)

$$s = \sqrt{s^2}$$

   % Coefficient of variation

$$\%CV = \frac{s}{x} \times 100$$

Relative centrifugal force (rcf)

Measures force of centrifugation acting on blood components and allowing them to separate. Can be used to calibrate centrifuges.

$rcf = 1.118 \times 10^{-5} \times 4 \times n^2$
r = rotating radius (centimeters)
n = speed of rotation (revolutions per minute)

Solutions

Specific gravity (sp g):

$$sp\,g = \frac{wt\ of\ solid\ or\ liquid}{wt\ of\ equal\ volume\ of\ H_2O\ at\ 4°C}$$

Temperature
  Celsius or Centigrade

$°C = K - 273.15; °C = °F - 32 \times 0.555$

  Kelvin

$°K = °C + 273.15$ or $\frac{5}{9} (°F) + 255.35$

  Fahrenheit

$°F = (°C \times 1.8) + 32$

Volume

deciliter (dL) = $\frac{1}{10}$ of a liter
10 dL   = 1 L
centiliter (cL) = $\frac{1}{100}$ of a liter
100 cL   = 10 dL = 1 L
milliliter (mL) = $\frac{1}{1000}$ of a liter
1000 mL   = 100 cL = 10 dL = 1 L

APPENDIX

■

Answers to Self Study Questions and Cases

OVERVIEW: SELF STUDY ANSWERS

CHAPTER 1

1. a, b, c, d
2. a, b, d
3. a, b, c
4. a, b, c
5. a, b, c, d
6. b, d
7. a, b, c
8. a, b, c, d
9. b, c, d

7. b
8. c
9. d
10. b, c

CHAPTER 3

1. a, b, c
2. a
3. a, c
4. a
5. c, d, e
6. a, b, c, d
7. c
8. b
9. d
10. a, b, c, d

CHAPTER 2

1. a, b, c
2. c
3. b
4. a, b, c, d, e
5. a, b
6. a, b, d

I. OVERVIEW:
CASE STUDY: ANSWERS/DISCUSSION

CASE STUDY: CHANGING ROLES IN PHLEBOTOMY PRACTICE

1. Trends in hospital restructuring are aimed at improving the quality of health care, eliminating unnecessary costs and redundancy, performing duties as a coordinated health care team rather than as individual specialists, and becoming more sensitive to patient's individual needs. Also, laboratory technology has enabled testing to be performed closer to the point-of-care or at the patient's bedside.

   Ms. Sanborn can learn more by asking administrators in her area about these changes, by reading about trends in the industry in newsletters and professional journals, by attending continuing education seminars to learn new technical skills and how to deal with change, and by networking with colleagues in other locations.

2. Ms. Sanborn already has very positive personality traits and work habits that should contribute to the team concept in a productive manner. She should remember the following skills needed for effective teams:

   - Understand the mission of the organization.
   - Know basic skills for group process and team dynamics (e.g., active listening, setting norms, etc.).
   - Understand relevance and commitment to team goals.
   - Be reliable and dependable in work assignments.
   - Be able to communicate ideas and feelings.
   - Actively participate in decision making.
   - Learn how to be flexible in decision making.
   - Constructively manage conflicts.
   - Contribute to the cohesion of the team.
   - Contribute to problem solving strategies.
   - Support and encourage other team members.

3. Ms. Sanborn has numerous positive attributes that will help her in her new role. These are efficiency in blood collection, her willingness to provide assistance, her attention to details, and her ability to communicate effectively with patients. These types of traits and work habits are universally beneficial no matter what type of health care setting she is in.

CASE STUDY: COLLECTION FROM THE DORSAL SIDE OF THE HAND

1. *Dorsal* (proximal) refers to the back of the hand in this case. The anterior hand or wrist should NOT be used for venipuncture.
2. *Supine* means lying on the back, face upward.
3. An orthopedic floor is for patients with bone and joint disorders.

II. SAFETY PROCEDURES: SELF STUDY ANSWERS

CHAPTER 4

1. d
2. b, c, d
3. b, c
4. a, b, c, d, e
5. b
6. b
7. c
8. c
9. b, c, d
10. b

CHAPTER 5

1. c, d
2. a, b, d
3. b, c, d
4. a, c, d

5. a, b, c, d
6. b
7. c
8. b
9. b

CHAPTER 6

1. a, b, c, d
2. a, b, c, d
3. a, c, d
4. a, b, c
5. a, b, c, d
6. b
7. a, b, d
8. a, b, c, d
9. a
10. c

II. SAFETY PROCEDURES: CASE STUDY ANSWERS/DISCUSSION

CASE STUDY: ACCIDENTAL INJURY

1. Even though Sally was tired, she had a job to do. Her fatigue might have contributed to her inability to draw blood from Mr. Johnson on the first try, however, there is no way to substantiate that. She probably did the procedure correctly except she should have discarded the first needle and holder immediately after she used it. At that time she would have noticed that the biohazard container was full, and she could have notified the appropriate person for a replacement. *She should not have stuffed the other needles into the full biohazard container!!* However, she took the appropriate action by notifying her supervisor immediately of her injury.
2. Sally would have to review the exposure control plan, OSHA standards, universal precautions for hepatitis and HIV, and safety procedures for disposing of contaminated waste.
3. Aside from a thorough review of the procedures mentioned in Question 2, Sally would benefit from going to classes on the importance of being rested and healthy for work. In addition, it appears she needs additional practice on patients who are difficult to draw.

CASE STUDY: TRANSPORTING SPECIMENS FROM HOMEBOUND PATIENTS TO THE LABORATORY

1. Larry seemed so pleased that he successfully communicated with Mr. Gonzales that he forgot to be meticulous about checking the specimen integrity. He should have carefully placed each specimen in a leakproof plastic container in an upright position in the carrying container. He should have securely locked the container, and placed it in a safer place in his car, perhaps the floor.
2. Larry should be careful not to touch the contaminated area. He should report the spill immediately and find out the appropriate procedures for spill cleanups.

III. EQUIPMENT AND PROCEDURES: SELF STUDY ANSWERS

CHAPTER 7

1. a, b, c
2. d
3. a
4. b
5. b
6. a
7. a, b, c,

CHAPTER 8

1. b, c
2. a, b, d
3. b
4. a, c, d
5. b, c
6. b, d
7. d
8. a
9. a, b, c, d
10. a, b

CHAPTER 9

1. a, b, c
2. b, d
3. c, d
4. a, b, c, d
5. b, c
6. b, c, d
7. b, c
8. b
9. a, b, c, d
10. c

CHAPTER 10

1. a, c, d
2. b, d
3. a, b, c, d
4. c
5. c
6. b
7. b
8. a
9. a
10. a, b, c

III. EQUIPMENT AND PROCEDURES: CASE STUDY ANSWERS/DISCUSSION

CASE STUDY: AMBULATORY HEALTH CARE COLLECTIONS

1. Under normal blood collection procedures with an evacuated tube system, the health care provider did use the proper order of draw for Mrs. Ragsdale's laboratory tests. The light blue–topped tube containing citrate should be collected prior to the red-speckled tube (gel separator tube). When using a blood collection set, however, the tubing in the assembly contains air and will *underfill* the first evacuated tube, leading to erroneous protime result.

2. The health care provider used the proper collection procedure. A 21- or 23-gauge needle is better, however, than a 25-gauge needle because the small diameter of the 25-gauge needle may lead to hemolysis of the collected blood and erroneous laboratory tests' results.

3. The proper blood collection procedure was used for obtaining blood from Mr. Sadler. Often, hemophiliacs have sclerosed veins due to so many blood collections and transfusions. Thus, a butterfly needle assembly used on the hand or lower arm is appropriate. A "complete" assembly set, however, should be used rather than pieces from, most likely, different manufacturers. Mismatched medical equipment has led to 50 percent of mucocutaneous blood-borne pathogen exposures* of health care workers to HIV-positive and/or HCV infected patients.

CASE STUDY: VENIPUNCTURE SITE SELECTION

1. The preferred site would be the dorsal side of the left wrist, below the IV site. The preferred phlebotomy method would be to use a winged infusion set in combination with evacuated tubes that could handle a short draw in case of difficulty.

2. The right arm of Mrs. McDonald should never be used for venipuncture because of her partial mastectomy. This type of surgical procedure often results in removal of lymph nodes resulting in edematous areas. Since she is a diabetic, foot veins should be eliminated because of an increased likelihood of complications. Since the left arm had an IV located below the anticubital area, this location could not be used for venipuncture due to contamination with IV fluid. The area below the IV site is acceptable for tourniquet application and venipuncture. The winged infusion system is most effective for the smaller veins of the wrist. It is also less painful for the patient.

3. It would be helpful to the clinical laboratory and other members of the health care team to document that the blood sample was drawn from below the IV site since the patient was diabetic, had a mastectomy on the right side, and had an IV located in the left arm.

4. Site selection can be facilitated by the following: proper positioning, use of a pillow or towel under the wrist, rotation of the patient's arm, palpation, warming the site, and dangling the arm for a short while to increase blood flow to the area.

*Ippolito G, Puro V, Petrosillo N, et al. *Prevention, Management & Chemoprophylaxis of Occupational Exposure to HIV.* Virginia: Advances in Exposure Prevention Publisher; 1997.

IV. SPECIAL PROCEDURES AND POINT-OF-CARE TESTING: SELF STUDY ANSWERS

CHAPTER 11

1. a, b
2. b, d
3. a, b, d
4. c
5. a, d
6. d
7. b
8. a, b
9. a, b, d
10. c
11. b, c
12. b, d

CHAPTER 12

1. c
2. c
3. d
4. a
5. d
6. c
7. a
8. b
9. a
10. b

CHAPTER 13

1. c
2. d
3. b
4. c
5. d
6. b
7. b
8. a
9. a
10. c

CHAPTER 14

1. b
2. b
3. c
4. c
5. c
6. b
7. b
8. c
9. b
10. b

CHAPTER 15

1. b
2. a, b, c, d
3. a, b
4. b
5. b
6. a, c
7. a, b, c, d
8. a, b, c, d
9. b, d
10. a, b, c

IV. SPECIAL PROCEDURES & POINT OF CARE TESTING: CASE STUDY ANSWERS/DISCUSSION

CASE STUDY: HOME CARE COLLECTION

1. | *Laboratory Assay* | *Color of Blood Collection Tube Top* |
   | --- | --- |
   | Calcium, ionized | green |
   | APTT | light blue |
   | CBC count | purple |
   | Protime | light blue |
   | Chemistry screen | red or red-speckled |
   | Digoxin | red or red-speckled |
   | Plasma potassium | green |

2. The order of draw was incorrect for blood vacuum tube collections. The correct order should have been red, light blue, green, and purple. The correct order prevents contamination of nonadditive tubes by additive tubes, and minimizes cross-contamination between the different anticoagulants.

3. The order of draw was incorrect for the syringe method. The green-topped tube should have been filled first so that the blood could immediately be mixed with the anticoagulant to prevent clotting. Then, the remaining blood should have been placed in the red or red-speckled tube to clot.

CASE STUDY: BEDSIDE GLUCOSE TESTING

1. The problem in this bedside glucose testing case is that the patient's meter was reading outside the control confidence limits. Thus, the glucose results are out of control and not considered accurate or reliable.

2. The phlebotomist, the nurse, and other health care providers involved in the bedside glucose testing for this patient should troubleshoot for
   a. Correct timing of the analytic procedure
   b. Reagents and controls stored at correct temperature and within appropriate expiration dates.
   c. Instrument blotting or wiping technique performed according to manufacturer's directions.
   In this case, the control solution had expired March 2, 1998.

CASE STUDY: NEWBORN NURSERY COLLECTION

1. Blood collected from a baby for a bilirubin determination should be collected in an amber microcollection tube or a tube covered with foil so that the microcollection tube is not exposed to light. Light breaks down bilirubin.

2. Because bilirubin breaks down in the presence of light, the longer a blood specimen is exposed to light, the more bilirubin is broken down. Thus, the bilirubin value will be falsely decreased.

3. Probably, the phlebotomist who collected Baby McPherson's blood on Sunday morning collected the blood in a clear microcollection tube and allowed it to remain in direct light for an extended period prior to delivering it to the clinical laboratory.

V. QUALITY, COMPETENCY, AND LEGAL ISSUES: SELF STUDY ANSWERS

CHAPTER 16

1. a, b, c, d
2. a, b, c, d
3. a, b, c
4. a, b, c, d
5. a, c, d

CHAPTER 17

1. b
2. e
3. b
4. d
5. c
6. d
7. c
8. d
9. d
10. b

V. QUALITY MANAGEMENT AND LEGAL ISSUES: CASE STUDY ANSWERS/DISCUSSION
CASE STUDY: COMMUNICATION

1. The phlebotomist should check with the floor nurse to determine whether Ms. Garcia speaks English and/or whether she has a hearing disability. If the patient speaks only Spanish, an interpreter or a written description of the phlebotomy procedure should be available in Spanish to assist in this situation. If the patient has a hearing disability, efforts should be made to write down instructions for the patient.

2. If a patient has a hearing disability, writing tools should be kept at the bedside of the patient. If a large segment of the patient population speaks another language, the hospital should provide interpreters who know the basic use of that language. Also, instruction sheets on phlebotomy steps should be made available in other languages for patients who do not speak English.

3. The patient has not consented to the venipuncture, nor did she appear to understand the verbal communication. The efforts mentioned in the above answers will facilitate seeking consent and minimize risk of legal or financial loss to the hospital. Above all, these efforts will provide a cooperative, professional interaction for the patient and health care worker.

Index